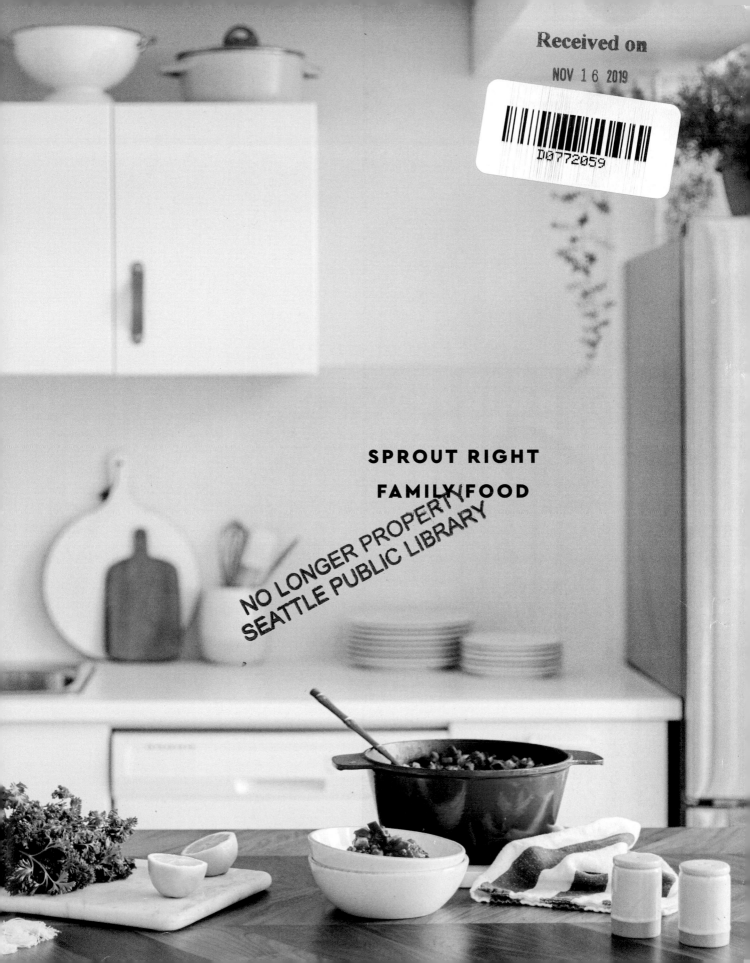

SPROUT RIGHT

FAMILY FOOD

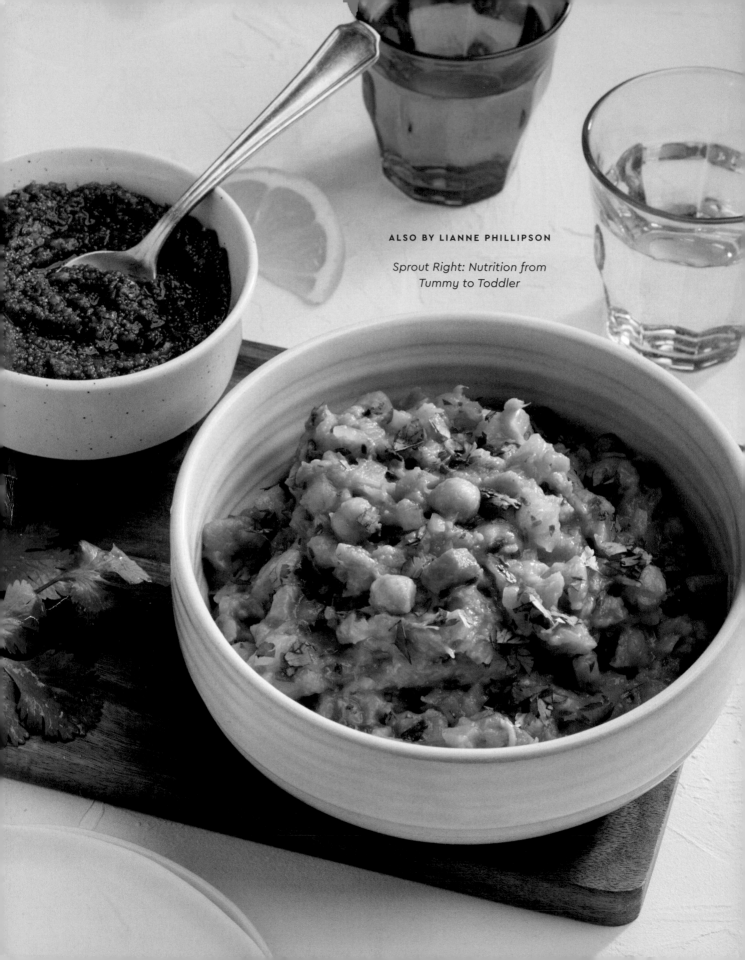

Sprout Right Family Food

Good Nutrition and Over 130 Simple Recipes
for Baby, Toddler, and the Whole Family

Lianne Phillipson

REGISTERED NUTRITIONIST

PENGUIN

an imprint of Penguin Canada, a division of Penguin Random House Canada Limited

Canada • USA • UK • Ireland • Australia • New Zealand • India • South Africa • China

First published 2019

LIBRARY AND ARCHIVES CANADA CATALOGUING IN PUBLICATION

Phillipson-Webb, Lianne, author
    Sprout Right family food : eat right from the start with good nutrition and healthy recipes for baby, toddler, and the whole family / Lianne Phillipson.

Issued in print and electronic formats.
ISBN 978-0-7352-3605-9 (softcover).—ISBN 978-0-7352-3606-6 (electronic)

    1. Nutrition. 2. Families–Health and hygiene. 3. Infants–Nutrition.
4. Toddlers–Nutrition. 5. Cooking. 6. Cookbooks. I. Title.

TX361.C5P48 2019   641.5'622   C2018-905430-1
                                             C2018-905431-X

Cover and book design by Lisa Jager
Cover and interior photography by Dan Robb for Sprig Creative
Food and prop styling by Dan Robb for Sprig Creative

Printed and bound in China

10 9 8 7 6 5 4 3 2 1

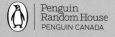

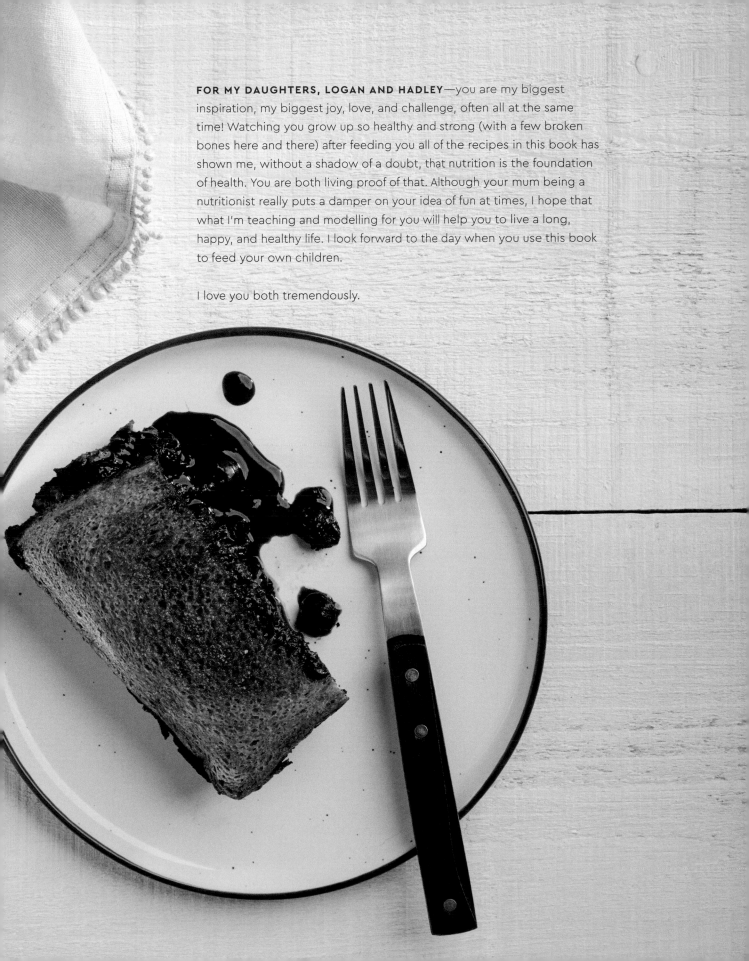

FOR MY DAUGHTERS, LOGAN AND HADLEY—you are my biggest inspiration, my biggest joy, love, and challenge, often all at the same time! Watching you grow up so healthy and strong (with a few broken bones here and there) after feeding you all of the recipes in this book has shown me, without a shadow of a doubt, that nutrition is the foundation of health. You are both living proof of that. Although your mum being a nutritionist really puts a damper on your idea of fun at times, I hope that what I'm teaching and modelling for you will help you to live a long, happy, and healthy life. I look forward to the day when you use this book to feed your own children.

I love you both tremendously.

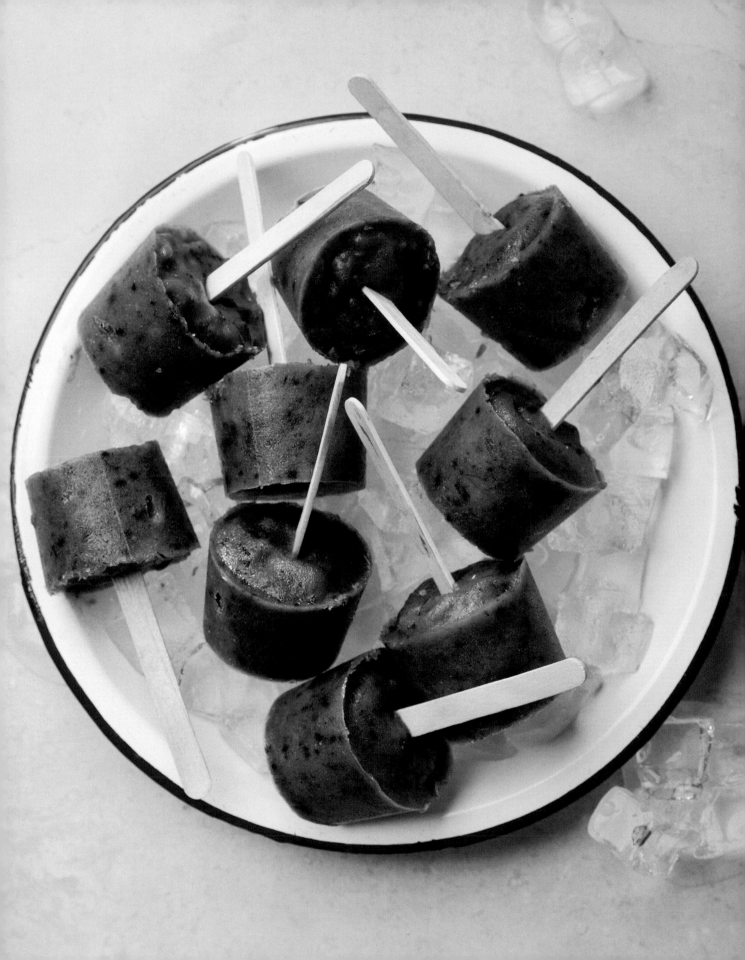

CONTENTS

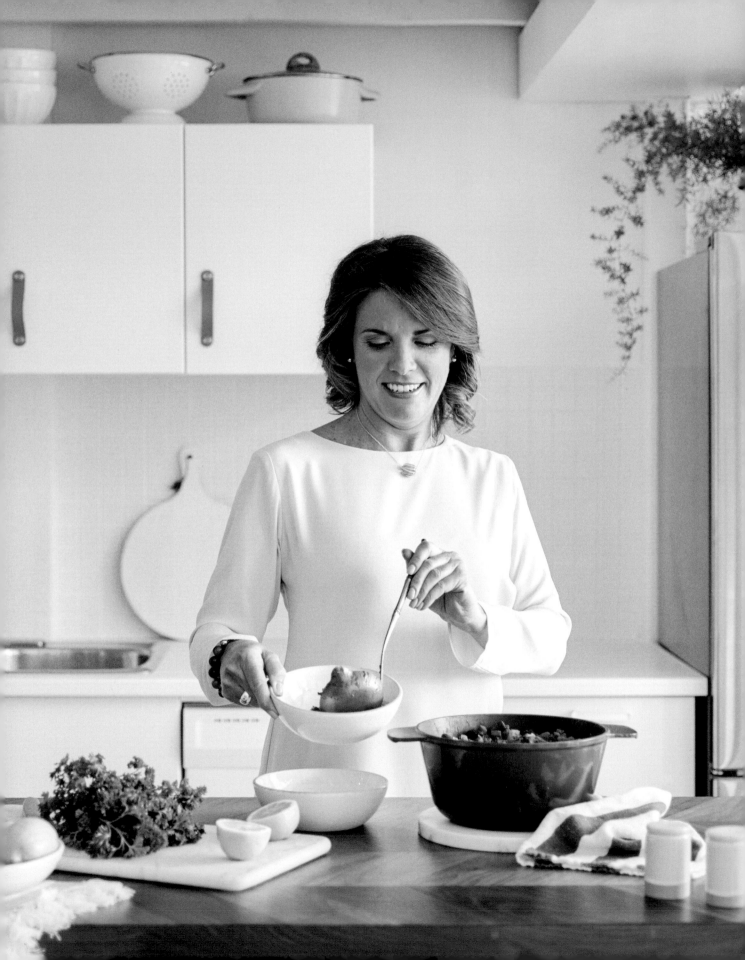

INTRODUCTION

Congratulations on entering this next stage in your life and becoming a parent (or grandparent, aunt, uncle, cousin, or caregiver in a little one's life). As with every new stage and phase of life, questions are bound to come up. Every parent I have ever met wants to do the best possible job nurturing her or his children, but wanting to do what's best can also bring great pressure. I found that becoming a parent brought me to a place of uncertainty and challenge like no other. My body instinctively knew what to do in growing, nourishing, and birthing my child, but when we got home from the hospital and it was my turn to take over, I suddenly became aware of all the choices I had—and all the things I didn't know. It was scary and exciting at the same time!

Because of my nutrition training and because I grew up in a household where home cooking was modelled for me, making meals for my family just like my mum did for hers felt completely natural to me. Not only did my mum cook from scratch, but she canned, pickled, and bought half a cow many times, using every morsel of it (yes, tongue sandwiches in grade 5 was a real thing). I understood that food prep was normal, and that stuck with me. I believe that this is something we need to model for our kids so they don't fall into the trap of not knowing how to cook and relying on processed and store-bought options.

Knowing that food is the most influential aspect of health is what made me choose to head back to school and become a nutritionist in the mid-1990s. I was living in England at the time and was fortunate to learn from forward thinkers at the Institute for Optimum Nutrition (ION) in London and to embark on their three-year program. I graduated in 1999 and began my new journey of focusing on food. I moved back to Toronto in 2001 and discovered that organic food, nutrition, and health weren't as much of a focus there as they were in England. After my first daughter was born in 2003, I started my company Sprout Right, speaking with parents all over the city in workshops on how to feed their babies, themselves, and their growing families. I taught my Mommy Chef cooking classes for eight years and began working in television and radio.

Being approached to write the first edition of *Sprout Right* in 2009 was a dream come true. I had always wanted to share what I had studied and taught in workshops and cooking classes with even more people across the country, and I certainly didn't know how that would ever happen—until it did! After *Sprout Right* was published, I received so many emails, comments, and messages from parents who told me that my book had become their "bible"—certainly not what I had been expecting, but incredibly humbling and thrilling to hear! I love teaching good eating practices and helping people introduce nutritional changes into their family life, whether through intimate to large speaking engagements, regular TV and radio segments, or interviews for print and online articles. Inspiring new parents to feed their babies well, and to see a change in their own eating and well-being as a result, is powerful. It makes me feel like I'm doing what I am meant to.

In large part, it's thanks to the feedback from readers of the first edition of *Sprout Right* that you'll find a lot of new information in this edition. There's also continual evolution in the scientific and medical research, which affects recommendations and trends in the diet and health arena. There's always more to learn when it comes to nutrition. Because you could be reading this book years after it was published, I encourage you to take charge of and responsibility for your family's health and decide if the recommendations here are right for you. If you don't agree with some of my suggestions, that's okay. Not everything is going to make sense for you and your family. But if I get you thinking, push you outside your comfort zone, and get you into the kitchen, then I have done my job. In some of the recipes you might encounter a food that you don't like, and don't think your baby will either. Try it—both of you! You never know when something unfamiliar will become your new favourite.

My daughters continue to be my inspiration, and now that they are teens and cook for themselves, they make many of the recipes in this book, including Apple Crumble (page 226), Go Faster Granola Bars (page 231), Chocolate Chip Cookies (page 311), and Sinless Chocolate Almond Brownies (page 228). Over the years, recipes like these have become classics in our home, but we've also developed some new favourites along the way. As my family grew and changed, our nutrition needs changed as well. *Sprout Right Family Food* includes a chapter on Family Meals. As a working mom, I know the stress of packing school lunches and getting a healthy meal on the table for my family, and I wanted to share some of my foolproof recipes and nutrition tips with you. I hope some of the favourites from my recipe catalogue become yours as well.

As in *Sprout Right*, I've included everything I know here. If you still feel like you need more information, you can find me at SproutRight.com. I'm grateful when parents reach out for additional support to deepen what they've learned, and I'm most grateful to teach, inspire, and support you through your food journey.

Bon Appetit!

HOW TO USE THIS BOOK

My intention as I sat down to write this book, both in its first edition and in *Sprout Right Family Food*, was to gather information about the most important aspects of health and combine that with the practical side of feeding your growing family. I believe that having a strong foundation of knowledge is like having a superpower. Once you know the basics, you can navigate your way through any situation with confidence. That's one thing parents often lack—the confidence to make choices. When you're unsure, doubt and worry can overrule common sense, and at times you may offer foods you never imagined you would, just to get a child to eat. *Sprout Right Family Food* will give you the building blocks you need to understand what a good diet is, why it's worth the effort, and how to make homemade food—with leftovers—that your kids will eat with ease.

In this book, I will guide you with chapters that detail nutritional needs at every stage from birth to school age. Chapter 1 delves into the needs of a new mom and her newborn baby. In Chapters 2 and 3, you'll find everything you need to know about breast and formula feeding, and Chapter 4 is dedicated to baby poo. (It may seem like I've written a lot of words on seemingly simple topics, but when you're going through this stuff, you'll need them.) Chapter 5 takes a close look at allergies and the immune system, and Chapter 6 introduces the idea of making homemade baby food. Chapters 7 to 10 will guide you through starting your little one on solids, baby-led weaning, and my Hybrid Feeding Method, as well as how to feed your toddler, your picky eater, and your school-age kids a nourishing breakfast, pack a stress-free lunch that will come home eaten, and cook a healthy family meal that will allow you to reconnect with your loved ones. Each of these chapters includes straightforward recipes to make feeding your family as simple as possible.

Through all of this, it's important for everyone to maintain a healthy balance of nutrients, healthy fats, and good bacteria in their body, but it's especially important for new mothers and infants, who have a lot of demands on their bodies. Supporting those demands with specific supplements is especially important, so throughout the book you'll find supplement recommendations for the whole family. Sometimes I indicate the amounts needed, and sometimes I recommend specific strains of probiotics or a type of a mineral. After years of recommending specific brands, I've now launched my own line of supplements under the Sprout Right name called *Take This*. I felt that I needed to know more about the products I was recommending, and that was becoming more difficult with mergers and takeovers of big brands. With formulation changes, some products don't offer the same benefits they once did. Products like those created by HMF will continue to help the masses, and I recommend them when appropriate. However, I've done a lot of research, put a lot of thought into my own formulations, and taken the best of all that I've worked with in the past and put it into my own product line. I will continue to support families with what I feel offers the best quality for their hard-earned dollars. In the book, you'll see mention of both my own line and other products, so you have options and choice. If you're looking for more in-depth information, you can always find it on SproutRight.com.

At times, while reading this book, you may need to read a chapter or two all the way through; at other times you'll find yourself skimming to find specific topics of interest or answers to your questions. Throughout, I've provided guidance that applies to specific situations, such as what to do if your baby has constipation and he's on formula. Or, maybe you've noticed that when you eat a certain food, your breast-fed baby won't settle. Has your toddler suddenly decided she hates everything she was eating last week? There's probably a good reason for that. And then there are the questions that plague all parents: What can I pack in my first-grader's lunch box that he will actually eat? And, what can I make for my family that's quick, healthy, and will be well liked? With over 130 recipes that cover every stage, we'll tackle it all.

I'm keenly aware of the rise in allergies and the difficulty and fear that this creates for parents and their kids, which is why I've included an entire chapter on allergies and the immune system. Because there are so many allergies that affect family meals, you'll find that most of the recipes in this book are free of common allergens. Just under each recipe title, I mention which allergens the recipe is free of. If a recipe is gluten-free, dairy-free, egg-free, nut-free, wheat-free, soy-free, or even vegetarian, it will be clearly marked so you can flip quickly through the book to see which recipes are suitable for your family.

HEALTHY EATING

Perspectives on what *healthy eating* means can be wide-ranging. In my philosophy, *healthy eating* means consuming a rainbow of fruits and vegetables each and every day (as in every colour of the rainbow, every day), along with either plant- or animal-based protein, whole grains, and a minimal amount of sugar and processed, fast, or junk food. Eating a diet made up of as much organic food as possible while being mindful of sustainability in farming of any kind—produce crops, fishing, or animal rearing—is ideal. Buying and eating organic is better for our planet and for us. If you can't stretch to all organic, see the section on buying organic on page 5 to learn how to be a savvy organic shopper.

EAT A RAINBOW OF FRUITS AND VEGETABLES EVERY DAY

I've been teaching both parents and children to eat a rainbow every day for as long as I've been a nutritionist. It's an easy way to organize eating a variety of colourful fruits and vegetables that are packed with water, fibre, carbohydrates, vitamins, minerals, and phytonutrients like anti-inflammatory bromelain found in orange and yellow foods, detoxifying chlorophyll in all green foods, powerful antioxidant curcumin in the orange root turmeric, and anti-aging resveratrol in red foods. That's some serious motivation to eat more colours.

To help keep everyone in your family on track, you may want to create a bit of healthy competition between family members. You can do this by creating a chart that the family contributes to every day. Write your names down the left side, add the colours of the rainbow across the top, and hang the chart on the fridge or a kitchen cabinet. Each time a person eats a fruit or vegetable, they can add a sticker, check, or scribble beneath the corresponding colour on the chart. If the chart isn't full by the end of the day, then you know what's for dessert.

During one of our first rainbow challenges, my daughters and I started making our own Rainbow Rice Wraps (page 292)—they are our favourite meal when we are on the go and would otherwise need to buy lunch out. I learned that they loved to create their own variations. They needed some guidance on getting all the colours into their wrap, so it allowed us to work together to create a colourful, healthy meal. This recipe is such fun to make and the perfect way to fill everyone's rainbow chart.

In case you need some new ideas, here are lists of fruits and vegetables you can ask your kids to choose from for the week ahead.

FRUITS
- Apples
- Apricots
- Avocado
- Banana
- Blackberries
- Blueberries
- Cantaloupe
- Cherries
- Currants
- Figs
- Grapefruit
- Grapes
- Guava
- Kiwifruit
- Lemon/lime
- Mango
- Nectarine
- Papaya
- Peach
- Pear
- Persimmon
- Pineapple
- Plum
- Pomegranate
- Raspberries
- Rhubarb
- Tangerine
- Tomato
- Watermelon

VEGETABLES
- Artichoke
- Asparagus
- Beans
- Beets
- Bok choy
- Broccoli
- Brussels sprouts
- Cabbage
- Carrots
- Cauliflower
- Celery
- Chinese broccoli
- Collard greens
- Corn
- Cucumber
- Dandelion greens
- Eggplant
- Endive
- Fennel bulb
- Garlic
- Herbs (fresh parsley, basil, cilantro, sage, thyme, rosemary, oregano)
- Kale
- Leeks
- Lettuce (mixed greens, romaine, green and red leafy)
- Mushrooms
- Mustard greens
- Okra
- Onions (red, yellow, green)
- Parsnip
- Peas
- Peppers (hot, green, sweet red and yellow)
- Radishes
- Rutabaga
- Snow peas
- Spinach
- Sprouts (sunflower, bean mix, Ancient Eastern blend)
- Squash
- Sweet potato
- Swiss chard
- Turnip
- Turnip greens
- White potato (Yukon Gold, russet, baby red)
- Yams
- Zucchini

BUYING FRUITS AND VEGETABLES

Shopping for what's best has become confusing with the movement toward buying local and organic. Which do you choose? If possible, I would try to get local, seasonal, and organic produce. Buying what's local and in season means that you're eating foods when they're at their peak for taste and nutrients—and also when they're in abundance, which means they'll cost less than when they're out of season.

ORGANIC

Organic foods are grown naturally without the use of synthetically manufactured chemical fertilizers, pesticides, herbicides, fungicides, antibiotics, hormones, or genetically modified organisms (GMOs). A staggering five to six billion pounds (two to three billion kilograms) of synthetic chemicals are applied throughout the world each year for everything from protecting crops to warding off malaria.[1] The Pesticide Action Network explains the health concerns associated with conventional foods: "Chronic health effects can result from low dose exposure to pesticides over time. Even extremely low doses of pesticides, particularly during foetal development, infancy and childhood, are linked to cancers, birth defects, developmental delays, asthma, and Parkinson's disease."[2]

I highly recommend buying as much organic food as you can find and afford. Introducing organic fruits and vegetables as your baby's first foods is especially important because the immaturity of your baby's developing systems leaves her vulnerable to chemicals. Eating more contaminated foods could increase the likelihood of intolerances and adverse reactions in susceptible babies. Organic farming is also better for the environment, as it uses compost and other natural fertilizers that make the soil rich with life and help keep the ecosystem healthy and alive. Below, you'll find the most important foods to buy organic, according to the Environmental Working Group (www.EWG.org). EWG's mission is to empower people to live healthier lives in a healthier environment, and its breakthrough research and education drive consumer choice and influence civic action in the United States and around the world. EWG has compiled lists of the most and least contaminated produce. I recommend you use these lists to help you become a savvy organic shopper.

EWG'S 2018 SHOPPER'S GUIDE TO PESTICIDES IN PRODUCE In 2018, EWG made some updates to its shopper's guide. The two lists below are taken from the EWG website and list the fruits and vegetables that contain the most and least amount of pesticides. I suggest that you always buy produce listed on the Dirty Dozen list organic, while produce listed on the Clean Fifteen list can be purchased conventional. The most worrying fact for me was that 97 percent of conventional spinach samples contained pesticide residues. A summer favourite of mine, strawberries, are another worry. One strawberry sample contained an astounding twenty-two pesticide residues, and one-third of all conventional strawberry samples contained ten or more pesticides. Hot peppers appear on the Dirty Dozen list not just because of the levels of pesticide residues they were found to be contaminated with, but because of the types of pesticides that are used on them, which were found to be toxic to the human nervous system.

DIRTY DOZEN[3]
1. Strawberries
2. Spinach
3. Nectarines
4. Apples
5. Grapes
6. Peaches
7. Cherries
8. Pears
9. Tomatoes
10. Celery
11. Potatoes
12. Sweet bell peppers + hot peppers

CLEAN FIFTEEN[4]
1. Avocados
2. Sweet corn*
3. Pineapples
4. Cabbages
5. Onions
6. Sweet peas, frozen
7. Papayas*
8. Asparagus
9. Mangos
10. Eggplants
11. Honeydew melons
12. Kiwis
13. Cantaloupes
14. Cauliflower
15. Broccoli

*A small amount of sweet corn, papaya, and summer squash sold in the United States is produced from genetically modified seeds. Buy organic varieties of these crops if you want to avoid genetically modified produce.

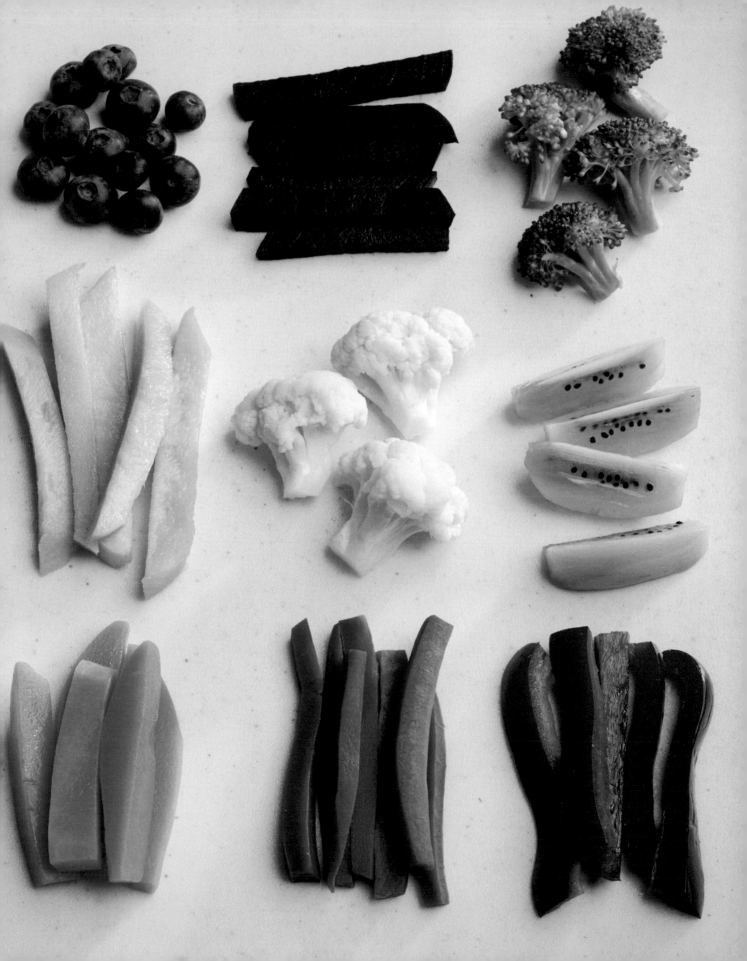

CONVENTIONAL

Conventional food is what you'll find at most supermarkets (that is, anything that's not labelled organic). It's produced using a variety of pest management techniques, including crop rotation, tillage, pesticides, and crop nutrients such as manure and synthetic fertilizers. Although organic offers many benefits, if you can't find organic, it's better to eat conventional fruits and vegetables than not eat them at all.

FROZEN

Frozen fruits and vegetables are convenient and are a great way to have out-of-season foods on hand without spoilage. Frozen produce has been picked and then flash-frozen to maintain its nutrients. If you grow fruits and vegetables in your garden, freeze them for future use. It may be worth packaging your harvest using a vacuum sealer to eliminate the chance of freezer burn.

CANNED

Use canned fruits and vegetables as a last resort. They're often high in sugar and salt and extremely low in enzymes and nutrients. Some cans are lined with bisphenol A (BPA), which can leach into your food. This is especially true of canned tomatoes. Canned beans (such as Eden Organic) usually have an enamel lining, so are safe to use and very handy.

PERFECTLY PREPARED FRUITS AND VEGETABLES

Always wash fruits and vegetables before consuming or cooking them, to clean off any bacteria, dirt, or water-soluble chemicals like pesticides.

- Wash your hands with soap and water before and after washing produce to avoid cross-contamination.
- Wash produce under clean, running water.
- Use a vegetable scrub brush or pot scrubber on produce with a firm skin like carrots, potatoes, melons, and squash.
- Always wash produce like squash, melons, and oranges, even if you don't eat the outer rind. Bacteria on the outer surface can be transferred to the inner flesh when the item is cut or peeled.
- When cleaning leafy greens, discard the outer leaves. Soak dense vegetables like broccoli, cauliflower, and Brussels sprouts in water for a few minutes to dislodge any dirt, then rinse thoroughly under running water.
- Soak herbs like parsley and cilantro in cold water for fifteen minutes, then rinse thoroughly.
- Soap, chlorine, and vinegar washes can leave residues and should not be used. Special produce washes remove chemical residues, which may remain on the produce, but they do not kill bacteria or moulds. Rinsing fruits and vegetables thoroughly under cool running water will help to wash them away.

STORING FRUITS AND VEGETABLES

Some fruits are better refrigerated than others. Some vegetables need to be stored in a cool, dark environment, and others can be stored in the fridge.

- Vegetables are best consumed fresh. Buy your vegetables every two to three days, if possible. Vegetables from farmers' markets were likely picked within days of purchase, so they may last longer.
- Wrap leafy vegetables in a tea towel or paper towel and then store them in a bag or container in the fridge.
- Washed fruits and vegetables store well in cloth bags (which breathe and are eco-friendly, unlike plastic), which helps lengthen their shelf life.
- Mushrooms are best stored in paper bags in the fridge so that they can breathe.
- Onions, garlic, and potatoes are best stored in a cool, dark, dry place.
- When you get home from shopping, wash all fruits so they are ready to eat, then place them in a bowl on the counter where they won't be forgotten and are easy to grab.

COOKING WITH WHOLE GRAINS, BEANS, AND LEGUMES

This is where your creativity gets to shine. All of the grains, beans, and pulses mentioned in this section are easy to cook and use creatively in your cooking once you know the ratio of water to grain, bean, or legume you should use. Creating dishes that incorporate different proteins (including plant-based proteins) along with vegetables, particularly greens and possibly tofu, makes for nutrient-dense meals.

PERFECTLY COOKED OATS, RICE, AND MORE

Grains provide many nutrients, including B vitamins and fibre, and give energy in the form of carbohydrates. If you eat whole grains that have been minimally processed—for instance, if you eat brown rice instead of white rice—you'll feel fuller for longer. Processed or white grains have had most of their nutrients and fibre stripped during processing and provide fast-releasing energy, called high glycemic, rather than slow and steady energy, called low glycemic.

When cooking grains, the general rule is to use one part dry grain to two parts water. All grains (except oats) need to be rinsed, especially brown rice and quinoa. Brown rice can have higher levels of arsenic (see page 119 for information on rice and arsenic), and quinoa has an outer layer that tastes bitter if not rinsed well. Placing grains in a sieve and giving them a thorough rinse works well in most cases. Ideally, prepare your grains by soaking them to reduce the amount of phytic acid before cooking. Eating grains without soaking them allows phytic acid to bind to minerals in the gastrointestinal tract, lessening absorption and leading to mineral deficiencies. Soak grains by placing them in a glass bowl and covering them with warm water. Then, for every 1 cup (250 mL) of water, add 1 tablespoon (15 mL) of acid—apple cider vinegar, lemon juice, or plain yogurt—and leave them to soak in a warm kitchen. Soak all grains except brown rice, buckwheat, and millet for twelve to twenty-four hours.

Brown rice, buckwheat, and millet have less phytic acid and need only seven hours for soaking. Drain any liquid and cook according to the chart below. Always bring water to a boil in an appropriate-size saucepan with a lid, then add in the rinsed or soaked grain and reduce heat to simmer with the lid on.

DRY MEASURE (1 CUP/250 ML)	WATER	COOKING TIME	YIELD
Amaranth	2½ cups (625 mL)	20 to 25 minutes	2 cups (500 mL)
Barley (hulled)	3 cups (750 mL)	1 to 1½ hours	3½ cups (875 mL)
Barley (pearled)	3 cups (750 mL)	50 minutes	3½ cups (875 mL)
Brown rice	2 cups (500 mL)	45 minutes	3 cups (750 mL)
Buckwheat (kasha)	2 cups (500 mL)	15 to 20 minutes	2½ cups (625 mL)
Bulgur wheat	1½ cups (375 mL)	20 minutes	2½ cups (625 mL)
Millet	3 cups (750 mL)	45 minutes	3½ cups (875 mL)
Oats (whole)	2 cups (500 mL)	40 to 45 minutes	2 cups (500 mL)
Quinoa	2 cups (500 mL)	20 minutes	2½ cups (625 mL)
Teff	1 cup (250 mL)	8 minutes	2 cups (500 mL)
Wild rice	3 cups (750 mL)	1 hour	4 cups (1 L)

PERFECTLY COOKED BEANS, PEAS, AND LEGUMES

Legumes like green peas work very well in soups. Yellow split peas have a milder flavour and pair well with rice or dal. Adding lentils to soups and stews is best, as they take on other flavours well. Beans contain large amounts of protein, carbohydrates, vitamins, and fibre. Before cooking, sort and clean the beans and remove any small pebbles or mouldy beans, then rinse well. Cover with water to about 2 inches (5 cm) over the beans and soak for twelve to twenty-four hours, adding 1 tablespoon (15 mL) of baking soda for every 1 cup (250 mL) of water. Drain and rinse beans well and proceed to cook according to the chart. Adding kombu seaweed or kelp to the cooking water imparts many minerals and flavour. Do not add salt to the water because it toughens the outer skin of the bean. Generally, 1 cup (250 mL) of dry beans equals 2 cups (500 mL) cooked. Canned beans are an easy option and are ready to eat—simply drain them and rinse well.

DRY MEASURE (1 CUP/250 ML)	WATER	COOKING TIME	YIELD
Adzuki beans	4 cups (1 L)	2 hours	2 cups (500 mL)
Black beans	4 cups (1 L)	1½ hours	2 cups (500 mL)
Black-eyed peas	3 cups (750 mL)	1 hour	2 cups (500 mL)
Garbanzo (chickpeas)	4 cups (1 L)	3 hours	2 cups (500 mL)
Great Northern	3½ cups (875 mL)	2 hours	2 cups (500 mL)
Jacob's Cattle	4 cups (1 L)	1½ hours	2 cups (500 mL)

DRY MEASURE (1 CUP/250 ML)	WATER	COOKING TIME	YIELD
Kidney beans	3 cups (750 mL)	1½ hours	2 cups (500 mL)
Lentils and split peas	3 cups (750 mL)	45 minutes	2¼ cups (550 mL)
Lima	2 cups (500 mL)	½ hour	1¼ cups (300 mL)
Pinto beans	3 cups (750 mL)	2½ hours	2 cups (500 mL)
Red beans	3 cups (750 mL)	3 hours	2 cups (500 mL)
Small white beans (navy, pea)	3 cups (750 mL)	2½ hours	2 cups (500 mL)
Soybeans	4 cups (1 L)	3 hours or more	3 cups (750 mL)
Yellow-eyed beans	4 cups (1 L)	2 hours	2 cups (500 mL)

MEAT, POULTRY, AND FISH

Meat and fish provide complex proteins, minerals, vitamins, and—in the case of fish and grass-fed beef—omega-3 fatty acids. Any naturally raised poultry is a better option than factory raised, both from an environmental aspect and because factory-raised chicken has the potential to harbour more bacteria. Dark meat poultry is not only cheaper, but also offers more iron, which is especially useful for babies, and has a more moist texture than breast meat as it's higher in fat. I recommend eating beef and lamb—preferably grass fed—in moderation. Some say that fish is a healthier source of protein than saturated fat-rich beef, but each food has its benefits and drawbacks. Fish can be contaminated with heavy metals from polluted waters and, if not wild caught, can contain even more.

FISH AND SEAFOOD

Try to eat fish that are high in omega-3 fats, such as char, herring, tuna, mackerel, salmon, sardines, and trout. The fish and seafood listed here are highest in omega-3 fats and usually have low mercury content:

- Anchovy
- Capelin
- Char
- Flatfish (flounder, sole, plaice)
- Hake
- Herring
- Lake whitefish
- Mackerel, Atlantic
- Monkfish
- Pollock
- Rainbow trout
- Sardines
- Salmon
- Smelt
- Turbot, Greenland
- Crab
- Mussels
- Oysters
- Shrimp

FISH AND MERCURY CONCERNS Fish higher in mercury include fresh or frozen tuna, shark, swordfish, marlin, orange roughy and escolar, King or Spanish mackerel, grouper, Chilean sea bass, and tilefish, as well as most canned albacore tuna. Generally speaking, albacore tuna is a larger species of fish that generally has higher mercury levels.

Around 2004, tuna consumption took a nosedive after Health Canada put limits on the amount of certain fish, those high in methyl mercury, that pregnant and breastfeeding women should eat because of their toxicity.[5] I wanted to know more about how to choose tuna that is safe to eat, as it's such a convenient food for the whole family and a good source of omega-3 fatty acids, so I spoke with Craig Cuffney, International Account and Partnership Manager at Safe Catch, about making a safer choice when buying tuna and salmon in cans. Safe Catch, for instance, uses technology to test each and every tuna. They only buy and use tuna that is well under the U.S. Food and Drug Administration's mercury action limit of methyl mercury measuring below 1 part per million (ppm). This limit isn't enforced but is recommended to be a safe amount. Safe Catch, unlike other companies I researched, ensures that all the tuna and salmon they can is well under this limit; their products average between 0.03 and 0.1 ppm. One in three fish don't pass Safe Catch's advanced screening, which means that other companies who do not undertake such rigorous testing can wind up canning fish with a much higher mercury content.

I've purchased many brands over the years, some sustainable and caught with admirable fishing practices, but I want to know that what I'm feeding my family has the lowest amount of mercury possible. I recommend that you do your own research to find the best product available in your area, as mercury isn't a heavy metal that any of us wants to consume.

It can also be helpful to get to know your local neighbourhood butcher and fishmonger. Your shopping experience will feel more positive when you are able to ask where the meat and fish you're buying comes from. You'll know that you can feel good about what you're buying for your family. Experts can help direct you to special cuts of meat and offer advice on how to cook it. If you want to try something new or are curious about the mercury or contaminant potential of a certain fish, your local fishmonger will likely know the answer. I've questioned many a fishmonger about their fish and ended up with something healthier than I expected.

NUTRIENTS FROM HERBS AND SPICES

Adding herbs and spices to any dish or meal that you prepare gives it an instant natural flavour boost. Herbs and spices are often overlooked as a good source of nutrition, so use them as often as you can!

HERBS

- Parsley is an excellent source of vitamins A, C, and K. It's also a good source of iron and folate.
- Cilantro helps control blood sugar, cholesterol, and production of free radicals. It helps stimulate digestion and is an amazing source of vitamin A, as well as lutein, which is necessary for good vision. Cilantro also contains calcium and potassium.
- Basil is an excellent source of vitamin K and a very good source of iron, calcium, and vitamin A. In addition, basil is a good source of dietary fibre, manganese, magnesium, vitamin C, and potassium.
- Oregano is a nutrient-dense herb with effective antibacterial properties. It's an excellent source of vitamin K and a very good source of iron, manganese, and dietary

fibre. In addition, oregano is a good source of calcium, magnesium, vitamin A, vitamin C, and omega-3 fatty acids.

- Rosemary contains substances that are useful for stimulating the immune system, increasing circulation, and improving digestion. Rosemary also contains anti-inflammatory compounds that may make it useful for reducing the severity of asthma attacks. In addition, it's been shown to increase blood flow to the head and brain, improving concentration. It's also a good source of the minerals iron and calcium, as well as dietary fibre. Fresh rosemary has 25 percent more manganese than dried rosemary (it's somehow lost in the process of drying) and 40 percent less calcium and iron, probably because of the higher water content.

- Thyme has a long history of use in natural medicine in connection with chest and respiratory problems. It is an excellent source of iron, manganese, and vitamin K. It's also a very good source of calcium and a good source of dietary fibre.

- Tarragon promotes the production of bile by the liver, which aids in digestion and helps speed the process of eliminating toxic waste in the body. It offers healing properties for the stomach and liver and is reputed to be a mild sedative. Amazingly, it's extremely valuable in fighting intestinal worms.

- Dill is an antibacterial herb and offers protection against free radicals and carcinogens. Dill seed is a very good source of calcium and a good source of the minerals manganese and iron.

- Sage is known as a memory enhancer and contains antioxidant and anti-inflammatory properties.

SPICES

- Cinnamon is good for relieving nausea and vomiting, as well as diarrhea and indigestion; it also stabilizes blood sugar and has anticancer properties. Its key nutrients include calcium; iron; magnesium; phosphorus; potassium; zinc; manganese; vitamins A, B1, B2, B3, B6, and C; folate; fibre; and 12 phytochemicals (plant nutrients with powerful health benefits).

- Coriander reduces gas and colic, relieves diarrhea (especially in children), and stimulates digestion and appetite. Its key nutrients include calcium; iron; magnesium; phosphorus; potassium; zinc; manganese; vitamins A, B1, B2, B3, B6, C, and E (in leaf only); folate; fibre; and twenty-two phytochemicals.

- Cumin improves digestion; relieves cramping, diarrhea, gas, colic, and headaches; and is an antioxidant. Key nutrients include calcium; iron; magnesium; phosphorus; potassium; zinc; manganese; vitamins A, B1, B2, B3, B6, C, and E; folate; fibre; and ten phytochemicals.

- Curry powder is a blend of spices that varies in different regions of the world. It's a digestive aid and appetite stimulant, it's good for treating dysentery and diarrhea, and it's antibacterial and antifungal. Key nutrients include vitamin B6, folate, calcium, magnesium, phosphorus, potassium, and copper; it's also a very good source of dietary fibre, vitamin E, vitamin K, iron, and manganese.

- Ginger alleviates nausea, morning sickness, vomiting, and motion sickness. It's antibacterial and anti-inflammatory, and it stimulates circulation, which helps relieve cramps, flatulence, dyspepsia, and colic. Key nutrients include calcium; iron; magnesium; phosphorus; potassium; zinc; manganese; vitamins A, B1, B2, B3, B6, C, and E; folate; fibre; and twenty-two phytochemicals.

- Turmeric is antibacterial and anti-inflammatory, increases blood circulation, decreases cholesterol, and acts as a digestive aid and liver stimulant. Key nutrients include calcium; iron; magnesium; phosphorus; potassium; zinc; copper; manganese; selenium; vitamins B1, B2, B3, B6, and C; folate; fibre; and seven phytochemicals.

- Paprika is anti-inflammatory and immune-boosting and a powerful antioxidant. Key nutrients are vitamins A, B2, B3, B6, C, and E; calcium; iron; potassium; phosphorus; magnesium; manganese; zinc; copper; selenium; pantothenic acid; folate; fibre; and phytosterols.
- Saffron is the most expensive spice. It acts as an antioxidant, an immune system stimulant, an expectorant, a pain reliever, and a digestive aid, as well as stimulating circulation and controlling blood pressure. Key nutrients are calcium; iron; magnesium; phosphorus; potassium; zinc; manganese; selenium; vitamins A, B1, B2, B3, B6, C, and E; folate; fibre; and six phytochemicals.

SPROUT RIGHT PANTRY AND FRESH ESSENTIALS: FOODS FOR A HEALTHY KITCHEN

Having a well-stocked pantry only leads to healthier eating. Even when the fridge is bare and you can't find time to shop, having dry goods, some frozen foods, and a rotation of fresh essentials on hand means you can pull off a dinner in no time. Keep in mind that some pantry items, like tetra packs of milk, and some condiments, like mustard or jarred pesto, will need to be refrigerated once opened. Always follow the storage instructions listed on the package. Many fresh essentials like bread and meat can be stored in the freezer for a number of months when packed in an airtight container. Use your freezer to ensure you always have the staples you need to whip up something healthy for your family.

GRAINS AND FLOUR
- Oats: whole, rolled, steel cut
- Rice: brown, wild, brown basmati/jasmine, Arborio
- Quinoa: grain, flakes
- Amaranth: grain
- Buckwheat: kasha, flakes
- Barley: whole, flakes
- Flour: gluten-free mix, whole wheat, brown rice

CEREALS
- Whole-grain cereals low in sugar, salt, and additives: Made Good Vanilla Brown Rice Crisps Cereal, Bob's Red Mill brand, Nature's Path brand

PASTA
- Whole wheat
- Brown rice pasta
- Kamut/spelt
- Amaranth/quinoa: GoGo Quinoa
- Soba or buckwheat: Eden Organic
- Lentil and chickpea

LEGUMES
- Lentils: red, green
- Beans: chickpeas, adzuki, kidney, cannellini, black, pinto
- Raw nuts: almonds, walnuts, pine, Brazil
- Seeds: sunflower, pumpkin, chia, flax, hemp

STAPLES

- Canned fish: salmon, tuna, mackerel (Safe Catch is low in contaminants)
- Tomatoes: canned or jarred
- Pasta tomato sauce
- Sundried tomatoes
- Salsa
- Almond butter, peanut butter, tahini, pumpkin seed butter, sunflower seed butter
- Apple butter

CONDIMENTS

- Tamari (wheat-free soy sauce)
- Vinegar: balsamic, apple cider, red wine
- Lemon and lime juice
- Organic miso paste
- Curry paste: Thai green or red curry, mild curry, butter chicken
- Dijon mustard
- Virgin coconut oil
- Extra virgin cold-pressed olive oil
- Sunflower oil

SWEETENERS

- Maple syrup
- Raw honey
- Brown rice syrup
- Barley malt syrup

MILK

- Unsweetened almond milk (without carrageenan)
- Brown rice milk
- Coconut milk, canned, full-fat, and tetra pack (watch out for sulphites)
- Cashew milk
- Oat milk

WHOLE-GRAIN BREADS

- Whole wheat
- Multigrain
- Pumpernickel rye
- Spelt
- Kamut

- Gluten-free
- Pizza crust
- Pizza dough
- Pita
- Naan
- Whole-grain crackers (Mary's Gone Crackers)
- Oatcakes

MEAT AND PROTEIN

- Whole chicken
- Chicken pieces: legs, thighs, breasts, ground
- Turkey: breasts, thighs, ground
- Fish: tuna (see Fish and Mercury Concerns, page 11), salmon, smoked salmon, mackerel, trout, sole
- Lean red meat (grass-fed or organic)
- Eggs, egg whites
- Tofu, tempeh (organic)
- Whey, bone broth, hemp, plant-based protein powder

DAIRY

- Yogurt: organic cow, goat, sheep's
- Cottage cheese
- Kefir
- Cheese: goat milk cheddar, organic cow's milk cheddar, mozzarella, sheep's milk pecorino, cottage cheese
- Organic milk: grass-fed, 2%, 3.8%, goat's, sheep's

OTHER

- Pesto: Sunflower Kitchen's Kale and Oregano, Basil, or Sundried Tomato and Olive
- Dips: Organic hummus, baba ganoush, tzatziki

ESSENTIAL TOOLS AND EQUIPMENT

Invest in a few good tools, and you'll be off to the races. The list below includes everything you need to make first baby foods and family meals. You might have some of these tools in your kitchen already, but if not, talk to friends to see which products they like, so you don't have to buy three peelers before you find one that works really well. I've detailed some of the specifics below, so that you'll know why I'm making these suggestions.

- Chopping boards: wood or plastic
- Chef's knife
- Carving knife (for slicing chicken, fish, and beef)
- Paring knife
- Peeler
- Bread knife
- Chicken shears (only to be used for cutting meat)
- Meat thermometer

- Saucepans from a small milk pan to a Dutch oven
- Rice cooker
- Frying pan (cast iron or non-toxic, non-stick)
- Cookie sheets of various sizes (for reheating as well as for roasting and baking)
- Roasting pan

- Stainless steel or bamboo steamer
- Large glass, stainless steel, or "safe" plastic bowl
- Hand blender, food processor, or high-speed blender
- Tasting spoons
- Serving spoon
- Ice cube trays that are BPA- and phthalate-free

- Freezer bags for storing food
- Casserole dish
- Colander
- Fine mesh sieve
- Garlic press
- Measuring cups
- Measuring spoons
- Lemon squeezer
- Tongs
- Spatula
- Wooden spoons

We all have our favourite tools and appliances for the kitchen. It's worth investing in ones that seem useful and passing on ones that do not.

CHOPPING BOARD

A large chopping board, either plastic or wood, is a must. Chopping boards made with food-grade plastic are safe and can be cleaned easily and sanitized by hand or in the dishwasher. Whichever board you use, make sure there are no deep grooves or cuts in them, as bacteria will make a happy home in these grooves and can transfer to your food. A good rule is to have one chopping board for raw meats and fish and one for only fruits and vegetables. I have a wooden one for fruits, veggies, and bread and a plastic one for raw meat and fish that I put in the dishwasher. Wash wooden boards with hot, soapy water, then sanitize when needed with a mixture of 1 teaspoon (5 mL) peroxide and 3 cups (750 mL) water. Rinse and air-dry completely after every use.

CHEF'S KNIFE, PARING KNIFE, AND PEELER

A chef's knife is essential for all cooking. You want to make sure it's a sharp knife that feels good in your hand, in terms of both the weight and its handle. If you aren't confident with a big 8-inch (20 cm) chef's knife, buy one that is less intimidating in size, between 6 and 7 inches (15 and 18 cm). It's worth checking out the knife section of a store such as Ikea to test a few before buying a new one. Contrary to what most people think, more accidents are caused by dull knives than by sharp ones, as you have to use more pressure with a dull knife and then—whoops!—the knife slips. A paring knife is also useful for slicing small fruit or cutting out the cores.

When you first make food for your baby, starting at around six months, you'll need to peel almost all the fruits and vegetables, as the peel could bring too much texture to a purée. I searched high and low for an excellent peeler for my Mommy Chef cooking classes, before someone gave me a Star brand peeler. The peeler blade runs horizontal rather than vertical, and it's the best peeler you'll ever find, so search it out online or at a home show. It's worth the effort.

STAINLESS STEEL STEAMER BASKET OR BAMBOO STEAMER

Choose a bamboo or stainless steel double boiler–type steamer. A double boiler steamer sits high above the bottom of the saucepan, allowing you to put a lot of water in the pot, so there's less chance of your saucepan boiling dry. For this reason, I don't suggest the "flower"-type baskets that sit inside a saucepan—you can't fit enough water underneath them to steam carrots for thirty minutes. Steaming is preferable to boiling, baking, or microwaving because it helps to retain more nutrients and, if the food's not over-steamed, the water content of the produce will remain high (especially compared to baking).

BOWLS

Mixing bowls are a must-have item in the kitchen. They can be used for preparing ingredients and for serving food. When making baby food, once you've steamed your fruits and veggies, you'll put them in a bowl and purée them. Glass, stainless steel, or "safe" (BPA-free) plastic bowls are best. Glass bowls are preferable—they have a great shape and are really durable. Plastic might get stained from carrots, beets, and blueberries, and stainless steel bowls can be loud when used with a hand blender.

HAND BLENDER

A hand or immersion blender is fast and effective and can be used for many foods, including purées. When trying out purées with different textures, a hand blender makes it easier to introduce a range of consistencies, as you can blend for a shorter period of time and mash the harder lumps in the dish. It's a cinch to clean and easy to travel with, too. If you have a high-powered blender like Vitamix or Blendtec, you certainly can purée in seconds using that!

BABY FOOD STORAGE TRAYS AND CONTAINERS

Whatever ice cube trays you use, make sure that they're durable and contain no BPA, polyvinyl chloride (PVC), or phthalates. There are silicone trays of many sizes, some larger than the usual 1-ounce (30 g) size, which work great for bigger eaters. You can also store food in glass containers or jars—just be sure to leave enough room for the food to expand, or the glass can break.

FREEZER BAGS FOR STORING FOOD

Once you've frozen your baby food in either trays or individual containers, pop it out and store each batch in a freezer bag, making sure to label and date the bag. Try to get as much air out of the bag as possible to reduce freezer burn. The food can be kept in a fridge freezer for up to three months.

1 · NUTRIENT NEEDS FOR MOM AND BABY

After the marathon of labour and growing another human over forty weeks or so, moms' nutrition needs to be top notch. It can be a tricky thing at a time when making super-nutritious meals is likely low on the priority list. In the weeks and months after your baby is born, sleep deprivation and the new routine that you're not always in charge of can throw off eating patterns. It can make breakfast happen closer to lunch, lunch nearer to dinner, and dinner before you go to bed, if at all. Even with the best of intentions, feeding yourself and your family may just become another stress in your day. This is a time to call in the troops for meal making, batch cooking, vegetable chopping, and grocery shopping. To anyone who offers to do anything, please say YES! Baby's dad, mother or grandma, friends, work colleagues, extended family—to pretty much anyone who's willing to make you some healthy meals and snacks, say thank you and ask them to keep them coming. This chapter goes into detail about the needs of both mom and baby from birth onward.

KEY NUTRIENTS AND SUPPLEMENTS FOR NEW MOMS

Breastfeeding mothers need more of certain nutrients to keep up with breast milk demands once baby arrives. Calorie intake should increase by 500 calories a day from your diet during pregnancy (for example, 2 tablespoons/30 mL of hummus with carrot sticks, about 20 almonds or cashews, and a 1¾-ounce/50 g piece of cheese) to produce enough breast milk for your baby without leaving you zapped of energy. I hear your concerns about eating more while wanting to lose the weight gained during pregnancy, but trust me, you'll still lose weight if you stick to that number.

It took nine months to put on your pregnancy weight, and it might take a little longer than that to lose it. Please don't set your expectations too high, and understand that your body has changed during pregnancy and your hormones are calling the shots. Now is not the time to diet, but you *can* make better choices about what you eat. Eat healthily instead of indulging your cake or cookie craving, and the weight will come off slowly and steadily. I know that's not what you want to hear (and that your favourite jeans are calling to be worn again). Exercise is crucial to slowly shedding some pounds and gaining strength for carrying your baby and that car seat all over the place. Exercise also helps to increase energy, improve mood, and strengthen your bones, which may be weaker after lovingly donating calcium to your baby's bones. Plenty of fitness companies offer stroller fitness, indoor aerobics, and boot camp classes with baby in tow if you want faster results than waiting for your pre-pregnancy shape to return on its own.

MULTINUTRIENTS

In an ideal world, we would all eat freshly picked fruits and vegetables, have a plentiful supply of the most nutritious whole-grain cereals and bread on hand, eat only fresh-caught fish, buy naturally farmed and fed poultry and red meat . . . and have it all cooked for us! And while we're at it, somebody else would wash the dishes after dinner and fold the laundry while we try to get some sleep. Well, that just isn't reality. So, where are you going to get the vitamins, minerals, proteins, carbohydrates, and fats you need? This is where a good-quality multinutrient comes in handy. Your baby took all of the vitamins and minerals she needed from you while in utero—calcium, iron, zinc, and vitamin D, to name a few—and has left you deficient in one or more. A multinutrient will help ensure that you're getting a base level of nutrients daily. Even if you do manage to eat a healthy, balanced diet, your body needs to keep up with the nutrient demands of making breast milk. If you're not breastfeeding, you still need three to six months to replenish the stores of minerals and fats that were nabbed from you during pregnancy.

What should you look for in a good-quality multinutrient? First, I'd suggest finding a health food or supplement store or asking a nutritionist or naturopath what brands she likes and why. Although a few chain drugstores and big-box retailers carry some higher-quality natural products and supplements, you won't get the same level of help in choosing a quality product. Always look for a multinutrient in capsule rather than tablet form. Capsules typically break down more easily, leading to better vitamin and mineral absorption.

Here's a rundown of the key vitamins and minerals your body needs every day, along with their most important functions.

FAT-SOLUBLE VITAMINS—VITAMINS A, D, E, AND K These vitamins all have different roles in the body, from supporting healthy mucous membranes to maintaining bone health, ensuring good heart function, and providing normal blood clotting. All of these vitamins are stored in the liver and fatty tissues of the body, and their absorption is helped by eating fat at the same time as taking a supplement. Excessive amounts of any fat-soluble vitamin can be toxic. Double-check with a nutritionist or naturopath for safe supplement levels.

WATER-SOLUBLE VITAMINS—B VITAMINS, INCLUDING B1, B2, B3, B5, B6, AND B12; FOLIC ACID; BIOTIN; AND VITAMIN C These vitamins are needed every day: they are taken into the body and used, and anything left over is then excreted. (Vitamin B2 is the one that makes your urine turn bright yellow.) B vitamins are important for many functions in the body but are best known for supplying energy. Be careful not to take more vitamin B6 than what's in your multinutrient while breastfeeding, as too much can lower your breast milk production. Vitamin C is also used for an incredible number of processes in the body but is perhaps recognized most often for its immune-boosting properties. Vitamin C has an antihistamine effect (great for treating allergies) and is needed for cardiovascular health, skin, and wound healing. It's used up quickly in times of stress, which—let's face it—most of us go through, so make sure you're getting enough; about 2000 mg per day is good (in divided doses, 1000 mg with breakfast and 1000 mg at another time in the day). If you're breastfeeding, you need all of these water-soluble vitamins in your diet, from your multinutrient or a stand-alone supplement, so they can pass into your breast milk.

MACRO MINERALS, OR BIG MINERALS—INCLUDING CALCIUM, MAGNESIUM, PHOSPHORUS, POTASSIUM, AND SODIUM Calcium is well known for building strong bones but is also needed to maintain your body's alkaline balance (see Building Strong Bones: It's More Than Just Calcium, page 36). Magnesium is important for muscles, bones, the immune system, blood sugar balance, stress busting, and heart function. Both calcium and magnesium are calming minerals—taking them before bed can ensure a good night's sleep. Calcium requires phosphorus to help absorption and contribute to bone and teeth strength, kidney and heart function, and nerve and muscle activity. Potassium is crucial for heart function, nerves, muscles, kidneys, and blood. And sodium, which has a bad reputation because it's overused, is actually important for keeping fluid levels in the body just right as well as maintaining a healthy heart.

MICRO MINERALS, OR TRACE MINERALS—THE MOST IMPORTANT BEING IRON, ZINC, MANGANESE, CHROMIUM, AND SELENIUM Micro minerals are needed in smaller amounts than macro minerals in our bodies. Iron is essential to the development and growth of babies and children and is used in the production of hemoglobin and by the immune system. Zinc is another incredibly important mineral that's involved in more than three hundred enzyme processes in the body. It's used by the immune system; along with vitamin B6, it aids in production of hydrochloric acid in the stomach for digesting proteins and carbohydrates; it helps wound healing; and it supports growth and development of the reproductive organs. Manganese is needed to make strong bones, synthesize fats and cholesterol, protect your body from free radical damage, and help with balancing blood sugar levels. Chromium works with manganese to balance blood sugar levels. Selenium is an important anticancer mineral, it helps the body use vitamin E, and it helps build healthy cell membranes.

All of the vitamins and nutrients discussed above are available in a wide variety of foods, but to get enough you need to eat a varied diet every day—and that doesn't always happen. In addition, aiming for as many organic foods as possible lessens your exposure to chemicals, and so less is shared with your baby while breastfeeding. To keep up with the requirements of your body at this stage, you'll need to take a good-quality supplement with a variety of vitamins and minerals, and even add an extra 2000 to 3000 mg of vitamin C; 1200 mg of calcium in the citrate, malate, or amino acid chelate form; and 600 to 800 mg of magnesium in the glycinate, malate, citrate, or amino acid chelate form per day. If your blood sugar balance is up and down (as most of the population's is), include an additional 200 to 400 mcg of chromium daily. White spots on your fingernails indicate zinc and other mineral deficiencies; add about 20 mg of zinc every day and even a tissue salt mélange that has all twelve essential minerals in it, until the spots fade. Supplements are really the only way to correct deficiencies. A nutritionist or naturopath can help you identify what you might be deficient in and advise you on how to correct it.

DHA FOR MOMMY BRAIN

Forgetfulness, an inability to concentrate, and on some days, forgetting where the car keys are *and* where you parked the car can be blamed on mommy brain (finally, a valid excuse!). The phenomenal development and growth rate of baby's neurological system and brain from the third trimester until she's three months old while breastfeeding demands a higher level of docosahexaenoic acid (DHA), the important brain- and memory-boosting part of the omega-3 fatty acids that most commonly come from eating fish. The best source of dietary DHA is oily fish: salmon, tuna, herring, mackerel, sardines, and trout. The DHA stored in mom's brain and tissues passes through the bloodstream to baby while in the womb. Amazingly, the mom's DHA reserves provide the fuel needed to make another brain and nervous system. So, she deserves a break if she can't remember where the diapers went! Sleep deprivation compounds the problem, and although a full week of eight hours of sleep a night might improve her functioning, it still won't help with the DHA deficiency in the brain.

DHA deficiency could increase the chance of postnatal depression or postnatal blues—in fact, low levels of DHA are linked to depressive disorders in any individual. Having a baby is transformational enough without the added risk of depression and even suicidal thoughts. Media attention has increasingly been directed toward postnatal depression and its treatment with antidepressants. That certainly is one way to go; however, I suggest women try taking omega-3 fish oils rich in DHA. I've received feedback that these oils have a positive effect. If mom's not a fish eater, there are other ways to get this important nutrient. I have a friend who couldn't take fish oil in the liquid form (which yields a much higher amount per teaspoon) I had recommended, no matter where she put it—in a smoothie, in salad dressing, or down the hatch with her nose plugged. Instead, she ended up taking handfuls of eicosapentaenoic acid (EPA)/DHA capsules every day. It was what she could manage, and although this was a more expensive way to take DHA, she was pleased that she'd made the effort and commented many times that her mommy brain was significantly less of a problem with her second child than with her first, born five years earlier.

A vegetarian or vegan source of omega-3 and DHA is algae—after all, it's what fish eat to become such rich sources. Vegans and vegetarians have a hard time getting enough DHA in their diet and have to take handfuls of algae DHA, which typically comes in 100 to 200 mg capsules, to get the recommended 600 to 1200 mg per day. In a study measuring DHA levels in breast milk, mothers following vegetarian and vegan diets had 50 to 70 percent less DHA than fish-eating moms.[6] Other sources of omega-3 fats that vegetarians and vegans could benefit from eating include walnuts and pumpkin, sunflower, flax, chia, and hemp seeds, but I wouldn't recommend relying only on these food sources during pregnancy or breastfeeding, as the body's ability to digest or break down these fats to usable DHA is poor.

You need 1200 mg of DHA daily from the third trimester until your baby is three months old while breastfeeding. After three months, you can reduce the amount to 600 to 800 mg per day. If you're not breastfeeding, 1200 mg a day for the first three months should top up what was taken from you during pregnancy. A cost effecitve way to get a high level of DHA is in a liquid oil, which usually yields a higher level—as mentioned above, most omega-3 capsules yield less than the necessary 1200 mg a day. At least 600 mg per day should be taken for six months after baby weans (or after baby is three months old if you've formula-fed since birth) to nourish your brain and build up your stores of DHA, especially if you plan to have more children.

When choosing an omega-3 or DHA supplement, always read the label to make sure that it contains DHA. If the omega-3 isn't broken down or predigested to DHA (look for a milligram amount on the label), your body can use up the omega-3 before it breaks down to DHA, leaving you deficient. As with your multinutrient, buy your DHA supplement from a reputable vitamin or health food store, and ask about different products. Try my *Take This* Omega Power; Genestra, Nutra Sea, and Nordic Naturals are also good brands. It's worth comparing the price versus yield of DHA in various products.

IRON AND ANEMIA

Amazingly, our bodies increase the uptake of iron from foods when our levels are low. Iron is supplied by our diet, and deficiency may be due to numerous reasons: eating too few iron-rich foods, poor absorption of iron, pregnancy, menstruation and heavy periods, long-term blood loss from peptic ulcers, long-term Aspirin use, and certain cancers or malignancies. When supplementing to correct iron deficiency, try to choose a non–ferrous sulphate supplement—a ferrous gluconate, chelate, or fumarate form. Studies have demonstrated that ferrous sulphate supplements (the most common form of iron, as it's inexpensive) didn't show the expected increase in iron levels. The absorption rate of ferrous sulphate is 10 percent, meaning that if you need to get 10 mg of iron per day, the label of your supplement should read 100 mg of ferrous sulphate. That's a very high level of iron that wouldn't be prescribed and would likely lead to instant constipation. Vitamin C increases the uptake of iron, so take the two together to optimize absorption. Also, take iron supplements between meals to lessen the chances that other minerals will hinder its absorption. Iron should be supplemented only after a deficiency is confirmed by a blood test. Iron in high doses not only can be toxic, but also competes with other minerals such as calcium, magnesium, and zinc for absorption, possibly leading to deficiencies in these other important minerals.

What Hinders Iron Absorption?

- Calcium and dairy products
- Bad bacteria, yeast, and parasites in the gut
- Black tea and some herb teas (peppermint, chamomile)
- Coffee and cocoa
- Oxalates found in some dark leafy greens

Signs of Iron Deficiency

- Pale skin
- Fatigue
- Irritability
- Dizziness
- Weakness
- Shortness of breath
- Sore tongue
- Brittle nails
- Decreased appetite (especially in children)
- Frequent respiratory or intestinal infections
- Pica (wanting to eat nonfood items such as dirt or ice)
- Headache (front of head)
- Itchiness

PROBIOTICS

Billions of bacteria, both good and bad, are found all over our bodies, inside and out. What I'm focusing on here are those that live within humans' digestive tracts or, more specifically, the intestines. For overall health, a strong immune system, and effective digestion and detoxification of what we ingest, we need high levels of good bacteria.

To explain this further in a visual way, think of a backyard or park. Picture a lovely green, lush, healthy lawn with few or no weeds. In the intestines, the lovely lawn without many weeds is what we'd like to see along the lining of our intestines—an abundance of good bacteria creates a healthy colonic environment. When the weeds, or bad bacteria, take over, the environment changes, leading to a not-so-green-and-lush lawn, or suboptimal health. This healthy environment must be cared for by supporting the proliferation of good bacteria with supplements called probiotics.

The benefits of a healthy digestive system and a strong population of good bacteria are far-reaching and include the following: lessening the potential for allergies; protecting against the ill effects of bad bacteria taking residence in the gut; better digestion of sugars (lactose); creating B and K vitamins in the gut; detoxifying and positively transforming many unsavoury substances, such as heavy metals of lead, mercury, and cadmium, and releasing helpful substances from foods that slow cancer growth.

Unfortunately, antibiotics have a similar effect on your intestines as weed killer has on a lawn. Although antibiotics are designed to kill the bad bacteria, or weeds, in your gut (or elsewhere in your body), a side effect is that they also destroy a large amount of the good bacteria. When the lush, green, healthy grass is destroyed, this is an opportune time for the weeds to come back strong and take over. For instance, if you tested strep B positive before delivery, you would have been given antibiotics during labour to kill the strep B bacteria and keep them from harming your baby. Although both mom and baby have benefited from killing the strep B, the beneficial bacteria in mom's intestines as well as those that the baby would take from the birth canal may have been wiped out. The immune-boosting effects of the beneficial bacteria for the newborn are now deficient, allowing any unfriendly bacteria to proliferate. Researchers attribute the rise of allergies in the developed world partly to the overuse of antibiotics. Because it's well known that an intestinal environment colonized with predominantly beneficial bacteria can help reduce the risk of allergies by a whopping 57 percent,[7] taking probiotics is crucial for anyone who has been on antibiotics.

DO YOU NEED MORE GOOD BACTERIA? Think of how gassy you are, or how smelly the bathroom is after you've had a bowel movement. That's a sign that your digestive system is off balance on some level. Do you have symptoms of thrush? Do you have alternating diarrhea and constipation? Have you taken antibiotics recently or for a longer period in your life? Do you get frequent colds, infections, or have allergies? Answering yes to any of these questions could mean that you would benefit from a huge boost of good bacteria from probiotics.

WHAT MAKES A GOOD PROBIOTIC? When you're looking to buy a probiotic, quality really does matter. A reputable company will have high standards for the manufacturing process as well as excellent quality control. When you are deciding on a probiotic, it's all about the numbers. How many billions of bacteria is it supplying? Which strains of bacteria are you getting? Is it a human strain of bacteria (much more effective for colonizing the gut)? Look for a probiotic that lists *Lactobacillus acidophilus* and *Bifidobacterium bifidum* and/or *B. lactis* on the label along with human strains called human microflora, for starters. Probiotics for infants under one year of age should contain *Bifidobacterium* strains. If you've just been on antibiotics, you need to take a very high-powered probiotic to ingest a hundred billion or more good bacteria per day for at least seven days after finishing the course of antibiotics. Continue taking probiotics at a dose of twenty-five billion during the three months that follow. If you find yourself gassy while taking probiotics, look for one without fructooligosaccharides (FOS), a prebiotic that's fuel for the probiotics. It sounds great in theory, but for anyone who has a history of yeast symptoms, including yeast infections, thrush, sinusitis, urinary tract infection, or cracks in the corners of your mouth, FOS may not be your friend. The rest of the probiotic profile is important, and you can find human strain probiotics without FOS that are effective.

If you're suffering from symptoms of thrush, ingesting at least fifty billion total bacteria a day should be your minimum. For overall health and to support your immune and digestive systems, any mixed strains above twenty-five billion per day is a good level. When you start taking probiotics, you could experience an increase in gassiness, perhaps a bit of diarrhea, or even constipation for the first three days. I suggest starting with lower amounts than those listed above, taking your probiotics after food (unless the label says otherwise), and taking them in the evening. If you're giving probiotics to your baby, start her on her own probiotic in the morning so that any gassiness won't cause discomfort and wake her up in the night.

Because probiotics are live bacteria, ideally they should be purchased from the fridge and kept refrigerated at home. Some probiotics are shelf stable for several months, but you'll lose some of those good guys the longer they're kept out of the fridge. With that said, do take your probiotics on holiday with you, even if they won't be refrigerated—it's better to take them and lose a few in your supplement than to not take them at all. See Chapter 5 for more information about probiotics for infants and the immune system and page 43 for a table listing the quantities of supplements, including probiotics, you need.

MOMMY MEALS

Here are some basic tips for the new mom:

- Drink plenty of water! Aim for more than 8 cups (2 L) of filtered water a day.
- Every morning, make a mug of hot water with a squeeze of lemon and add 1 or 2 tablespoons (15 or 30 mL) of apple cider vinegar; drink this before you have anything else. It starts your digestion working and stimulates the kidneys and liver, improving overall good health and giving you extra energy.
- If you're breastfeeding and think your baby may be reacting to something in your diet, keep a food diary of what you eat and drink. Write down the symptoms your

baby is experiencing. Look back over twenty-four to forty-eight hours in your diary and try to figure out what may be the problem. If you can't see a pattern, reach out to a nutritionist or naturopath for help.

- Try to eat something about every two and a half to three hours. Ideally, you should eat three meals and two to three snacks each day. Eating regularly will help keep your blood sugar and energy balanced.
- Make sure you eat protein at each snack and meal. Increase your protein intake at breakfast, especially by eating eggs, cottage cheese, or protein powder in a smoothie. I like to add hemp protein powder some days, and a cold-processed whey protein powder or bone broth protein powder on other days, to get a high level of protein. Hemp also offers extra omega-3 and fibre.
- Increase your intake of fruits and veggies. A handful of almonds or a tablespoon (15 mL) of almond butter with an apple is an excellent fast snack, giving you fibre, carbohydrate, protein, essential fats, tons of nutrients, and long-lasting energy.
- Be sure to have at least five servings of fruits and veggies every day.
- Watch the amount of wheat and dairy you're eating. These are the two most common food sensitivities. Try to switch up the grains you eat from wheat to spelt, kamut, oats, rice, or quinoa. Add rice or almond milk to your smoothie for a change from dairy milk.

Don't Forget to Feed Yourself

As a new mom, on some days you're probably lucky if you shower, brush your teeth, and get out of your PJs. Eating takes a back seat to caring for your bundle of joy. But if you're a breastfeeding mom, your nutritional requirements are higher than when you were pregnant. Feeding yourself is an extra task that you don't always have time for. Let's make it simple.

- You may need to become a snackaholic during the day to keep yourself going if making meals other than dinner is difficult.
- You must have raw fruits and vegetables on hand, as they're healthy and fast, with little prep time. Think baby carrots, cucumber, apple, banana, and fresh berries.
- When you cook, always prep two meals at once. Make larger batches to save leftovers for the next day's meals. For example, grill four chicken breasts or thighs instead of two and add some to your salad or wrap for lunch the next day, or mix them with some frozen vegetables and rice for the next night's stir-fry.
- Stash dried fruit like pineapple, figs (Golden California figs are my favourite), dates, or raisins in your car and around your house for a quick energy boost. Ideally, combine these with a handful of good fat and mineral-rich nuts like almonds or walnuts.
- Stock up on meals that freeze well for fast and easy dinners (with extra for leftovers). See the meal suggestions on pages 28 to 29, for more ideas.

BREAKFAST

- A piece of fruit and Mini Frittatas (page 257)
- A smoothie made with rice, almond, coconut, or cow's milk (see Mom's Super-Powered Smoothie on page 29)
- Overnight Oatmeal (page 259) with rice, almond, or cow's milk; ground nuts and seeds (flax, chia, hemp, sunflower, or pumpkin); and fresh or frozen fruit
- Low-sugar or Crunchy Granola (page 263) with organic Greek yogurt or milk
- Fibre-rich cereal with nuts and seeds or an egg
- Poached or scrambled egg on toast (kamut, spelt, rice, or whole wheat bread) or in a wrap with veggies
- Overnight French Toast (page 260) with fresh fruit and raw honey or maple syrup
- Toast with almond, peanut, or hazelnut butter and fruit spread (sweetened with fruit juice instead of sugar)
- Organic Greek yogurt with fruit, Crunchy Granola (page 263), and chia seeds, ground or whole nuts, and seeds
- Chia Pudding (page 259) made with almond or coconut milk, vanilla extract, and a splash of maple syrup or raw honey
- Blender Pancakes (page 255) served with fruit spread, almond butter, or peanut butter
- Egg and Avocado Wrap (page 258) or egg and avocado on toast

LUNCH OR DINNER

- Large green salad of kale or baby kale, spinach, arugula, and/or romaine lettuce; half an avocado; and protein of choice: nuts, seeds, fish, chicken, tofu, falafel, beans or chickpeas, cottage cheese, or egg
- Sandwich or wrap with fish, chicken, egg, cheese, nut butter (almond butter is good), or hummus and sprouts (see Roasted Veggie Tagine on page 279)
- Any other grains, such as buckwheat, quinoa, amaranth, or brown rice (try my Coconut Rice on page 308), with tofu, chicken, or fish and vegetables—cooked together in a saucepan or as a stir-fry
- Pasta with meatballs (see Super Burgers, Meatballs, or Meatloaf, page 217) and marinara sauce
- Baked potato topped with Veggie-Packed Chili (page 211), cottage cheese, or tuna and corn
- Falafel with hummus and salad
- Pesto Fish (page 289), Super Simple Baked Trout (page 284), Garlic Maple Salmon (page 283), Chicken Souvlaki (page 273), or Golden Grilled Curried Chicken Thighs (page 274), served with two colourful vegetables
- Mixed Bean Salad (page 303) with a leafy green salad on the side
- Quesadilla (like the Bean and Veggie Kamut Quesadillas on page 220) and Pure Green Hummus (page 309)
- Sweet Potato and Coconut Soup (page 215) or Corn, Coconut, and Ginger Soup (page 295), served with whole-grain bread or crackers and Hummus (page 182)
- Egg and vegetable frittata with greens like broccoli, kale, baby kale, spinach, and arugula or my Mini Frittatas (page 257)
- Mixed nuts or seeds on top of anything

- Beans or pulses, such as chickpeas and lentils, with a salad or grains
- Salmon or Tuna Melt Sandwich (page 285) or Salmon Burgers (page 286), served with a side of greens and Salad Dressing (page 304) (Safe Catch is a low-mercury brand of fish)

SNACKS
- Spelt, kamut, or sprouted grain bread with nut or seed butter and fruit spread
- Crudités (vegetable sticks) with nut butter, guacamole, Hummus (page 182), nuts, or seeds
- Air-popped popcorn drizzled with olive oil, herbs, and spices with nuts or seeds
- Oatcakes (page 318), rice cakes, Ryvita crispbread, or crackers with Hummus (page 182), a mixture of tahini (sesame seed paste) and honey, cottage cheese, avocado dip, or dairy, goat's, or sheep's milk cheese
- Beany Green Dip (page 181), Yummy Carrot Spread (page 180), or Pure Green Hummus (page 309) with carrot, celery, or zucchini sticks; Finger Food Pancakes (page 178); or Mary's Gone Crackers or low-sodium pretzels
- Organic baked corn chips with Hummus (page 182) or salsa
- Mom's Super-Powered Smoothie (recipe below)
- Fruit with nut butter, such as banana or apple with almond butter
- Granola bar (see my Go Faster Granola Bars on page 231) or whole-grain bar such as MadeGood, Kind, CLIF Nut Butter Filled, or CLIF Kid ZBar Filled

---

Mom's Super-Powered Smoothie MAKES ABOUT 1½ CUPS (375 ML)

This smoothie is packed with nutrients for every member of the family. If you're pregnant or breastfeeding, add fish oil to get beneficial omega-3 fats and DHA to you and your baby. Switch up the fruits to include mango, peach, melon, or other berries for different nutrient profiles. The banana masks most flavours, so this is a great place to hide some not-so-favourite foods or tastes.

1. Blend all ingredients in a high-speed blender until smooth. Serve immediately.

1 cup (250 mL) milk of choice (unsweetened almond or coconut)

1 ripe banana

½ cup (125 mL) frozen wild blueberries

½ pear, core removed, or ½ cup (125 mL) mango

Handful of sunflower sprouts or baby spinach

1 tablespoon (15 mL) flax or hemp oil

2 tablespoons (30 mL) whey, bone broth, hemp, or rice protein

1 tablespoon (15 mL) almond butter, peanut butter, or sunflower seed butter

1 tablespoon (15 mL) black strap molasses (optional)

NUTRITIONAL INFORMATION This smoothie is high in fibre, antioxidants, omega-3 fats, and protein to keep blood sugar stable.

NUTRITION FOR BABIES: AN IN-DEPTH LOOK AT THE NUTRIENTS YOUR BABY NEEDS

Now that your baby has arrived, let's lay the groundwork for what you need to know about vitamins and minerals, fats, and oils in the first six months to one year of your baby's life, before you start baby on solids. Most new parents probably have some knowledge of these nutrients, but here I'll expand on why they are important and how to ensure that your baby is getting what she needs. At the end of the chapter, I sum up the nutrient requirements for mom and baby by situation and age.

VITAMIN D: THE SUNSHINE VITAMIN

Vitamin D, known as the "sunshine vitamin," has been getting a lot of attention in recent years as research has shown its role in preventing numerous diseases, including multiple sclerosis, type 1 diabetes, and cancer in adults and children. Vitamin D is important for mom during pregnancy as well as breastfeeding to ensure that baby has adequate amounts.[8]

Full-term babies are born with vitamin D stores taken from mom that will last for about the first two months of their lives. However, premature babies had less time in utero to take vitamin D (and other nutrients) from mom before birth. If you're deficient in vitamin D—perhaps you were pregnant during the winter, you remained inside on bed rest, you're dark-skinned, you wore clothing covering most of your body, or you just weren't in the sun—there likely will have been less to give to your baby. If this is the case, you can improve your baby's levels by supplementing yourself if you're breastfeeding, as vitamin D is one of the nutrients that passes to your baby through breast milk.

Studies show that babies who were exclusively breastfed from birth to six months and have adequate exposure to sunlight are not at risk for developing vitamin D deficiency or rickets.[9] After the first two months, as stored vitamin D starts to run out, you'll need to rely on other sources for your baby, including sunlight or ultraviolet B (UVB) rays and breast milk or vitamin D–fortified formula. Vitamin D in breast milk is easily absorbed and acts more effectively than that in formula or foods. It's bound to water-soluble proteins that aid its absorption, which is why it's important for mom to supplement with adequate vitamin D to pass to baby. According to the Public Health Agency of Canada, from July 2002 until December 2004, 104 cases of vitamin D deficiency resulting in rickets were confirmed among children living in Canada, mostly in the northern territories.[10,11] The majority of those cases involved infants and toddlers with intermediate and dark skin who had been exclusively breastfed without vitamin D supplementation. See page 43 for supplement recommendations.

A DOSE OF VITAMIN D AND SAFE SUN EXPOSURE In recent years, the association between exposure to sunlight and cancer has had us applying sunscreen liberally on ourselves and our children, limiting the amount of vitamin D our bodies can generate by 95 percent. Sunscreen isn't recommended for babies under six months of age because absorption of the chemicals found in sunscreen can be harmful. Instead, Health Canada advises that for the first year, babies stay in the shade and wear protective hats, sunglasses, and clothing. Although these recommendations are a safe way to avoid sunburn and other negative effects of UV rays, they can have detrimental effects on vitamin D levels.

I recommend that a breastfeeding mother supplement her diet with 3000 to 5000 international units (IU) of vitamin D daily. Some of this can be attained from cod liver oil, which also supplies vitamin A and DHA and is one of the most absorbable sources (check the label of your product to see how much it offers). Vitamin D supplementation during the summer months may not be as necessary, depending on how much you're out in the sun. If you're outside only on weekends, this may not be enough.

A formula-fed baby who's usually covered up in the sun should be given a supplement of at least 400 IU of vitamin D per day. Some recommendations are double that. Cod liver oil is an excellent source of vitamins A and D in a natural ratio that's easy for the body to use: give 1 mL for every 4.5 kg (10 pounds) of weight. For example, if you weigh 59 kg (130 pounds), you'd need to take 13 mL of cod liver oil a day, which works out to almost a tablespoon. The oil can also be applied by rubbing it on baby's skin. Otherwise, look for a supplement without flavouring, sugar, or colouring. My *Take This* Sunshine D + K2 is a liposome spray for super-fast and efficient absorption with vitamin K2, which increases vitamin D absorption even further. Carlson makes a product called Ddrops that contains nothing artificial and no sugar. Both are very easy to give to your baby. Breastfed babies may not need to be supplemented if mom is taking at least 2000 IU of vitamin D per day or is out in the sunshine daily. Supplement your baby if he's formula fed, if you're not taking a vitamin D supplement, or if you can't get out in the sunshine every day. See the Resources page on SproutRight.com for a list of good supplements for mom and baby.

What's the Best Form of Vitamin D?

Vitamin D3 is the most absorbable form of vitamin D. Margarine and soy products are fortified with vitamin D2, a less absorbable form.
Read the label of your supplement to ensure that it's a source of vitamin D3.

IRON FOR BRAWN, BLOOD, AND BRAINS

Your baby will have stocked up on iron while in utero. This essential mineral supports the development of baby's brain for cognitive and behavioural maturity and makes hemoglobin, the protein in red blood cells that delivers oxygen to the body's organs, muscles, and tissues.

Iron deficiency anemia, a lack of adequate red blood cells caused by too little iron, affects about 50 percent of pregnant women and can be a concern for premature and low birth weight (less than 2.25 kg/5 pounds at birth) babies. Although iron requirements during pregnancy more than double, even if mom was anemic during pregnancy, an interesting study has shown that baby won't be predisposed to having low iron stores.[12]

YOUR BABY'S BUILT-IN IRON STORES Healthy, full-term babies have enough iron stored to last for at least the first six months of life. Many parents worry that their babies will suddenly run out of their iron stores and become anemic at six months, but current research has shown that they should last between six and twelve months, perhaps longer in exclusively breastfed babies. So, breathe a sigh of relief and don't worry as much while you're figuring out the introduction of solids or why your baby isn't terribly interested in eating. There appears to be a strong link between low iron levels and birth weight. Preterm babies born with a low birth weight—less than 2.5 kg (5 pounds, 8 ounces)—are likely to have low iron. A low-for-gestation birth weight (same as above) or preterm baby would benefit from delayed clamping of the umbilical cord at birth to allow more maternal blood to flow to the baby. Blood drawn from an infant for testing can also contribute to low iron levels.

Your baby is also at risk of iron deficiency during times of rapid weight gain that last for a month or more (not to be confused with the common growth spurts at three and six weeks and three and six months, when your baby drinks more than usual). You may see a jump in the weight percentile on your baby's chart, and although this may ease your worry about baby's low weight, it will use up more of baby's already low stores of iron. If your baby was born close to her due date at a birth weight above 3 kg (6 pounds, 10 ounces) and breastfeeds or formula feeds well, she's unlikely to have low iron. Unless there has been blood loss for some reason, you don't need to be overly nervous about iron deficiency.

Babies at Increased Risk for Low Iron Levels
- Premature babies, as babies take on most of mom's iron during the last trimester
- Preterm babies born less than 2.5 kg (5 pounds, 8 ounces)
- Babies born to mothers with poorly controlled diabetes during pregnancy
- Babies fed cow's milk instead of breast milk or formula during the first year

AVOIDING THE SIDE EFFECTS OF IRON SUPPLEMENTS Constipation is the most common side effect of iron supplementation. If you're giving iron to your baby— perhaps your baby was premature or had blood tests in early infancy—watch for constipation and fussiness as signs that he's not tolerating it. If I see this, I recommend that Ferrum Phos tissue salt be given alongside another form of iron. Dosage depends on the individual. Most infant iron supplements are also full of sugar and flavouring, so do read the label before choosing one. Iron can also be a double-edged sword when it comes to our immune systems. It's important for fighting infection, but it's also food for bad bacteria such as *Escherichia coli*, *Salmonella*, *Clostridium*, *Bacteroides*, and *Staphylococcus*. Because iron contained in formulas feeds these unfriendly bacteria, it's essential to give infant probiotics to your baby when formula feeding. Read more about formula feeding and iron in Chapter 3.

Iron Absorption from Breast Milk, Formula, and Infant Cereal

Iron has the highest absorption rate from breast milk—the vitamin C and high level of lactose in breast milk, as well as the proteins lactoferrin and transferrin, help to increase its absorption.

The absorbability of iron from different food sources is as follows:[13]

- Breast milk: 50 to 70 percent
- Iron-fortified dairy formula: 3 to 12 percent
- Iron-fortified soy formula: 1 to 7 percent
- Iron-fortified cereal: 4 to 10 percent
- Cow's milk: 10 percent

IRON ON YOUR PLATE: HEME AND NON-HEME SOURCES Two types of iron are found in food: heme and non-heme. Heme iron makes up about 40 percent of the iron found in meat, chicken, and fish. The remaining iron in these animal sources—as well as all non-meat foods, including dairy, eggs, fruits, and vegetables—is called non-heme iron. Heme iron is more readily absorbed by the body, at 15 to 35 percent. The amount of non-heme iron that's absorbed varies from 2 to 20 percent or more, depending on the other food and drinks you consume at the same time. You can increase the absorption of non-heme iron in foods by eating them with vitamin C–rich fruits and vegetables and cooking with cast iron cookware. For example, a bowl of whole-grain cereal or toast with almond butter (an iron source) with a kiwi or berries (a vitamin C source) will boost your iron intake. Cooking tomatoes in cast iron especially increases the uptake of iron from the pan due to the tomatoes' acidity.

Iron-Rich Foods

MEAT AND SEAFOOD	BEANS, LENTILS, AND VEGETABLES	GRAINS AND CEREALS	FRUIT, JUICE, AND OTHER
Beef (4 ounces/115 g),* 3.5 mg**	Beans (½ cup/ 125 mL), 2 mg	Pasta (4 ounces/ 115 g), 1.5 mg	Dried apricots (10 halves), 1.6 mg
Lamb (4 ounces/115 g), 2.5 mg	Chickpeas (½ cup/ 125 mL), 2 mg	Bagel (1 ounce/ 28 g), 1 mg	Figs (5), 2 mg
Pork (4 ounces/115 g), 1 mg	Potato (1 with skin), 2.5 mg	Bread, whole wheat (1 slice), 1 mg	Raisins (4 ounces/115 g), 1.5 mg
Veal (4 ounces/115 g), 1.5 mg	Pumpkin (4 ounces/ 115 g), 1.7 mg	Iron-fortified cereal (1 ounce/ 28 g), 4–8 mg	Prune juice (8 ounces/ 227 g), 3 mg
Chicken liver (4 ounces/115 g), 10 mg	Peas (4 ounces/ 115 g), 1 mg	Quinoa flour (½ cup/ 125 mL), 8.5 mg	Nuts (1 ounce/28 g), 1 mg
Beef liver (4 ounces/115 g), 6.5 mg	Lentils, cooked (½ cup/125 mL), 3.3 mg	Quinoa, dry (¼ cup/ 60 mL), 3.9 mg	Tofu, firm (3 ounces/ 85 g), 3.5 mg
Chicken, light meat (4 ounces/115 g), 1 mg	Sweet potato (4 ounces/115 g), 1.7 mg	Amaranth (½ cup/ 125 mL), 7.4 mg	Blackstrap molasses (1 tablespoon/15 mL), 3.5 mg

Chart continues

MEAT AND SEAFOOD	BEANS, LENTILS, AND VEGETABLES	GRAINS AND CEREALS	FRUIT, JUICE, AND OTHER
Chicken, dark meat, roasted (1 leg and thigh), 2.3 mg	Tomato paste (4 ounces/115 g), 3.9 mg	Amaranth flour (½ cup/125 mL), 8.5 mg	Sunflower seeds (2 tablespoons/30 mL), 1.9 mg
Turkey, light meat (4 ounces/115 g), 1.6 mg	Tomato sauce (4 ounces/115 g), 0.8 mg		Pumpkin seeds (2 tablespoons/30 mL), 4 mg
Turkey, dark meat, roasted (3 slices), 2 mg			Infant formula (8 ounces/227 g), 3 mg
Clams (4 ounces/115 g), 3 mg			
Oysters (4 ounces/115 g), 8 mg			
Shrimp (4 ounces/115 g), 2 mg			

*Serving size **Iron content

RECOMMENDED DAILY ALLOWANCE (RDA) OF IRON* FOR WOMEN AND CHILDREN[14]	
7 to 12 months	11 mg
1 to 3 years	7 mg
4 to 8 years	10 mg
Pregnant women	27 mg
Breastfeeding mothers	9 mg
Non-anemic, non-breastfeeding women	18 mg

*Recommended as an overall daily intake from both food and supplements.

BABY SMARTS

As your baby grows, so does her brain. During the first three months of life, the DHA concentration in your baby's brain will triple, allowing for growth and development of the spinal cord, the neurological system, and, of course, the brain. You will see this growth at each doctor's visit, because along with weight and height, the doctor will measure your baby's head. The increase in head circumference shows that your baby's brain is growing proportionately. DHA makes up 11 percent of the dry weight of the brain, and arachidonic acid (AA) accounts for 8 percent; so, together these equal almost 20 percent of the brain's weight. This is a crucial time to ensure that your baby is getting adequate levels of both DHA and AA. An overwhelming amount of research supports the link between higher intake of DHA and an increase in cognitive function and neurological development, a lowered risk of hyperactivity and attention deficit disorders, and a higher IQ for baby. And did I mention a reduction in severity of allergies? Getting adequate levels of DHA sounds like a no-brainer (sorry, I couldn't resist!).

AA is also essential for development and works with DHA to enhance its beneficial effects. Formula companies have begun fortifying their products with AA as well as DHA. It's not necessary to supplement with AA, as it's present in our diets worldwide. Arachidonic acid is found in saturated fat, mainly red meat, full-fat dairy products, and fried foods. Most adults typically eat too much of this type of fat. Saturated fat has been linked to an increased risk of cardiovascular disease, including high cholesterol, stroke, and heart attack; Alzheimer's disease; and other age-related diseases. Our bodies do need a small amount of AA, but not at the levels found in most Western diets. In short, babies need it, but adults, not so much.

FISH OIL DHA If your baby was born preterm and you're breastfeeding, I recommend that your DHA intake increase to between 1200 and 1800 mg per day. Babies experience massive brain growth of 400 to 500 percent in the third trimester, so your preterm baby didn't get the chance to finish his brain growth spurt; therefore, you need higher levels of DHA in your cells to pass along through breast milk. Preterm and formula-fed babies can be supplemented with DHA only at a level of 200 mg per day. DHA-only supplements may be difficult to find; Genestra's Super Neurogen DHA is a great algae-based DHA supplement. For a full-term baby, mom can take up to 1200 mg of DHA a day until three months postpartum, at which point she can drop that level down to 800 to 1000 mg per day. You can get this amount by taking high-dose cod liver oil or an EPA and DHA supplement, or by eating fish 24/7. To reach the higher level of DHA from fish, you would need to eat about 2 pounds (900 g) of oily fish, such as sardines, mackerel, herring, or wild salmon, every day—and more if you eat only whitefish. Now, I love fish, but I can honestly say there's no way I would be able to eat that amount every day, even if Jamie Oliver cooked it for me—not to mention that I'd set the fishmonger up for life financially! As well, because new moms are notorious for not having as good of a diet as they could (they're a bit busy keeping up with the demands of this new life), 2 pounds (900 g) of fish daily is probably not on the menu, so either recommendation above is your best option.

As your baby continues to build her brain cell by cell, providing good levels of DHA and AA supports the best possible outcome. I've come across plenty of new moms who were unaware of how crucial these fats are and didn't take DHA during pregnancy, or with earlier babies, and who are now worried about the implications. Most likely, the baby took these fats from mom during pregnancy and used them for as much brain building as possible. This may lead to a different outcome, but not necessarily a negative one. But, of course, you want to do your best to help your baby reach her full potential, so start with a DHA supplement if breastfeeding or give a supplement to your baby or child as soon as possible. Supplementing will still have beneficial effects no matter when you start, even at one year of age.

Your baby needs 100 to 130 mg of DHA daily. DHA is stored in the body, so if you don't give that amount every day, not to worry. However, the accumulated level still needs to be reached, even if a supplement isn't given every day. DHA is present in breast milk, even more so if mom is supplementing with it. Some formula companies fortify their products with DHA and AA. If you're giving your baby DHA/AA-fortified formula, I would recommend only 100 mg of DHA daily on top of what your formula label quotes. Once a formula container is opened, the nutrients, including fats, start to oxidize and leave less available for absorption. Unfortunately, I don't have a crystal ball to say what will happen if you don't take your DHA, but after studying nutrition for more than twenty years, I can honestly say that I have only ever seen positive results from taking essential fatty acids in all forms. As I specialize in pregnant women, new moms, and their children, not a day goes by that I don't talk about or recommend DHA to mom or baby, and I also take it myself and give it to my children daily (and they love it!). See the Resources page on SproutRight.com for supplement recommendations.

BUILDING STRONG BONES: IT'S MORE THAN JUST CALCIUM

When your baby is born, he has about three hundred bones, some of which are made up of soft, flexible cartilage. As your baby grows, the cartilage is slowly replaced by bone, and the bones grow and fuse together to eventually form 206 adult bones that reach full size by age twenty-five. Your baby accumulated a total of about 30 g of your calcium during pregnancy, mostly during the third trimester, nabbing between 200 and 350 mg a day.[15] That's a huge amount of calcium taken from your stores (oh, what we do for our babies!), and following a calcium-rich diet while breastfeeding should make up for what you lose within a few months after you stop nursing.

Bones store calcium and phosphorus and, in the bone marrow, make blood and immune cells and store fat as an energy source. Bones are made up of a matrix of 25 percent water, 25 percent fibre, and 50 percent mineral salts. Mineral salts of calcium, magnesium, fluoride, and sulphate are deposited between the protein fibres of collagen, crystallize into salts, and make the bone hard. Bones that are too mineralized are brittle and can break easily. As your baby grows, his bone is destroyed and reformed again and again to eventually reach its full adult shape. Some bone cells eat up the bone, and others rebuild it.

Minerals of calcium, phosphorus, magnesium, boron, and manganese and vitamins D, K2, C, A, and B12 are all used in the complex action of making of bone. Vitamin D increases the absorption of calcium from food but also promotes the removal of calcium from bone. Vitamin K2 is an unsung hero and crucial for sending calcium into bones to strengthen density. Vitamin C is essential to the collagen matrix, where the calcium is deposited. A deficiency may lead to decreased collagen production, slowing bone growth and delaying the healing of broken bones. Vitamin A is involved in breaking down and building up bone, and therefore a deficiency may lead to stunted growth. Finally, vitamin B12 is involved in building up bone after it has broken down. Human growth hormone (hGH) is the head honcho when it comes to growth of all tissues, including bone. Too much or little of this hormone can cause overgrowth or undergrowth of bones. Bones need to be stressed to remain strong. So, as your little one grows, remember that walking, running, and jumping are all activities that stress the bone, which in turn keeps the breakdown and buildup of bone in perfect balance.

CALCIUM AND BONES Despite all the minerals and vitamins that go into building bone, only one usually makes the news—calcium. Calcium is one of the most talked-about minerals and one that I constantly speak about with new moms with regards to when to introduce foods to their babies and toddlers. The co-factors involved in calcium absorption all need to be in place for overall health.

Dairy products are only one source of calcium; other foods, including nuts and seeds, deliver more calcium than milk (and in a more absorbable form, since they're often raw), with sesame seeds offering 2200 mg of calcium per cup (250 mL) versus milk offering 228 mg per cup. You probably would never eat a cup of sesame seeds at one sitting, but even if you had one-tenth of a cup, or 1½ tablespoons (22 mL), you would get the same amount of calcium as in 1 cup (250 mL) of milk. Tahini, or sesame seed butter, is an excellent addition to anyone's diet and is found in hummus, but be careful when introducing it to your baby, as it can be allergenic. Almonds are a powerhouse of calcium, but peanuts offer the least amount of calcium of all nuts and seeds (technically, peanuts are a legume). Salmon and sardines (with bones) rank high in calcium, as do soy, navy beans, blackstrap molasses, amaranth (see pages 150 and 168 for yummy recipes), broccoli, and kale. In fact, almost any green leafy vegetable is high in calcium. Milk, however, loses about 50 percent of available calcium in the pasteurization process. Low-fat and skim milk offer even less because the milk fat is used for transportation and absorption of calcium.

CALCIUM STRIPPERS So, now you know what to eat to get calcium, but on the flip side, it's important to understand the factors that can diminish levels of this mineral in the body.

- High-caffeine coffee, tea, soft drinks, and chocolate increase calcium excretion in the urine.
- Sugar has the same effect as caffeine, and when a food containing calcium and sugar, such as sweetened yogurt, is eaten, the absorption of calcium in the intestines is greatly reduced.[16] Sugar also decreases the amount of phosphorus in the blood.
- High phosphorus intake from meat, grains, and soft drinks can take calcium from bones. Phosphorus and calcium need to be in particular balance to have a positive effect on bone mineralization. Having too much or too little phosphorus in circulation can have a negative effect on calcium status.
- Salt has the same effect on calcium as caffeine and sugar.
- Low levels of vitamins D and K2 can lead to low levels of calcium absorption and use.
- A high-fibre diet, with most of the fibre coming from wheat and gluten, can lead to lowered calcium absorption, as this fibre binds to calcium and is excreted from the body.
- Protein eaten in excess depletes calcium substantially in two ways. When protein is eaten, it has an acidic effect on the body, requiring alkaline minerals to buffer the acidity. Calcium, an alkaline mineral, comes out of the bones (along with a few other minerals) to buffer that acid. Junk foods, refined foods, and most cooked foods also have this acid-forming effect on the body. Protein acts as a diuretic as well, causing the kidneys to send calcium and other minerals out in the urine. This is called a negative calcium balance. In her book *Allergies: Disease in Disguise*, Carolee Bateson-Koch notes that eating too much protein causes more calcium depletion from the bones than consuming too little calcium. Once again, it's all about balance.

A breastfed or formula-fed baby is getting the right amount of protein in her diet from her daily milk intake, so an emphasis on protein in her daily diet may not be needed.

There is 0.9 g of protein in 3½ ounces (100 mL) of breast milk, and as breast milk intake decreases, the protein content increases. It's hard to tell, however, how much a breastfed baby drinks in a day. If you're feeding your baby formula, read the nutritional composition to see how much protein is in it. Similac Advance, for instance, has 1.4 g of protein per 3½ ounces (100 mL) of formula. Most formulas will have a similar value, as manufacturers must follow guidelines for specific ranges of protein and nutrients.

Calculating Protein Requirements

To calculate how much protein your baby needs, multiply weight in pounds by between .36 to .50 (as an average range, so you aren't number crunching all day) to get the daily protein requirement in grams. Pregnant women need an extra 10 grams of protein a day, and lactating moms need 12 additional grams per day.

As we've seen, calcium is important for strong bones, but bone health isn't just about calcium and vitamin D intake. It's also closely related to the hormonal balance of breaking down and building up bone, and to making sure there are limited stressors to calcium. A diet high in protein can be more of a concern, as the body uses calcium to buffer the acidic effect of protein, leading to a negative calcium balance, where what is excreted is more than what is taken in (this also applies to diets high in dairy, wheat, and refined, processed, and packaged food). Food for thought!

DAILY CALCIUM REQUIREMENTS[17,18]	
Birth to 1 year	400 mg
1 to 3 years	500 mg
4 to 8 years	800 mg
Pregnancy, lactation, and adolescence (9 to 18 years)	1000 mg
19 to 50 years	1300 mg
51+ years	1200 mg
Individuals at risk for or with osteoporosis	1500 mg

PEARLY WHITES: THE START OF HEALTHY BABY TEETH

When your baby is born, her teeth are already hiding in the gums. Well, that's part of the picture. Pediatric dentist Dr. Shonna Masse explains how it all happens:

Your baby is born with teeth already formed in the jawbone underneath the gums. Baby teeth start to form as early as six weeks in utero, and permanent or adult teeth begin formation as early as five months in utero. The tooth bud goes through many developmental stages and eventually the tooth enamel is calcified, making the outer surface of the tooth hard prior to it erupting through the gums (teething). Calcification of baby teeth begins at about the fourth month in utero, and calcification of permanent teeth begins at birth. It's busy

in that little mouth! Wisdom teeth (third molars) formation starts at about five
years of age and usually completes formation by age eight or nine, but these
teeth may never erupt into the mouth. At each stage of dental development,
be it in utero or postpartum, problems that lead to dental abnormalities can
occur, such as in the number of teeth (too many or too few), the size or shape
of the teeth, the structure of the enamel, the colour, or the eruption pattern.
It's important to arrange for your child's first dental examination as early as
the arrival of the first tooth. This is especially necessary if your child is faced
with any dental abnormalities. Your dentist will recommend the appropriate
treatment or management of the issue.[19]

Good nutrition is essential during pregnancy to support healthy tooth formation. As with bones, minerals of calcium, phosphorus, and vitamins A, C, D, and K2 are all used for building teeth. Fluoride is needed in trace amounts to balance mineralization and demineralization when the teeth are exposed to acid. Your baby will have strong teeth before fluoride is introduced in her diet. Your baby's teeth may tell your dentist a story or two about your pregnancy. Dr. Masse explained to me that if there is some kind of illness, trauma, fever, infection, or even use of medication during pregnancy, it can show like a timestamp in the enamel of the tooth that you will see once the tooth erupts. I found that really interesting and wondered what story my first daughter's teeth might have told Dr. Masse, since I broke my wrist when I was five months pregnant with her!

WHAT ARE TEETH MADE OF? Teeth are made from the same tissue as fingernails, hair, skin, and glands in utero. This tissue then becomes a calcified connective tissue, called dentin, which gives the tooth its basic shape and rigidity. Dentin is covered by enamel made up primarily of calcium phosphate and calcium carbonate. Enamel is the hardest substance (as hard as diamonds) in the body, protecting teeth from the constant wear of chewing. It also protects dentin from dissolving in acids that occur in the mouth after eating. The mouth is an alkaline environment with a high pH level, and tooth decay is possible only in the acid environment—at a low pH level. This pH changes after food or drink is ingested. Dental caries (cavities or tooth decay) happen when bacteria in the mouth act on sugars, found in all carbohydrates, including breast milk, formula, milk, juice, and food, and give off acids that break down or demineralize the enamel. Plaque is formed from bacteria, sugars, and particles that stick to the teeth, covering them and preventing the alkaline saliva from protecting the surface of the teeth from the bacteria. Brushing or rubbing away this plaque from the surface and flossing between tight molars help get rid of plaque, allowing the saliva to once again protect the teeth from bacteria.

A DENTIST'S TIPS FOR HEALTHY TEETH
• Don't let your baby fall asleep on the breast, as the sugars in breast milk will sit in the mouth, and when babies fall asleep, saliva production stops.
• Never allow your baby to go to bed with a bottle of juice, milk, or formula. Water only.

- Start brushing teeth from the first eruption. Wipe early teeth with a cloth or gauze, or brush with an appropriate-size toothbrush.
- Floss between back molars if they are close together. If there is sufficient space between the teeth, food will come out with brushing.

THE FIRST DENTIST VISIT Going to the dentist doesn't have to be a worry. Get your baby or toddler used to going to the dentist by taking him with you when you go. Let him see what it's all about and how mommy or daddy does it, or let older siblings show younger ones how it's done. Find a pediatric or general dentist, who should have all sorts of kid-friendly names for the tools they use. One of my favourites is "Mr. Thirsty," who sucks out the saliva in the mouth. Some dentists recommend a first visit at about age three, and pediatric dentists like to see the little teeth as they come in, so visit by age one. After taking my daughters to the dentist regularly, I understand why some dentists recommend a slightly older first visit—often children are scared or shy when someone they don't know looks in their mouth. At the same time, good oral health and cavity prevention start early, so the more you know as the teeth erupt, the better equipped you'll be. When you visit the dentist and either you or your child needs a filling or sealants to cover the teeth, ask questions about what is in the product they will be using and do your homework before you go ahead with the procedure. If x-rays are needed, see if your dentist does digital ones, which give off 90 percent less radiation. Ask about the composite used to fill or seal teeth and any harmful chemicals it may contain. Dentists commonly suggest sealing teeth, especially those with deep grooves in them. Although there has been a movement away from amalgam or mercury fillings because of the known negative neurotoxin effects, the white or composite fillings may contain bisphenol A (BPA), a chemical also known for its potentially harmful effects on the nervous system as well as its link to cancer and other health issues. Remember this if you need any dental work while breastfeeding, as the toxins may get into your breast milk and thus into your baby at a crucial time of development.

THUMB SUCKING AND SOOTHERS Some parents worry about thumb sucking because a thumb isn't as easy to take away as a soother or pacifier. For some babies, self-soothing with fingers or a thumb is comforting, and that's something that shouldn't be discouraged. I recall my second daughter sucking her fingers as a newborn, and it was a beautiful thing when she soothed herself back to sleep on many occasions (although that habit didn't last long!).

Dentists don't seem to be too worried about the use of a thumb or soother, until the age of three, anyway. In my interview with dentist Dr. Dana Colson, she said that she's not opposed to either, as both help develop the open airway that's so important for good sleep.[20] Use an orthodontic soother, which lessens the likelihood of changing the angle of the upper teeth.

Have you ever put your baby's soother in your mouth after it dropped on the floor to "clean" it? This practice concerns Dr. Masse, who explains, "Oral bacteria can be spread between parent and child. It may be done by something as innocent as sharing a utensil or a kiss, but the bacteria are microscopic and transfer easily. If there is an infection or cavity-causing bacteria in mom or dad's mouth, then it can be shared with the baby and may lead to oral health issues, namely cavities for the child."[21] So, hang on to the soother until you can wash it somewhere other than with your mouth!

TRICKY TEETHING Teething is painful for everyone involved. Your baby is unhappy while you try to figure out what you can do to help her weather the erupting tooth. Teething can happen without a tooth making an appearance for months. Your baby might show signs of teething—drooling, fussiness, chewing on anything and everything, low-grade fever, pulling on her ears, diarrhea or constipation, lack of appetite for food, bum rash usually close to the anus, and red cheeks—for months before a tooth breaks through the gums.

Babies can start teething at a young age, when you probably wouldn't attribute any of the symptoms listed above to teething. Your baby may sail through the first tooth but have more symptoms with the next one. Signs of teething come and go and can be worse at night, followed by long days of clinginess and irritability. Your baby may want to nurse more for comfort, chew on your knuckles, and be held all day long.

Your mission is to try to help your baby, and yourself, through these teething episodes. Offer your baby a clean baby face cloth that has been dampened with water and chilled in the freezer; a hard toy to chew on; a large, cold whole carrot (so it won't break off and become a choking hazard); or even an ice cube wrapped in a cloth to numb the teeth. A common misconception is that teething biscuits help babies with teething. Not only do they not help, but they're often full of ingredients that baby hasn't tried yet; they may contain wheat flour and sugar, which suppress the immune system at a time when baby's more susceptible to sickness. I've even seen one product sweetened with honey, which is on the avoid list for babies under one year of age. As well, when your baby is teething, he usually loses his appetite for solid foods but not for breast or formula milk. Symptoms of diarrhea are more common than constipation, but bowel movements can change either way depending on your baby. Her stool and urine can become more acidic, leading to red bum cheeks and soreness that sometimes can become raw and bleed. A protective barrier cream, especially a natural one, or even coconut oil is perfect for this kind of rash. I have also seen eczema flare up with teething episodes in some babies.

Homeopathy, a safe, alternative medicine based on treating the symptoms of ailments, offers various remedies that can make a world of difference for your baby's teething symptoms, and you'll often see fast results. Consult a homeopath or naturopath to match your list of teething symptoms to particular remedies, or try store-bought remedies like Boiron's Camilia. If it works, you'll know after the first couple of doses. If you don't see an ease in some symptoms, it's not the right mix of remedies. Try another teething remedy by a brand like Hyland's or a liquid remedy called Unda 22, to help calm the nervous system. Medication is often a last resort to help everyone sleep for more than an hour or two, and sometimes parents will use teething gels. But be careful with these gels (other than homeopathic ones), as they can numb not only the gums but also the tongue and lips. Be sure to read the label carefully when giving any medication to your baby, and consult the pharmacist if you have questions.

Is It a Cold or a New Tooth?

It's easy to confuse teething with the start of a cold, as symptoms can sometimes seem similar: runny nose, low-grade fever (less than 38°C/100°F), ear pulling, and fussiness. When teeth are starting to erupt, the immune system can get confused, see the teeth as a foreign invader breaking through the skin, and send out the immune army to deal with it. While the immune system's busy, your baby may be prone to colds, infections, and flare-ups of eczema. Support his little body with immune-boosting probiotics, homeopathic teething remedies, and a lot of comfort.

BRUSHING AWAY THE BUGS Start brushing your baby's teeth with a cloth or piece of gauze wrapped around your finger as soon as they erupt. As the teeth continue to erupt, it becomes more important to wipe or brush them daily. Once the premolars come in at around one year of age, and then molars at about two years, those bite surfaces need to be brushed well to remove any debris. And don't forget to brush in between those teeth, too—it's a common area for plaque to build up and bacteria to live. The three dentists I spoke with all agreed that toothpaste isn't necessary for your baby, and two of them said that you never need to use it. Toothpaste can be something sweet to entice your baby or toddler to brush, but it isn't really necessary (they usually just suck it off, anyway). If you do want to use toothpaste, find one that is fluoride-free and read the ingredients. Most toothpastes, even those sold in health food stores, contain sodium lauryl sulphate, a chemical foaming agent also used in skin care and bath products. And if you don't want to offer blue bubble gum–flavoured toothpaste, look anywhere other than the pharmacy. Search for safe products on the Skin Deep website (www. cosmeticsdatabase.com). All dentists recommend avoiding fluoride toothpaste until about age three or until your child is able to spit out the toothpaste during brushing, as ingesting fluoride is not recommended.

JUICE VERSUS WATER Giving juice at bedtime is a definite no-no, but even offering juice throughout the day can leave sugars hanging around in tooth crevices and in between the teeth. As dentist Dr. Robert Penning explains, "As a dentist, I tell parents that after milk and water, most other beverages are largely entertainment. Much of the decay I see would likely disappear if other beverages were eliminated."[22] If you do give juice, which I don't recommend until after two years of age, dilute it by more than half with water and give it with a meal or in one sitting rather than all day long.

To sum up the nutritional nuts and bolts that you and your baby need, here's a handy reference chart.

Summary of Supplements for Mom and Baby

	VITAMIN D*	IRON	DHA*	CALCIUM/ MAGNESIUM	PROBIOTIC
Pregnant woman	2000 IU or sun exposure daily	27 mg	600 mg in first and second trimesters and 1200 mg in third trimester	1300 mg/600 to 800 mg	25 billion colony-forming units (CFU), including *Lactobacillus acidophilus* and *Bifidobacterium*, once or twice daily***
Breastfeeding mom	3000 to 5000 IU or more than 2 hours of sun a week	9 mg	1200 to 1800 mg until the baby is 3 months old, then 800 mg per day	1300 mg/600 to 800 mg	25 billion CFU, including *L. acidophilus* and *Bifidobacterium*, once or twice daily***
Non-breastfeeding mom	2000 IU	18 mg	600 mg	800 mg/400 mg	10 to 25 billion CFU, including *L. acidophilus* and *Bifidobacterium*, once or twice daily***
Preterm baby	400 to 800 IU	2 to 4 mg/ kg/ day**	1200 to 1800 mg taken by mom while breastfeeding, or 200 mg of DHA only for baby	Not generally supplemented	10 billion CFU, including *L. acidophilus* and *Bifidobacterium***
Breastfed full-term baby	None if mom is supplementing, but 400 to 800 IU if mom is not supplementing	None	None if mom is taking the above	400 mg/200 mg	10 billion CFU, including *L. acidophilus* and *Bifidobacterium***
Formula-fed full-term baby	400 to 800 IU if not exposed to sunlight	None	100 mg	400 mg/200 mg	10 billion CFU, including *L. acidophilus* and *Bifidobacterium* and galactooligosaccharides (GOS)***

Vitamin D and DHA can also be obtained from cod liver oil while breastfeeding only. It's not suitable during pregnancy. Use ¼ teaspoon (1 mL) for every 4.5 kg (10 pounds) of weight. For example, if you weigh 59 kg (130 pounds), you would need to take 13 mL of cod liver oil a day, which works out to almost a tablespoon.

**Should be prescribed by a doctor.*

***Preferably a human microflora strain.*

2 · THE WHITE STUFF: BREAST MILK AND FEEDING

Whether to breastfeed your baby or not is often a hot topic before you give birth, and, as usual, everyone has their own advice and experience to offer. Understanding the benefits of breastfeeding for both you and your baby can help you decide whether to give it a try. If you took prenatal classes, you may have talked about breastfeeding but nothing really prepares you for the actual experience.

Breast milk or formula is your baby's main source of nutrition for the first year of life, and it's her only source of nutrition for the first six months before she starts on solids. It's amazing that just the white stuff will provide all the nourishment needed for the remarkable growth that happens during this early period of life.

For some, the thought of breastfeeding is foreign, and the decision to breastfeed or not is a real struggle. Unfortunately, it's not for everyone. Others decide that they are going to breastfeed exclusively and are devastated when it doesn't work out. Feeding your baby may not go as smoothly as you'd hoped for a multitude of reasons, whether you are breastfeeding or formula feeding. But I've heard some wonderful success stories from new moms who, with great determination and excellent support, worked through the challenges of breastfeeding. In my own early days of nursing, I had different challenges with the latch. I found that both of my daughters reacted to foods I had eaten—dairy, wheat, sugar, and chocolate were the worst. Although I follow a healthy diet most of the time, I'm not a saint. Every time I ate something I wasn't supposed to, a rash, constipation, or discomfort would show up in my babies. I felt like the worst mother in the world for being so weak as to eat something I knew might cause a reaction. Although we all try to do the best we can for our children, we are still human.

THE BENEFITS OF BREASTFEEDING

Anyone who thinks that breastfeeding is the most "natural" thing for a new mom to do is only partly right. Breastfeeding does not come naturally or easily to every new mom. Yet everywhere you turn, you're told that breast is best. Well, it is, but it also may be more challenging than you thought. Breastfeeding is a new skill that both you and your baby need to learn. Even if this is your second baby, you might need a bit of practice to get it right. If you're having difficulty, it's crucial that you seek help from a lactation consultant, breastfeeding clinic, or your midwife.

Mastering the latch of your baby's mouth to your nipple can be a challenge. But once your baby does latch on, he'll receive the appropriate amount of colostrum (the first fluid delivered to your newborn) or milk. A poor latch can lead to your baby having insufficient nutrition; dehydration; inefficient clearing of bilirubin, leading to prolonged jaundice; or a lack of bowel movements, including meconium (the first, tarlike poo), and urination. In mom, an improper latch can cause low milk production from lack of nipple stimulation and sore or cracked nipples while nursing. These are the many reasons why it's essential to master a good latch as quickly as you can and to get help when you need it.

Breast milk is the perfect food—the gold standard—for both mom and baby. One study reported that women who breastfed for one year or more over their lifetime were less likely to develop high blood pressure, diabetes, high cholesterol, breast cancer, or cardiovascular disease than were women who never nursed.[23] It's associated with a lower incidence of necrotizing enterocolitis and diarrhea during the early period of life and with a lower incidence of inflammatory bowel diseases, type 1 and 2 diabetes, and obesity later in life. It's also associated with a reduction in the risk of acute otitis media, nonspecific gastroenteritis, severe lower respiratory tract infections, atopic dermatitis, asthma (young children), childhood leukemia, and sudden infant death syndrome. Scientists have studied breast milk for years to try to uncover every aspect of what it does, how it does it, and why. I'll share as many of its benefits as I can here, so that you'll find out more than just a few well-known facts.

IMMUNITY

Breast milk provides antibodies for your baby to protect her body from foreign invaders until her immune system has matured. Colostrum, the first milk your baby receives after birth, is loaded with secretory immunoglobulin A, or sIgA (see Chapter 5 for more details). This antibody guards the mucosal entranceways to the body—the nose, eyes, mouth, and, most importantly, digestive system—by binding to bacteria and viruses and quashing them. Amazingly, sIgA is found in higher levels in the milk of mothers of preterm babies; these babies, with their premature immune systems, are even more susceptible to bacteria and viruses.[24] Babies who are born vaginally take on good bacteria, *Lactobacillus* and *Bifidobacterium*, from the birth canal as well as not-so-good bacteria that live around the anal area of the digestive tract. I know it's not a nice thought, but baby taking on immune-challenging bacteria in this crucial step stimulates the newborn immune army to start working toward balancing itself. Your skin also offers good and bad bacteria to your baby's digestive system through his mouth, from the first skin-to-skin contact and breastfeed. You provide your own sIgA to your baby through colostrum and breast milk, giving your baby a head start in protecting himself from the bad bacteria that you, and the world around him, shares with him.[25] Also, sIgA allows for the colonization of friendly bacteria, *Lactobacillus acidophilus* and *Bifidobacterium*, in the intestines without mounting an attack—another key aspect of developing a strong immune system.

Breastfeeding increases the size of baby's thymus, a gland in the immune army.[26] The thymus is where immune cells, called T cells, including killer T cells, mature before heading out into the battlefield of the body. The larger the thymus, the more T cells are produced and the stronger the immune army is. The more your baby breastfeeds, the larger the size of his thymus.

DIGESTIVE HEALTH

The digestive system benefits greatly from breast milk. Breastfed infants' intestines are typically dominated by *Bifidobacteria*, unlike those of adults. These bacterias are commonly used as probiotics and are beneficial to infants in many ways: higher resistance to bad bacteria or pathogens, better responsiveness to some vaccines, and better-functioning gut barriers. *Bifidobacteria* also appear to enhance the immune army and reduce inflammation. Infant-type *Bifidobacteria* present during weaning to solid food may help the immune system tolerate new foods and avoid them becoming an allergy.[27] Breastfed newborns can carry a more stable and uniform population of beneficial bacteria when compared to formula-fed babies.[28]

VITAMINS AND MINERALS

Breast milk contains the most absorbable forms of all vitamins and minerals, especially iron and zinc. Although iron concentrations are low in breast milk, this iron provides maximum absorption. Zinc blood levels are higher in breastfed babies than in formula-fed babies, even though the concentration level of zinc is higher in formula milk.[29]

Once again, it all comes down to absorbability. Water-soluble vitamins (B vitamins and vitamin C) are taken from mom's diet and passed on to baby. Fat-soluble vitamins A and E are found in the hind milk, or fatty milk, in perfect proportions and are taken from your stores, rather than from your diet or supplements.[30] Vitamins are directed to the mammary glands, away from use by your own body[31]—all the more reason to take your pre- and postnatal vitamins and eat a nutrient-rich diet.

NOURISHMENT

Breast milk has the right proportions of fats, protein, and carbohydrates for your baby's growth and development. Here's a look at the specific components of breast milk, in some detail and with a bit of science thrown in, as it's fascinating to see what makes up breast milk.

FATS Essential fatty acids docosahexaenoic acid (DHA) and arachidonic acid (AA) are found in abundance in breast milk. They are extremely important for the development of the brain, retina, and neurological system and may even help decrease the potential for allergies. Mom doesn't need to supplement with AA since her diet easily supplies what her baby needs. DHA, on the other hand, is needed in such large quantities that mom usually needs to supplement with fish oils containing DHA. Hindmilk has twice the level of fat as foremilk (the first, carbohydrate-rich milk your baby gets).[32] Breast milk contains not only these two fats, but also a host of other lesser-known essentials, including lauric, myristic, palmitic, stearic, oleic, linoleic, and linolenic acids.[33] In a clever twist, breast milk also contains lipase, a fat-digesting enzyme that's essential to the digestion of these important fats because a newborn baby's digestive system isn't mature enough to produce its own enzymes.[34] Lipase then stays in the digestive tract, furthering the digestion of all fats found in breast milk.

PROTEIN Whey and casein are the main proteins found in breast milk. The immune protein sIgA and the binding proteins lactoferrin, folate, and cobalamin (vitamin B12) are also components of breast milk and help with baby's absorption of iron, folic acid, and vitamin B12.[35] Lactoferrin has many other important functions, such as providing antiviral effects against fungus such as *Candida albicans*, lowering the risk of urinary tract infections, promoting the growth of *Bifidobacteria* in the digestive tract, and helping the growth of the mucosal lining of the intestines.[36]

CARBOHYDRATES Lactose is the primary carbohydrate that gives your baby energy for every bodily process. It also enhances the absorption of calcium, iron, magnesium, and manganese.[37] The largest solid component in human milk is oligosaccharides. These carbohydrates are fuel for the beneficial bacteria in the digestive tract. They also take up residence in the walls of the intestines, where, like posters put up on a wall, they cover as much space as possible so that other pathogens or bad guys can't move in and cause an infection or illness.

Water makes up 87.5 percent of breast milk.[38] Hint, hint—how much water have you had to drink today? My midwife always told me to drink a glass of water every time I breastfed. This was great advice and I recommend you do the same.

LOWERED RISK OF OBESITY

An appetite-regulating hormone called leptin is found in breast milk.[39] This hormone also stimulates the immune army and its hard-working soldiers. (I talk more about the immune army in Chapter 5.) With the rise in obesity in recent years, medical research linking the potential of lowering obesity rates to the milk that a baby is fed is beneficial for everyone. The presence of this hormone in breast milk seems to have a significant protective factor against obesity and could be the reason for its decreased incidence in breastfed babies later in life.[40,41]

GROWTH

Breast milk contains nucleotides that cow's milk and dairy formula do not. Nucleotides are the building blocks needed by DNA and RNA to support the growth and development of all systems in the body, including the immune system.[42]

HEALTHY MOUTH

Breastfeeding encourages healthy muscle development through the suckling action of the jaw and mouth, which is different from the action of a baby fed from a bottle. However, for healthy teeth, dentist Dr. Dana Colson suggests, "Try not to let your baby fall asleep on the breast, as the sugars in the breast milk sit in the mouth and, when baby falls asleep, saliva production stops. Saliva protects the teeth from the acidity of the sugars."[43] This is good advice, although sometimes it's easier said than done.

HEALING

Using breast milk to treat eye infections, nasal congestion, baby acne, or other skin issues your baby has is like applying magic to the skin. No fancy creams needed. Express a bit of breast milk into a cup and use a dropper to squirt it up the nose, apply it to the skin, squirt it in the eye, or use it on a rash.

MAKING THE GOOD STUFF BETTER: WHAT CAN YOU DO?

If you're a nursing mom, you'll need a good-quality daily prenatal or postnatal multinutrient or an extra boost from a concentrated food source supplement. Although not all vitamins and minerals in a multinutrient will be passed on to your baby, it will cover the extra demands on your own nutrient stores. Supplements in capsule or liquid form have far better absorption than hard tablets. Food source concentrate supplements in the form of powders and liquids offer higher nutrients than you're able to eat. The labels of some better-quality multivitamins might suggest taking two to four per day because they just can't fit all those nutrients into one capsule!

Your dietary or supplemental iron intake does not have a direct influence on the level of iron in breast milk. Ensuring that you're not iron deficient is important for your well-being, but breast milk uses the iron stored in your body to nourish your baby.[44]

Vitamin D levels can be increased with supplementation and sun exposure. It might take about two weeks to influence the level of vitamin D in breast milk, but it can increase dramatically while providing the appropriate amounts to your baby, whatever level you are exposed to or taking orally.[45]

Water-soluble vitamins, including the B family of vitamins (B1, B2, B3, B5, B6, folic acid, and B12) and vitamin C, increase in breast milk when present in mom's diet, either from food or supplements. Vegan and some vegetarian mothers are more at risk for vitamin B12 deficiency because B12 is found in eggs, fish, dairy, and meat. If you're deficient, your baby can be as well, so if you're following a vegan diet, be sure to supplement with adequate vitamin B12. A word of caution about vitamin B6: taking more than what's found in your multinutrient could cause a decrease in breast milk production.

Although the probiotics *Bifidobacterium* and *L. acidophilus* that you may be taking in your daily capsule don't go directly into breast milk—they live in the digestive tract and don't reach the bloodstream—they do enhance certain immune components in your body. Those components then pass into breast milk from your bloodstream and have a positive immune-enhancing effect in your baby.

The essential fats DHA and AA are taken from your body, from either red blood cells or tissues such as the brain (you'll feel that as mommy brain!), to support the development of your baby's brain, retina, and neurological system. Taking 1200 to 1800 mg of DHA in the last trimester and for the first three months of your baby's life has far-reaching benefits, including a much lower risk of postpartum depression and increased IQ and development in your baby (see the table on page 43 for a list of which supplements to take and when).

Any saturated or unhealthy trans fats you eat also make it into breast milk, so it's advisable to avoid fried foods and lessen your intake of red meat and prepackaged fatty foods as much as possible. These fats are associated with cardiovascular disease.

As we've seen, many elements of what you ingest reach your baby. This also applies to medication. Before taking any medication, contact www.motherisk.org or refer to *Dr. Jack Newman's Guide to Breastfeeding*.

> ### Begin Probiotics at Birth
> I believe that if all babies were exposed to probiotics at birth, we'd have a healthier next generation! With that said, I highly recommend giving your baby her own supplement of *Bifidobacterium animalis* and *Lactobacillus salivarius* starting at birth. They are both found in my *Take This* Bio Boost Baby product.

BREASTFEEDING CHALLENGES

As mentioned earlier, breastfeeding is not without its difficulties. These can include serious situations of pain or infections in mom. In the past years, I've become more and more aware of babies with tongue- and lip ties; when these conditions are recognized and treated, both mom and baby do so much better on every level. Here's what can happen and how to avoid it.

CRACKED NIPPLES

Most nursing moms, sadly, will end up with cracked nipples, caused by stretching as baby draws the breast tissue into her mouth. Cracked nipples can happen because of an incorrect latch, when the baby doesn't take enough of the areola into the mouth and mainly sucks on the nipple. Diagnosing a tongue- or lip tie, correcting the latch with support from a lactation consultant, or ensuring that you get all of the areola into your baby's mouth with the bottom lip visibly curled away from the breast should ease this often excruciating condition, which can lead to bleeding or infection. Natalie Rogers, a childbirth educator who specializes in lactation and holistic nutrition, suggests, "When cracks appear, a frequent recommendation is to rub a little expressed breast milk onto the nipple after each feed (breast milk has antibacterial and healing properties!); as well, the application of aloe gel, lanolin, calendula ointment, and/or olive oil is thought to be healing for cracks."[46] You can try a nipple shield temporarily to let the cracks heal, then go back to nursing without it. I was given a tincture with St. John's wort and calendula to dilute and drizzle on my cracked nipples, and it healed them right away. Consult an herbalist for the right product.

TONGUE-TIE

I've seen many clients whose babies have been diagnosed with tongue-tie and heard stories of it not being diagnosed fast enough or at all. I asked Dr. Dan Flanders, MD, FRCPC, FAAP, and owner and director of Kindercare Pediatrics in Toronto, about his thoughts on tongue-tie. He does not believe tongue-ties are more prevalent in recent years, but he does believe there is an increased awareness of the problem, and a corresponding spike in diagnoses. Diagnosing a tongue-tie seems to be dependent on the professional assessing the need for treatment. For many, including myself, cracked nipples—a symptom of tongue-tie—seem pretty normal at the beginning of breastfeeding.

Bottle feeding doesn't present the same feeding difficulties for babies with tongue-tie that breastfeeding does, because the mechanics are very different and extension of the tongue doesn't play as big a role in bottle feeding.

If tongue-tie is diagnosed, treatment is a frenectomy: the frenulum is cut to allow the tongue more movement. The earlier this is done, the easier it is for baby to learn how to use his tongue in the right way. It's not a nice procedure to think about, but it should be quick and easy. It seems that one of the most important aspects to this treatment is that parents are taught how to stretch after the frenectomy. The mouth heals very quickly, and it's common for the tongue-tie to re-attach itself, which means another cut must be done. There is the option of having laser treatment, but both treatments have the desired effect.

It's important to find a pediatrician or dentist to support you and provide a diagnosis if there is an issue. There are many Facebook groups that can offer support and direction. I've heard that dealing with tongue-tie is a specialty that not everyone masters, in terms of both treatment and follow-up, so doing your research here is key. In some cases, it takes months to have tongue-tie diagnosed and, by that time, baby has stopped breastfeeding. To help find someone for support, visit the Tongue-Tie & Lip-Tie Support Network at www.tt-lt-support-network.com.

BLOCKED DUCTS

Blocked ducts can happen at any stage of breastfeeding. They're most common in women with adequate milk supply but inadequate breast drainage during feeds. This can lead to milk stasis, or clogging of milk in the ducts, resulting in painful, localized swelling around the affected duct that's sometimes visible as a tiny white plug on the nipple or a palpable, tender lump.[47] Nursing with your baby's chin pointed toward or in line with the blocked duct aids in releasing the blockage. The strength of sucking is more powerful from the lower jaw than from the upper jaw, so try new positions to pull that blockage through while compressing your breast with your hand to drain it toward the nipple (for visual help, visit the Newman Breastfeeding Clinic at www.ibconline.ca).

MASTITIS

Mastitis is a bacterial infection of the breast. The first symptoms are fatigue, localized breast tenderness, and a flu-like muscular aching, followed by fever and swelling and redness of the affected breast. Factors contributing to mastitis include plugged ducts, stress, fatigue, cracked or fissured nipples, bra constriction, tongue-tie, engorgement or milk stasis, and an abrupt change in frequency of feedings.[48] Mastitis can happen at any stage of breastfeeding. Treatment usually includes frequent nursing of the affected breast, application of moist heat (such as a hot face cloth or shower), increased fluids, bed rest, and antibiotics if the infection does not resolve within two to four days. If you do take antibiotics, remember to follow up with probiotics, both for yourself and for baby, during and after the treatment, as antibiotics can lead to candida or thrush.

YEAST, THRUSH, OR CANDIDA INFECTIONS

I've talked many times about good bacteria and bad bacteria. Well, this is one of the bad guys. Classed as a fungus, *Candida albicans* is present in all of us, but the problem arises when we have higher levels in the digestive tract, usually after a course of antibiotics. According to *Dr. Jack Newman's Guide to Breastfeeding*, the shooting or burning pain of thrush can begin late in the feeding or afterwards, it's usually worse in the evenings, and it's felt throughout the breast and sometimes in mom's shoulder or back, lasting for minutes or hours and starting at any age of the baby. A common first treatment of thrush is a purple liquid called gentian violet, which is applied around the nipple and areola and in the baby's mouth on a Q-tip. It's a messy affair. Antifungal medications are often prescribed; Dr. Newman recommends grapefruit seed extract. Genestra's Candicin capsules have worked wonders for many of my clients, as have tongue-tie revisions. I've seen homeopathic remedies provide fast and safe help for both mom and baby. Giving probiotics to both mom and baby in higher doses is also imperative.

BABY'S REACTIONS TO BREAST MILK

Some of the foods or drinks you consume may not agree with your baby. Common symptoms include gassiness, fussiness, diarrhea, constipation, rashes, runny nose, and spitting up. I've seen remarkable improvement in babies when mom removes certain foods from her diet. I recall a mom in one of my Mommy Chef cooking classes who cut dairy out of her diet to help her son's skin rash. This cleared up the rash, and to her amazement he stopped spitting up. She'd had no idea that her dairy intake could affect him—her doctor had told her that some babies are "spitter-uppers" and to just live with it.

Common foods that may upset your baby are dairy products, including milk (usually the worst), cheese, yogurt, and cottage cheese; chocolate (sorry); caffeine (again, sorry); melons; cucumbers; peppers; citrus fruits and juices; and spicy foods. Gas-forming foods, such as cauliflower, broccoli, Brussels sprouts, cucumbers, red and green peppers, onions, beans, and legumes, can also be a contributing factor. These are the most likely culprits, but not all of them may affect your baby.

A milk allergy in your baby may show; although he's not yet drinking cow's milk, the reaction may come from your own dairy intake. This allergy often presents itself as discomfort such as gassiness, colic-like symptoms, and pulling up the legs while crying; skin reactions such as eczema; or, even worse, blood in the stool. Most doctors will suggest removing dairy from your diet in the case of bloody stool. Soy should come out of your diet as well. Both are highly allergenic foods. While soy might seem like a viable milk alternative, many babies that have dairy issues will also have issues with soy.

This may seem like a very limited diet, but start eliminating by looking at what you're eating in the largest quantities. Often, it's wheat and dairy because they're easy to grab and found in most quick and easy foods (other than munching on a banana or cucumber). There are many alternatives to these foods, so you won't go hungry, and I wouldn't suggest restricting your diet too much, as you need nutrients and calories for your body and breast milk production. With the help of a nutritionist, you can eat a super-healthy diet without the foods that are upsetting your baby. Start by keeping a food diary and writing down your baby's reactions next to the foods you've eaten to see what might be a trigger. Remember, though, that it may take some time for the food you've just eaten to get into your breast milk and be digested by your baby, so with any reaction you'll need to look back a meal or two, and maybe even at what you ate yesterday. Next, eliminate any suspected foods to see if this has a positive effect on your baby. Think about whatever you eat or drink every day or more than once a day and see if removing it from your diet for at least two weeks helps. Food sensitivity tests also can be done to determine what you or your baby is reacting to.

After my first daughter ended up with a scarlet-red bum rash when she started on solids, I consulted a naturopath, sent us for food-sensitivity testing. My results showed my own sensitivities, and my daughter's list showed some of the same sensitivities and more! I now had two lists to follow. Out went gluten, dairy, sugar, some fruits, and even goat's milk products. I followed a very limited diet for a few months, and then we were retested. Slowly, my daughter's "safe foods" list expanded as her skin problems cleared up.

BREAST MILK APLENTY

Breast milk production is all about supply and demand. A good latch in the early days, especially in the first hours of baby's life, ensures that prolactin, the hormone that produces breast milk, is stimulated to keep it flowing. Support is essential to get that latch just right so that you don't suffer nipple pain, cracking, or infection (see Tongue-Tie on page 51).

Many mothers have told me that they began formula feeding because of a lack of breast milk—or because they thought they weren't producing enough milk. However, before giving up on nursing, I would suggest consulting with an expert such as a lactation consultant to uncover the reasons behind low milk supply and to confirm that there is, in fact, an issue. Softer breasts, compared to the feeling in the first weeks that they might explode, may make you think that you aren't producing as much milk, but your body has regulated its production and your breasts aren't as full as in the early days. There's usually plenty of milk there to nourish your baby. Make an appointment with a breastfeeding clinic or lactation consultant as early as you can, even before the birth, just to make sure you're on the right track, and learn how to improve the latch or hold and check for a tongue-tie.

Some medications, such as estrogen in birth control pills, may reduce milk production, and fertility hormones, if you're working on baby number two or three, may also decrease supply. Breast augmentation, especially breast reduction, may lead to lower production. In his *Guide to Breastfeeding*, Dr. Jack Newman notes, "There is no doubt that some women are unable to produce enough milk, just as some people do not produce enough insulin or thyroid hormone. But this does not mean that these mothers cannot, or should not breast feed."[49] Dr. Newman supports the use of a lactation aid to keep milk production going as well as continuing to try feeding from the breast. He's of the opinion that if you're producing less breast milk than your baby requires, some is better than none, and you shouldn't stop. He opposes giving formula in the first 24 hours of a baby's life, as it can be detrimental to mom's milk supply and baby loses out on colostrum.

Try these tips to increase your milk supply:

- Make sure you're getting enough calories in your diet. While breastfeeding, you need to eat an additional 500 calories—for example, 1 cup (250 mL) of Mom's Super-Powered Smoothie (page 29). Dieting is not advised, as your breast milk may decrease with a lower calorie intake. Dieting also liberates stored toxins and waste products that can get into your breast milk. I highly recommend seeing a nutritionist, who can help you deal with your weight challenges while maintaining a healthy diet for you and baby. There are snack ideas in many of the later chapters of this book, including Chapter 10 (pages 315–319), and in Mommy Meals (pages 26–29). Breastfeeding actually speeds up weight loss without a calorie-restricted diet. That sounds much better than running on a treadmill, doesn't it?

- Drink enough water. Dehydration will zap your energy and is detrimental to overall health, so aim to drink 2 to 3 quarts (2 to 3 L) of water per day. Your body needs water to make breast milk, and preference goes to the baby, as usual, so you might suffer from low energy, dry skin, or constipation if you don't drink enough water.

- Check how much vitamin B6 you are taking. The level in your multinutrient should be fine, but too much vitamin B6 can reduce breast milk production. Avoid taking extra vitamin B6, such as in a B-complex supplement.

- Try the herbs fenugreek and blessed thistle. Dr. Jack Newman recommends taking fenugreek until you can smell it on your skin (or three capsules each of fenugreek and blessed thistle, taken three times a day). He notes that you'll usually see an increase in breast milk within the first 24 hours after taking these herbs. If you don't see a difference after a week, they may not be for you.

- Try to get more sleep. Call on friends and family to come over and watch baby for a couple of hours so you can have a nap, or go to bed early two to three nights a week.

- Reduce your stress. Having a baby can be stressful without all the other usual demands of life, and stress can impede breast milk production. Plan some relaxation time for yourself—ask someone to watch your baby while you take a long bath, head to a yoga class, meditate, get a massage, or curl up with a good book! Get in the habit of taking walks in nature and calling on friends to talk with. Joining a moms group is an excellent way to know that you're not alone. Sharing your feelings is very important in combating the loneliness that some new mothers feel.

- Consult your doctor for medications that may help, or see the Newman Breastfeeding Clinic website (www.ibconline.ca) for helpful breastfeeding information sheets.
- Try milk-producing tea like Mother's Milk by Traditional Medicinals and eat complex carbohydrates like in the Lactation Cookie (recipe below).

Lactation Cookie MAKES 24 COOKIES

DAIRY-FREE • EGG-FREE • GLUTEN-FREE • VEGAN • VEGETARIAN • WHEAT-FREE

This cookie makes for a great snack, in addition to providing the nutrients needed for increased breast milk production. You can also use two eggs in place of the flax eggs, but flax is good for breast milk production.

2 tablespoons (30 mL) freshly ground flaxseed

6 tablespoons (90 mL) filtered water

1 cup (250 mL) gluten-free old-fashioned rolled oats

2 cups (500 mL) almond flour

5 tablespoons (75 mL) brewer's yeast

½ teaspoon (2 mL) baking powder

½ teaspoon (2 mL) baking soda

½ teaspoon (2 mL) cinnamon

¼ teaspoon (1 mL) sea salt

1 medium overripe banana

½ cup (125 mL) coconut oil

½ cup (125 mL) pure maple syrup

2 teaspoons (10 mL) pure vanilla extract

½ cup (125 mL) vegan mini dark chocolate chips or chunks

1. Preheat the oven to 325°F (160°C). Line a baking sheet with parchment paper and set aside.

2. In a small bowl, make the flax eggs by mixing together the flaxseed and water for 5 minutes.

3. In a medium bowl, mix together the oats, almond flour, yeast, baking powder, baking soda, cinnamon, and salt.

4. In another medium bowl, mash the banana and then mix in the flax egg, coconut oil, maple syrup, and vanilla.

5. With a spatula, gently fold the dry ingredients into the wet ingredients until just combined. Do not overmix. Fold in the chocolate chips.

6. Spoon the dough onto the prepared baking sheet in 1-tablespoon (15 mL) measurements.

7. Bake for 15 minutes or until golden and cookies spring back when touched. Cool to room temperature on a wire rack and store in an airtight container for up to 5 days. These cookies are suitable for freezing for up to 1 month.

NUTRITION INFORMATION Oats are a very good source of iron and since low iron levels can decrease your milk supply, iron-rich foods are important. Brewer's yeast is known as a galactagogue and is great for energy. Almonds are full of protein and calcium, which are both needed for healthy breast milk production.

GET THE MILK FLOWING: WORDS FROM A LACTATION CONSULTANT

Low breast milk production is almost always tied to poor technique and insufficient nipple stimulation. The more nipple stimulation there is, the more the hormone prolactin is produced, and the more milk the breast makes. But if the latch isn't working, there's a tongue-tie, or he's not on one breast for long enough to drain it completely, the body will start to slow down production. Newborn babies need to be awakened if they fall asleep at the breast, especially if they have come through a medicated labour and delivery (epidurals make them sleepy). It's not always understood that babies need to feed often to build up mom's milk supply in the first few days. There is an optimum time for mom to get baby to the breast after birth, within the first half-hour to hour after birth, to set up the hormones that ensure adequate milk supply. That's not to say that you can't build up a good milk supply if you can't breastfeed right away, but it is an added advantage.

Nighttime is the optimum time for baby to have unrestricted access to the breast. Weaning baby off night feeds too early can result in reduced milk production because prolactin levels are higher at night. Stress is a big factor when it comes to having enough milk for baby. Mom's stress and difficulty in feeling relaxed interferes with the "let-down" reflex while nursing and affects how much milk the baby gets. Physiological issues that can affect milk supply are breast surgery where milk ducts have been severed or removed or an actual deficit in breast glandular tissue, which is very rare. Other than that, it's pretty much technique and frequency.[50] – Natalie Rogers, CBDE, RHN (Childbirth Educator)

BREASTFEEDING AND SOLID FOOD

When your baby is around six months of age, it's time to start him on solid food. Some mothers decide to put off giving their children solids and only breastfeed for the first year. I have yet to hear of any health concerns in any children who were exclusively breastfed in their first year, but it's uncommon to wait that long. Your baby has been exposed to many different tastes and flavours through your breast milk—when you eat spicy food, for instance, or garlic and onions. Most babies enjoy the flavour and spice, but it can also go the other way. You may recall a time when you ate a spicy curry or Thai meal and it didn't agree with baby, and so everyone was up all night! Exposure to moderate spices not only helps everyone sleep at night, but is also a good start to the new experience of eating food. When your baby first starts solids, her breast milk intake shouldn't change. As her appetite for solid food increases to two or three meals a day, she might nurse less, although you may not even notice at first. She'll nurse a few minutes less here and there, until she drops a feeding altogether. But go easy on the amount of food you offer your baby—you don't want to take away the great nutrition of breast milk by offering too much food too quickly. Remember that everything your baby needs is in breast milk, especially in comparison to a few tablespoons of purée. Natalie Rogers notes that "as the baby breastfeeds less when solid foods are introduced, the milk becomes more concentrated in some minerals and proteins."[51] It's nature's way of making sure that baby is still getting what he needs. I find that remarkable.

PUMPING AND STORING BREAST MILK

Pumping in the early days is usually an easy task and will give you milk to store for feedings when you're not around. Milk can be pumped and frozen in ice cube trays free from bisphenol A (BPA), phthalate, and polyvinyl chloride (PVC) or in safe, sterile plastic bags designed for breast milk. These bags have lines to indicate the amount of milk and a space to write down the date so you can use the oldest milk first and know how long it's been in the freezer. Natalie Rogers gave me the rundown on storage: milk can be stored in amounts that the baby will use in one feeding, and pumped milk should be refrigerated within six hours and consumed within two to five days (shake to remix it). If milk is frozen in a fridge freezer, use within one month; if frozen in a deep freezer, use within six months. Discard any thawed and warmed milk that's left over from a feeding. Warming should never be done in a microwave, as it creates hot spots and kills many of the delicate nutrients, immune components, and proteins. Try placing a milk-filled bottle or container in a bowl of very warm tap water or thawing it under running tap water, and warm it to skin temperature. Never thaw milk on the counter overnight, as this enables bacteria in the milk to multiply. Don't use a stove to warm the milk—overheating can destroy the vitamin C content and alter the proteins, including the sIgA.

WEANING FROM BREASTFEEDING

Breastfeeding can continue for as long as you want it to. I recommend breastfeeding for the first two years, and even longer if possible, or at least breastfeeding regularly for the first year. If you're heading back to work around the time your baby turns one, offer the breast first thing in the morning and before bed (but don't forget to start brushing those baby teeth). Keeping the morning and evening breastfeed provides a time of closeness that's especially precious with the new dynamic of mom being away from baby.

When you feel that it's time to stop breastfeeding, you need to provide an alternative until your baby is at least one year old. Some doctors recommend giving cow's milk if your baby stops breastfeeding between ten and twelve months, but I don't entirely agree. Switching to cow's milk as a full replacement for breast milk can come with many issues like ear infections, eczema, and cold-like symptoms of a constant runny nose, sickness, and cough. Because cow's milk is the most allergenic food, it's better to wait until at least one year before giving it to your baby as a replacement for breast milk. At ten months, your baby may still be drinking a lot, and four to six 8-ounce (225 mL) bottles of cow's milk is a lot to digest at this stage. The better option is to start baby on formula if you're weaning off breast milk before age one. This decision should also take into account the amount of solid food your baby is eating. See Chapter 9 (page 188) for suggestions of milks to move on to at age one.

Mothers who are heading back to work after maternity leave are often anxious about weaning their babies from the breast before the big day. The amount of breastfeeding at six months is very different from that at eleven months. Wait until closer to ten months to assess the situation, so you can see how much your baby is nursing then.

Trying to get your baby to take a bottle of anything can often be challenging, especially if mom is the one doing the feeding. Your baby might be wondering why she has to drink from a bottle when the breast is right there. It may work better to have dad start feeding with a bottle to get your baby used to it (so she won't smell your milk); a skilled child care worker should also be able to get a bottle or sippy cup full of some kind of milk into your baby—perhaps not on the first day, but it will come. I encourage good eating habits—if your baby is eating food with varied nutrients, you won't need to worry as much about the milk. Not all babies like the taste of milk or formula after breast milk, so if they won't take it, don't force it. If you're concerned about baby missing out on the nutrients and calcium in milk, be more aware of the nutrients in food and what should be on baby's plate to make up for the lack of milk (see Calcium and Bones on page 36 for calcium-rich foods). The babies I know who have refused the moo-juice have grown up healthy and strong.

To wean your baby off the breast, start to offer the alternative by replacing one feeding at a time about a month before you want to completely stop to balance your milk supply and to gradually introduce formula to baby's digestion. Don't be disappointed if you don't have instant success. Talk to your baby about what is coming up: "Mommy is going back to work and instead of nursing, this is what you are going to have when you are at _____, or when _____ is here with you." Although they can't talk, babies need to know what's going on and why. You might also try shortening the length of each nursing and offering substitutions of either food or water. Let your baby know he'll still be able to nurse when he wakes up and before he goes to bed. However, when your baby needs breastmilk for nourishment, of course offer the breast.

If breastfeeding is just for baby's comfort, try to distract her with another activity. Again, talk to your baby about what's going on by explaining that nursings (or whatever you call breastfeeding) are slowing down now, so here's what the alternative is. When my second daughter was finishing up nursing at twenty-six months, I talked with her about how she was just going to have a "little nurse" before bed. She would look up at me with those big baby-blue eyes and say, "Just a little nurse, Mama," and slowly it happened less and less often. Her dad got more involved in putting her to bed, so breastfeeding at bedtime wasn't an issue. And to stop the morning breastfeed, her dad would take her downstairs for breakfast, avoiding me and the usual morning routine.

3 · MORE WHITE STUFF: FORMULA FEEDING

Some moms choose not to breastfeed or to nurse only some of the time or for a shorter period. Others don't have a choice—they may not be able to offer any breast milk at all because of complications during labour and delivery; an earlier decision to have breast reduction surgery, which affects milk-producing capabilities; or many other reasons. Many babies who've grown up on formula milk are fit and healthy. Being informed when it comes to purchasing an infant formula can give you greater confidence in your choice and help alleviate the guilt that can overwhelm some moms. You'll find my breakdown of the challenges and the formula charts on SproutRight.com helpful when navigating formula feeding your baby.

In an ideal world, all babies would benefit from colostrum right after birth and then from breast milk for as long as possible. That doesn't always happen, for various reasons. Over the years I've met many mothers who wished they could breastfeed and tried everything to nurse their babies, but sometimes it just doesn't work out. A lactation consultant can offer incredible support and you should also familiarize yourself with tongue-tie (page 51). Even if you can't offer breast milk exclusively, don't despair—any amount of breast milk you give your baby will have him off to a great start. If you nursed for the first few days in the hospital and he received colostrum, well done! If you breastfed for six weeks, three months, or nine months, even better.

CHOOSING THE RIGHT FORMULA

With so many brands, types, and categories of formula on the market, browsing the formula aisle in the supermarket, drugstore, or even health food store can be overwhelming. Each brand is vying for your hard-earned dollars, so while you might think they have your best interests at heart, keep in mind that they have sales targets to reach and will do what they can to get their products in front of you in any way they can. The only way to know which is the best formula for your baby is to do your research, read the labels, and adjust your choice after you see how it works for your baby.

You need to know the ins and outs of formula before choosing which one is right for your little one—remember, every baby is different. Your doctor may recommend brands when you're thinking about starting your baby on formula. However, formula company salespeople inform doctors about their products, and your doctor might not know all that's available or might not have asked for the same information that you would have. I'd be overjoyed if some of these questions were answered: Does your product contain genetically modified ingredients? Should I be giving probiotics to my baby even though there's a prebiotic in the brand of formula I buy? How confident are you about the DHA source in this formula? I've heard that it can cause diarrhea in some babies. But that's not very realistic.[52] In fact, while I was researching this chapter, it proved difficult, if not impossible, to get responses to my own questions from the formula companies. Many things can influence your decision about which formula to purchase, and although health care professionals are the right place to start, it's best to keep searching until you're confident that you've made an informed choice that aligns with your values and also works for your baby.

Comparing formula to breast milk is unfair. It's unfair to the formula companies and unfair to breast milk. It's best to compare formulas to each other. There are about nine main formula companies in Canada and a few more in the United States, all of which use different ingredients that will either work for your baby or not. The addition of DHA, arachidonic **acid** (AA), and some beneficial bacteria—all of which, manufacturers note, makes their formula "closest to breast milk"—is good in theory, but formulas still aren't quite a match to breast milk and its complexity. You might be saying to yourself, "High in iron . . . that sounds good—iron is important, right? Prebiotics—I've heard of probiotics, so that brand looks better than the other. And that one has DHA and AA—I'm not sure what they are, but the formula companies know what they're doing so it must be okay . . . I think." Deciding on a formula for your baby should involve careful consideration. There are good reasons for choosing one formula over another, and it's not about the catchy labelling. Your baby may need a certain protein ratio or need the proteins broken down a bit (known as being hydrolyzed), you might prefer an organic formula (that would be my preference), a friend mentioned goat's milk formula to you, and you're unsure what any of it means or what might be right for your baby. So, let's start at the beginning and look at some of the most common ingredients found in formula.

FORMULA INGREDIENTS: THE GOOD AND NOT SO GOOD

PROTEIN

The protein source in dairy formulas is whey and/or casein. The ratio of whey to casein seems to differ among the formulas suitable for different age groups (see the chart on SproutRight.com). Newborn formula aims for a ratio of whey to casein similar to that in breast milk, and formulas for six-month-olds and older babies offer different proportions. If your baby is displaying any symptoms of allergic reaction—eczema, asthma, blood in the stool, vomiting, or hives—it's mostly caused by the beta-lactoglobulin protein in whey (only protein is associated with this type of allergy, called type 1 allergy; see Chapter 5 for more on allergies). Some babies and children, especially children with autism, have difficulty digesting casein. See the table comparing various formulas' ingredients on SproutRight.com.

Soy formula relies on soybean as its protein source. Soy formula is advised in cases of galactosemia (a rare genetic metabolic disorder) or an allergy to cow's milk (although hydrolyzed formula may be a better option). See page 66 for more on soy formula.

CARBOHYDRATES

Lactose, corn maltodextrin, corn syrup, corn syrup solids, glucose, sucrose, and brown rice syrup are carbohydrates added to formula for energy as well as sweetness. When milk is separated to extract the protein from everything else, a carbohydrate source needs to be added alongside the protein when making a formula. Because lactose is also found in breast milk, almost all babies will tolerate it well and it's the best choice of carbohydrate. Lactose also aids in the absorption of calcium and helps feed the good bacteria in the gut.[53-57] Corn syrup, maltodextrin, brown rice syrup, and sucrose are all used in place of lactose. Corn syrup and sucrose are worrisome: nonorganic corn syrup can contain genetically modified corn, and sucrose is a simple sugar known as table sugar—the white stuff you add to your tea or coffee.

In an interview I conducted with Jay Highman, founder of Nature's One, which manufactures Baby's Only Organic formula, he explained that lactose is naturally occurring in all milk powder used for formula unless it's taken out. "When lactose is listed in the ingredient declaration panel," Highman explains, "this means an additional amount of lactose has been added to complete the carbohydrate requirements of a baby. The added amount of lactose can overwhelm a baby's available supply of lactase, an enzyme found in the small intestine needed to break down milk lactose. If there is not enough lactase, then undigested lactose moves into the intestinal tract and produces bloating, cramps, diarrhea, and ultimately a very unhappy baby. Baby's Only Organic daily formula does not list lactose as an ingredient because it's naturally occurring. We complete the carbohydrate requirement by adding a complex carbohydrate, organic brown rice syrup. We believe that is the perfect balance." Formula manufacturers are required to list anything that's been added to formula. Nature's One formulas include brown rice syrup, an easily digested source of carbohydrates that's more complex than sucrose, for instance, in its carbohydrate structure; it enters the bloodstream slowly, as lactose does, but without stressing the lactase enzyme. This is called a low glycemic food, and it's preferable for everyone's blood sugar stability. A lot has been reported on arsenic and brown rice syrup, so I spoke with a Nature's One dietitian, Diane Wilson, who explains, "Nature's One uses the most advanced methodologies recommended by the World Health Organization to test its organic brown rice syrup. Our test results from an independent laboratory indicate the new organic-compliant filtration process used by Nature's One reduces arsenic found in brown rice syrup to less than detectable levels."[58]

FATS

Soybean, high-oleic (acid), sunflower, safflower, palm olein, and coconut oil are all found on the ingredient lists of formulas and make up the fatty acids your baby needs. Formula companies use a mixture of these oils to create a fatty acid profile closest to that of breast milk. It's important to understand the different fats, though. Research indicates that palm olein oil is not preferred because it's associated with constipation and lower calcium absorption from the formula for strong bones.[59] A study concluded that "healthy term infants fed a formula containing PO [palm olein] as the predominant oil in the fat blend had significantly lower BMC [bone mineral content] and BMD [bone mineral density] than those fed a formula without PO. The inclusion of PO in infant formula at levels needed to provide a fatty acid profile similar to that of human milk leads to lower bone mineralization."[60]

Avoiding palm olein oil might narrow down your choices considerably; I came across only three formulas that didn't have it—Similac, Kirkland, and Nature's One—one of which isn't available in Canada but can be purchased online from the United States. Other formulas listed "palm oil or palm olein," making it difficult to know for sure which oil is included. It irks me when manufacturers use "or." I understand that the supply of certain ingredients may be limited, so they're hedging their bets on what they can get, but especially in the case of formula, I want to know exactly what's in the product. If you do use formula with palm olein oil, counteract constipation with extra probiotics and flaxseed oil until you find an alternative (see Chapter 4 for more on constipation).

A new ingredient under the fat umbrella is milk fat globule membranes (MFGMs). Breast milk contains MFGMs, which have many bioactive components. It is suggested that supplementing infant formulas with bovine MFGMs may narrow the gap in health outcomes between formula-fed and breastfed infants and improve cognitive development; however, further studies are needed as of the time of writing.[61]

IRON

Formula must contain minerals within a set range, so you'll notice that the nutritional content of all formulas is roughly the same. One of the most important minerals during infancy is iron, as it's involved in brain development and cognitive function. All formula is fortified with between 0.7 and 1.8 mg iron per 100 mL. When deciding whether your baby needs a higher level of iron, you'll need to take your baby's history into consideration. For instance, was your baby premature? If so, look for a formula that's a bit higher in iron because preemies are more likely to have lower iron stores (they didn't have the time in utero to take what they needed from you). Note that there are formulas for premature babies that have an easier-to-absorb protein structure. If your baby was born at term and had a low birth weight (less than 2.5 kg or 5 pounds, 8 ounces), you may also want to consider a formula with a bit more iron. For all other babies, a higher-than-average iron-fortified formula isn't necessary.

The big concern with iron is its absorbability. Breast milk contains two proteins, *lactoferrin* and *transferrin*, that grab on to the iron, delivering it to your baby's bloodstream and keeping any bad bacteria in the intestines from making a meal of it (bad bacteria thrive on iron). Formula doesn't contain these key proteins, so you'll need to assess whether your baby is likely to have high levels of bad bacteria in her intestines (we all have a certain amount). Look back at your pregnancy, labour and delivery, and postpartum period if you were breastfeeding. If you took antibiotics during any of these times, it's possible that your baby will have lower levels of good bacteria to keep the bad guys in check. If your baby was given antibiotics or was born by Caesarean section, the same applies. When more bad bacteria are hanging around, there's less chance for your baby to absorb iron from the formula, so offer a human strain of probiotics or beneficial bacteria containing *Bifidobacterium* strains and *Lactobacillus acidophilus* at a level of at least ten billion bacteria, ideally with galactosaccharides, or GOS (found in Genestra's HMF Baby F for formula-fed babies). This can help to keep the bad bacteria at bay and therefore allow iron to be better absorbed.

ESSENTIAL FATTY ACIDS

Essential fatty acids—DHA and AA—are essential for the development of the brain, eyes, and nervous systems. Formula companies are marketing this addition as making their products that much closer to breast milk, leading parents to believe that formula is as good as breast milk, which is not the case. These added fats have also created controversy. In a 2008 report, the Cornucopia Institute, an organization that supports sustainable and organic agriculture, examined the use of these oils in formula.[62] The institute's concern is that DHA and AA are extracted from algae and fungal sources and processed using a toxic chemical, hexane. There is now a form of DHA that's produced without hexane and available in certain formulas like Nature's One. The main worry is that these oils can cause diarrhea in babies, leading to health complications. It's a tough decision whether to buy formula fortified with these essential fatty acids. I have suggested that parents purchase formula without DHA and AA and add the DHA themselves. Babies can use the other fats in formula to make AA in their bodies, but they can't do the same for DHA at the level they need for optimal brain and eye development. Of course, the exact composition of DHA and AA in breast milk may not resemble that added to formula. That said, some research conducted on small groups of children has shown an increase in IQ and visual acuity in babies fed formula fortified with DHA and AA.[63]

NUCLEOTIDES

Nucleotides are molecules that help make up the structure of DNA and RNA and are naturally found in breast milk. Some formula companies (mostly in the United States) have been adding nucleotides to their formula for several years. At a time of such rapid growth and cell turnover in your baby's digestive, immune, and metabolic cells, nucleotides are important factors; however, in the form that's added to formula, they are a chemical, so possibly they're not the best addition for your baby. They are not allowed in organic formulas because they are synthetic. In the coming years, I suspect we will find nucleotides listed as standard ingredients in all formulas.

BENEFICIAL BACTERIA

The *microbiome*—gut flora or the bacterial environment in the gut—is quite the buzzword now, and it applies to everyone, even your baby. Probiotics and prebiotics are essential for overall gut health and well-being. One of the newer additions to formula is a prebiotic called galactooligosaccharides (GOS). It's found in abundance in breast milk and helps the probiotics adhere or stick to the intestinal wall. It is a very important part of the process of colonizing the gut with good bacteria. One formula company (at the time of writing) has added in "natural cultures," or probiotics. Good bacteria are so important for your baby's digestive and immune systems, and although this formula contains only one strain, *Bifidobacterium lactis*, it's a good start. My concern is that most probiotics need to be refrigerated and will die off with any heat, so how much will be left after warming formula (especially if warmed in a microwave), or even after opening the tin, remains to be seen. I still recommend giving your baby a probiotic with at least ten billion colony-forming units (CFUs), with mixed strains and GOS, in it.

FORMULA CHOICES FROM AROUND THE WORLD

In recent years, formulas available only in Europe have become the go-to for some parents. There are different standards in the European Union, many of which are tighter or healthier than those in North America. Companies like HiPP Organic and NANNYCare in the UK and Holle in Germany have parents ordering products both from U.S. distributors and direct from each country. The ingredients are simple, with whey being the main source of protein, which suits more sensitive babies better. I've recommended goat's milk formula for years and have seen many symptoms like eczema, rashes, vomiting, spit-up, gassiness, diarrhea, and constipation ease considerably after switching to goat's milk formula. More work and cost is involved to get it, but for some, it's well worth it.

TYPES OF FORMULA
SOY FORMULA

Soy formula may be the only choice for some babies, such as those with the rare genetic disorder galactosemia or cow's milk allergy (although some babies who are allergic to dairy are also allergic to soy). The American Academy of Pediatrics states that "soy protein–based formula is a reasonable alternative for term infants who cannot tolerate cow milk–based formulas or lactose found in cow's milk formulas."[64]

When buying soy formula, go with an organic product. Conventional soy is typically genetically modified (GM) and may lead to negative health issues. GM soy (canola, cotton, and corn) is a product I advise all parents to avoid, whether in the form of tofu, tempeh, soy sauce, edamame (soybeans in their shells), milk, or formula. The potential health risks include a higher chance of developing allergies because the DNA structure of the food has been altered and becomes similar to other allergens or the GM food has been adulterated with part of a nut, such as Brazil nut in the case of some soy products.[65] Babies and toddlers have such fast growth rates in their first years that they have much greater susceptibility to health issues from eating GM foods.[66] Check out www.geneticroulette.com for research as well as up-to-date lists of which foods contain GM ingredients. Conventional or nonorganic dairy formula also has the potential to contain GM products from corn and from cows being fed GM feed, which will affect their milk. It takes a bit of research to find out which foods may contain GM products, but once you look into the issue, you'll understand why the extra effort is worth it. Another reason to be cautious about consuming any soy product, whether organic or conventional, is that soy contains a compound called phytate. Phytate binds with minerals such as iron, zinc, and calcium and interferes with their absorption by the body. Although soy formula is fortified with these minerals, as well as phosphorus, it's not recommended for premature babies, as it has been associated with a higher risk of low bone density (osteopenia).[67] But for other babies, soy formula may be the only option.

GOAT'S MILK FORMULA

Goat's milk formula and goat's milk is generally better tolerated than cow dairy. There are two main brands of goat's milk formula that I do regularly recommend to parents: Holle from Germany and NANNYCare Goat Milk Formula, with milk from New Zealand. The oldest on the market is NANNYCare, which is produced by the Dairy Goat Co-operative and available online and from health food stores and pharmacies in the UK. The ease of digestion is key because the protein structure of goat's milk is more similar to that of breast milk. I've seen all sorts of reactions, including eczema, spitting up, behaviour issues, and colic, improve when parents switch to goat's milk formula. The Holle goat's milk formula has a simple ingredient list with organic fats and goat's milk whey, which makes it easy on the digestion. You need to add DHA and probiotics to this formula yourself, which I always prefer.

Why is goat's milk formula better? NANNYCare notes on its website some benefits of this formula: it offers a protein source that's easier to digest (smaller curds), supports digestive health by reducing "leaky gut," contains absorbable fatty acids, is made from the milk of goats that are naturally raised without growth stimulants and hormones, has essential nutrients needed for growth, and, if you are so inclined, can even be used in cooking![68] I often recommend goat's milk as a substitute for dairy for toddlers over one year of age; it seems to be less reactive than cow's milk. But some babies still react, so it's not for everyone. Even if you can't manage to switch to goat's milk formula entirely, you could rotate it in for three days a week and use cow's milk formula for the rest of the week, depending on what your baby's symptoms are.

LACTOSE-FREE FORMULA

When I first heard of lactose-free formula, I wondered what on earth was going on. Breast milk contains lactose, so it's almost impossible for babies to be lactose intolerant. But after hearing from parents about how much better their babies did on lactose-free formula, I had to dig deeper. Lactose is the sugar, or carbohydrate, most commonly found in all milk, from both humans and animals. Not only is it an important carbohydrate source, but it enhances calcium absorption and helps the colonization of good bacteria in baby's intestines.

Lactose-free formulas replace the lactose with corn syrup, maltodextrin, sucrose, or brown rice syrup. As I mentioned earlier, the use of corn syrup is a concern because it can be made from GM corn, it's very sweet, and it has been associated with allergies. Sucrose also isn't the best choice because it's as sweet as purple grape juice and can lead to overfeeding.[69] Search out an organic formula that uses an alternative sweetener or carbohydrate.

WHEN SHOULD YOU USE A LACTOSE-FREE FORMULA? If you see that your baby isn't comfortable with the formula you're offering, try another. A lactose-free formula may ease digestive symptoms of gas and bloating, fussiness, discomfort with colic-like pain and diarrhea, loose stools, or even constipation.[70] Secondary lactose intolerance can be caused by digestive disorders such as celiac disease, gastroenteritis, or diarrhea (even from teething). There may be damage to the enzyme-producing sites in the intestines, or the lactase enzyme may be whooshed out in cases of diarrhea as the body tries to get rid of bacteria, a virus, or a parasite. In any case of diarrhea, whatever the cause, it's advisable to remove dairy from the diet immediately. If your baby is on formula, switch to a lactose-free, goat's milk or soy formula to avoid lactose intolerance and the symptoms described below. Once the diarrhea episode has passed, give probiotics to recolonize baby's intestines with good bacteria, and wait three days before returning to your baby's usual formula. If gassy symptoms start, even with probiotics, slowly ease back on to the usual formula, rather than making a straight switch back.

Lactose Overload

When parents think their baby is lactose intolerant, and the baby has been breastfed or is drinking formula already, it's likely that lactose overload is causing fussiness and gassiness that will improve with a lactose-free formula. Baby's lactase production may be unable to keep up with the amount of lactose ingested, such as when a baby quickly drinks large amounts of formula every day. That's where the term *overload* comes in. Any formula with lactose on the ingredient list has more than a naturally occurring level and may overwhelm the lactase enzyme; then digestion can't keep up. That's not a lactose intolerance; the situation is caused by lactose overload. Switching to a lactose-free formula means that the carbohydrate source is corn syrup, maltodextrin, glucose, sucrose, or brown rice syrup, which could help ease symptoms (although not all of these ingredients are ideal sweeteners

HYDROLYZED FORMULA

Formula that has had its proteins broken down or predigested to amino acids (amino acids are the building blocks of protein) is called *hydrolyzed* or *hydrolysate protein*. The point of this process is to break down proteins to make them more digestible, so hydrolyzed formula is often the product of choice for babies showing symptoms of milk allergy, blood in the stool, gassiness, skin issues like eczema, or failure to thrive. You may see it written in the ingredient list as partially hydrolyzed protein.

One concern with hydrolyzed formula is that the process of predigesting the protein to amino acids results in a bitter taste, so sweet-tasting ingredients are added to improve flavour (even then, it still doesn't taste great). During this process, lactose is removed and replaced with a carbohydrate source and a sweetener, usually corn syrup or sucrose, which can pose their own health concerns. In addition, the benefits of lactose in helping with the absorption of calcium and the replication of good bacteria in the intestines are lost. Hydrolyzed formulas are sometimes recommended in the case of family history of allergy or immune disease, and to prevent milk allergy, as it's the proteins in milk that usually cause the allergy. I suggest looking into a hydrolyzed formula if your baby has a higher potential for allergies because he has a sibling with an anaphylactic food allergy; he was premature or had a low birth weight; he wasn't breastfed at all; he was born by Caesarean section; you took antibiotics during pregnancy, labour, or delivery, or while breastfeeding; your baby has had antibiotics; or there's a family history of allergy in either parents or a sibling. Use hydrolyzed formula while you support the baby's digestive system with probiotics for at least one month, then switch to a non-hydrolyzed one.

Hydrolyzed formula isn't offered as an organic product, and it's usually more expensive than non-hydrolyzed formula. I've seen this formula help many babies who couldn't tolerate the other types, even partially hydrolyzed formula; babies who were once gassy and uncomfortable, waking throughout the night, sometimes sleep better, and eczema can improve (although infant probiotics often give better results). The consequences of using hydrolyzed formula for a prolonged period haven't been studied in depth, but some parents may have no choice but to use it.

PREMIXED VERSUS POWDER FORMULA

Premixed formulas may be a better option for premature babies because of the risks associated with not mixing powder formula properly or contaminating it with bacteria on mixing. Sterilizing your bottles; letting them air-dry; using filtered, boiled, and cooled water to make the powder formula; and double-checking your measurements should eliminate any problems with powder formula. Premixed formula might be a better choice if you're going away on holiday and can't guarantee the safety of the water where you'll be. Finally, although premixed formula can be convenient, it's usually more expensive.

Tips for Mixing Powder Formula

- To reduce the risk of bacteria contamination, sterilize your bottles and always wash your hands before preparing the formula.
- Let the bottles air-dry before filling them.
- Use filtered water that has been boiled and cooled. Reverse osmosis filtered water can be used straight from the tap or bottle (I'd suggest boiling it for preemies or newborns, though).
- Check the expiry date on the can.
- Carefully follow the instructions for quantity of water to powder, and once mixed, refrigerate and use the formula within 24 hours.
- If you're going out, bring a bottle with premeasured dry powder and mix it with water from a thermal mug (to keep it warm), rather than taking an already mixed bottle. That way, you don't need to keep the formula cool while you're out and about.
- Discard anything your baby doesn't drink from a prepared bottle immediately.

DO YOUR RESEARCH AND READ THE LABEL

STEP 1

Before choosing a formula, check for recent recalls or contamination information on the websites of the Canadian Food Inspection Agency (www.inspection.gc.ca) and the U.S. Food and Drug Administration (www.fda.gov). The last thing you want is to find out that your formula has been recalled or found to contain something that it shouldn't.

STEP 2

Consider whether to go organic or not and if goat or cow dairy is best for your baby. I highly recommend buying an organic formula, if possible. There are two on the Canadian market and more in the United States. I have had clients who had Baby's Only Organic formula delivered from the United States to their homes. Holle and HiPP Organic products can be ordered online or directly from Germany and the UK. Although some organic formulas' ingredient lists aren't perfect, buying organic lessens the possibility of exposure to the hormones, antibiotics, and GM feed given to cows and reduces the overall toxic load from herbicides and pesticides.

STEP 3

Speak with your doctor if your baby seems to have a problem with formula and shows any of the following symptoms: spits up or has diarrhea or constipation, eczema, or rashes; doesn't sleep well; seems restless and unsettled (different from poor sleep habits); or fails to develop or gain weight as expected. Then see the table comparing formulas on SproutRight.com or check the ingredient list on your formula. Don't discount the possibility that a health issue may be linked to formula. See what the sweetener or carbohydrate source is—lactose, corn, or something else (brown rice syrup is less likely to cause a problem). Then look at the protein source—whey, casein, or a mix of both. Breast milk is a mix of both proteins in a ratio of about 70 percent whey to 30 percent casein, so both are important. Goat's milk formula may be a better option for your baby. If your baby is suffering from constipation, look for palm olein oil on the label and try another brand. No extra iron is needed for babies born at term. If you don't use a formula with added DHA and AA, supplement with DHA.

STEP 4
No matter which formula you choose, always give probiotics, preferably one with galactooligosaccharides (GOS) in it. GOS is found in breast milk, but not in all formulas. The GOS helps probiotics to adhere to the intestinal wall, which is what we want. Probiotics help with iron absorption, reduce the risk of allergies, and support the maturation of the digestive system. They are suitable for any baby.

STEP 5
If your baby has no particular health issues, don't get too fancy. A standard formula (again, preferably organic) is just fine. Formula has been around for years, and dairy formula is the oldest and most trusted (although I prefer goat's milk formula). Unless absolutely necessary, avoid soy formula; but if you have to use it, buy organic.

STEP 6
Be a savvy shopper. Read the ingredient lists and shop around. Although there's a certain stigma to buying a chain store's generic brands or products, comparing their ingredient labels with those of the top brands may save you a lot of money. In my research on different formulas, I found out that one company manufactures formula products (especially the organic ones) for many retail companies, which then apply their own private labels. There can be up to $15 difference in price for the same product.

I believe that the greater incidence of allergy is partly to do with babies being fed formula with the new ingredients described in this chapter, some of which are from genetically modified sources, and this worries me a lot. We won't know for years what the negative effects of these new formulas might be, until there's an increase in a certain disease or a new illness that affects our children's generation. All you can do is make an informed choice by doing research, asking the important questions, and reading labels. Then, lift the weight of guilt off your shoulders, knowing that you've done the best that you can. That's great parenting!

FORMULA COMPARISON CHARTS
To compare Canadian, U.S., and International formula brands that are available to purchase in store and online, visit the detailed formula comparison charts on SproutRight.com.

4 · BABY POO: KNOWING THEIR "BUSINESS"

You may be thinking, "There's a chapter on baby poo? What is she thinking?" Believe it or not, baby poo is a hot topic among parents. Although some parents are embarrassed to talk about poo, it gives you a sneak peek into what's going on inside baby's little body. Bowel movements should be a daily occurrence, and although changing diapers isn't much fun, those baby poos are vital for a healthy body.

NEWBORN POO

The first poo is the dark, sticky, and tarlike meconium that baby passes soon after birth. It's a mixture of a buildup of skin cells, mucus, amniotic fluid, bile from the gallbladder, and water. Nothing has been ingested by baby yet, so meconium is bacteria-free and almost sterile. It should be completely passed by the end of the third day postpartum. Rub an oil such as olive or coconut on your newborn's clean bum so that the meconium will wipe off easily later.

Once the meconium has cleared, baby's poo becomes mustard yellow in colour, and the texture is quite liquid, with seedy white bits. Breast milk poo is unique in consistency as well as colour because most bacteria in breastfed babies' intestines are *Bifidobacteria*. If your baby drinks formula or has started eating solid food, stools will be more formed and brown or tan because of the change in the balance of intestinal bacteria away from predominantly *Bifidobacteria*.

Baby Bacteria

According to Dr. Nigel Plummer, a prominent microbiologist from the United Kingdom, only 22 percent of the fecal matter from a formula-fed baby will contain *Bifidobacteria* (good bacteria), with the remaining 70 percent containing the undesirable bacteria. In comparison, a breastfed baby's poo contains 95 percent *Bifidobacteria*. We want to encourage the colonization of the good bacteria to help support baby's immune system and digestive function, with the hope of reducing the chance of allergies and improving overall health. To foster the growth of beneficial bacteria, I recommend that all formula-fed babies supplement with a probiotic containing human strains of both *Bifidobacterium* and *Lactobacillus acidophilus* at a level of at least ten billion total bacteria, or colony-forming units (CFU) per day.

TYPICAL BREAST MILK POO

Breastfed babies can have bowel movements anywhere from one to six times a day. And on occasion, your baby may not poo for five days. Breastfed babies use most of what is in their milk, so sometimes, during a growth spurt or around six months when they are almost ready to start solids, there may not be much to eliminate and you won't see a bowel movement for a few days. This is common and not a huge concern. If your baby hasn't pooed for a week, discuss this with your doctor just to be sure that all is well.

Breast milk poo doesn't have a particularly offensive odour—a slightly acidic smell is distinct, with a hint of vinegar. The consistency is more liquid than solid, and it should always be mustard yellow. If it ever has a greenish tinge to it, your baby either isn't getting the hindmilk (the fattier breast milk toward the end of a feeding) or could have an infection of some kind. If it's the former, your baby might be fussier than usual. The foremilk (milk from the first few minutes of nursing) is more carbohydrate rich and doesn't have the more sustaining fat to keep baby going longer. It's a bit like eating a plain cracker—it doesn't satisfy you until you top it with fat-rich avocado, hummus, or almond butter. If you see green poo, try to nurse for as long as possible on one breast and then switch to the other. If your baby is the on-and-off type, keep offering the same breast for that feeding. If the stools are still green, see your doctor to ensure that your baby doesn't have an infection. (See Constipation: Hard Poo, page 77, for tips if your baby isn't pooing frequently.)

TYPICAL FORMULA POO

A formula-fed baby should be pooing at least once a day. Because bacteria in the digestive system of a formula-fed baby are more similar to those in an adult or in a baby who has started on solids, the poo will be similar in consistency, colour, and smell to adult stool. However, it shouldn't be formed or hard. The consistency should be like soft ice cream, and you'll need a few wipes to see a clean bum. Sometimes the stool reflects the smell of the formula. If your baby's poo smells particularly offensive, the odour lingering after you leave the change table, there may be more unfriendly bacteria than good guys present in the digestive tract. I always recommend giving babies probiotics containing *Bifidobacterium* and *L. acidophilus* to help balance the bacteria in the intestines with a better ratio of good to bad guys. It's common for formulas to lead to constipation, so don't hesitate to switch until you find a formula that doesn't.

DIARRHEA: WATERY POO

Diarrhea happens when the time it takes for food to travel from mouth to toilet or diaper is too fast, and so the digestion process can't complete its task of breaking down food particles into nutrients and absorbing water from the intestines. Diarrhea can be serious in an infant because of the potential for dehydration. The wateriness of diarrhea results from the fast transit time, which doesn't allow for reabsorption of water from the intestines. Water reabsorption in the intestines helps to balance hydration in our bodies. This water loss must be replaced orally for us to stay hydrated.

Diarrhea is commonly a symptom of the body trying to get rid of a bacterium, virus, or parasite from something that has either been ingested or passed from another person. Don't try to suppress it too quickly, but rather let the body try to rid itself of what it needs to. Newborns experiencing diarrhea should be seen immediately by a doctor, and the same applies to an infant or child who has had diarrhea for more than twenty-four hours. Diarrhea is also common during teething, when it's particularly acidic to a little bum. If diarrhea or quite loose stools last for a long time and don't seem to be related to a virus or bacteria from food contamination, it may be a sign of food sensitivity. There are a few common culprits, including dairy and wheat (see Chapter 5). The only way to treat chronic or long-term diarrhea, or even loose stools, is to dig until you find the cause. Your doctor might do stool tests to see whether the cause is bacterial or even a parasite, or you may need to remove suspected foods from your diet if breastfeeding. Think about changing formula if it has added docosahexaenoic acid (DHA), or figure out if the source is a food, if your baby's on solids. Keeping your baby hydrated is essential. If your baby has started on solids, expect him to refuse food during an episode of diarrhea or other sickness, whether the cause is bacterial, viral, or teething. It's better for his body to clear what it needs to before filling back up on food. Do keep up his breast milk or formula intake (lactose-free is appropriate here) to ensure that he's getting some nutrition. It can take up to two weeks after sickness, especially a gastrointestinal type, for the appetite to go back to normal. I always recommend that parents give probiotics to recolonize the intestines with good bacteria; in my experience, it has also helped return the appetite to what it was, faster. No matter what the cause of diarrhea, remove all dairy products from the diet. Milk and dairy products, as well as most formulas, contain a sugar called lactose. When diarrhea hits, the fast transit time clears not only any fibre, food, bacteria, and water from the intestines, but also the lactase enzymes, which digest lactose. With that enzyme missing, the body is unable to digest lactose in dairy products, especially milk or formula, which can lead to instant lactose intolerance, the inability to digest lactose. Lactose intolerance is more common in adults—usually it affects babies only in this situation or in very rare cases. Switch to a lactose-free formula (see the formula charts on SproutRight.com) for at least two weeks after the diarrhea passes to allow lactase to build up again and let the intestines heal. If you start back on a lactose formula too early, gassiness or abdominal discomfort may occur. If your baby was on solid food before the diarrhea, ease slowly back into the regular diet, offering simple foods such as applesauce, mashed banana, puréed vegetables, and whole-grain brown rice or potatoes. Don't start on anything new until bowel movements have gone back to normal. Avoid fatty foods and too much protein, as they are harder to digest and the intestines still need to recover. Probiotics can lessen the severity and length of diarrhea as they put the good bacteria back into the intestines, where they recolonize and heal the intestinal lining. Homeopathic remedies are often quick to resolve diarrhea, and some herbal teas, such as peppermint or ginger, can be soothing to the digestive tract. Pedialyte and similar rehydrating solutions contain sugar, salt, and water in a specific balance for maximum rehydration. Coconut water is also beneficial for rehydration. Be careful to avoid sugars from other drinks or food sources, as they can make the diarrhea worse.

Other Reasons for Diarrhea

For Breastfed Babies: Because what you eat passes to your baby through breast milk, some possible causes of diarrhea in your diet include getting too much vitamin C or magnesium from a supplement; using antacids containing magnesium salts; eating foods with sorbitol, mannitol, and xylitol; consuming milk or other dairy products; and eating spicy food.

For Formula-Fed Babies: Diarrhea is common in the case of an intolerance to dairy, whether it be protein or lactose. You may need to either switch to a goat's milk formula or rotate through a few formulas before you find one that eases this symptom. There seems to be a correlation between the DHA added to formula and diarrhea in some babies. If you've just started your baby on a new formula (with or without DHA), try a hydrolyzed or lactose-free formula.

CONSTIPATION: HARD POO

Constipation is a lack of or incomplete bowel movements, with hard-to-pass and very formed stool. Unfortunately, it's a common problem among infants and children. It includes straining to poo, eliminating a hard or formed stool, as well as passing infrequent or incomplete stool. Again, this situation can be quite different for breastfed and formula-fed babies.

BREASTFED BABIES AND CONSTIPATION

Constipation doesn't usually occur in breastfed babies. A lack of a daily bowel movement is common but is not to be confused with constipation because when breastfed babies do poo, stool is not hard and formed. In the early days, your newborn should be having two to three bowel movements a day, sometimes more. If twenty-four hours go by without a poo, seek help from the breastfeeding clinic or a lactation consultant, as your baby may not be getting enough milk as a result of an improper latch and possible tongue-tie (not because you're not producing enough milk). Breastfed babies can have between one and five poos a day. There doesn't seem to be any particular reason for having more or less. After two to three weeks of age, your baby may start skipping bowel movements for a day or two but will continue to be happy and healthy and to gain weight. This is normal. Breast milk is so absorbable and so highly used in the body that there may not be as much to eliminate. I've heard of babies going without a poo for a week or two—and in one case, almost a month. If you've had a few days or more of super-fast diaper changes (with no poo to clean) and your baby is content and shows no fussiness, gas, or pulling her legs up to her belly, you don't need to be overly concerned until that changes. Sometimes grunting or straining to have a poo doesn't produce results. If this is the case, you can help by putting your baby to the breast because as the milk goes into the stomach, it stimulates the digestive system lower down to start contracting and moving fecal matter along and out of the body. If that doesn't help, you might try to stimulate the anus, most commonly with a thermometer or well-oiled Q-tip. This should produce results immediately or soon after. Don't allow this to become regular practice, though, as there could be issues behind the constipation that need to be examined. When you've been waiting for a bowel movement for a few days or more and it finally vacates the bowel, be prepared for an explosion that can burst right out of the diaper and up baby's back, as far up as the neck. Unfortunately, as Murphy's law dictates, this never happens at home, where you could simply wash baby from head to toe. If your baby is having regular problems with infrequent bowel movements, look at what you're eating or drinking in case this is a reaction to a food or drink in the breast milk. See Baby's Reactions to Breast Milk (page 52).

FORMULA-FED BABIES AND CONSTIPATION

Unfortunately, constipation in a formula-fed baby is quite common. It occurs as a reaction either to ingredients in the formula or to the increased concentration of nutrients, minerals, and different fats, particularly palm olein oil.[71] Breast milk contains more water and nutrients and thus needs less digestion than formula. Unlike a breastfeeding baby, a formula-fed baby needs to poo every day. The digestion process sees formula more as a food than a drink, so there's enough to eliminate on a daily basis. The consistency of the stool will be unlike that of breastfed babies because of the different bacteria present in the intestines. If your baby becomes constipated on a new formula or while weaning onto formula, I'd suggest looking for an alternative. Parents often wonder whether the iron fortification in the formula causes constipation, but studies show that's not likely the culprit. Palm olein oil is used as a fatty acid source in most formulas and has been demonstrated to increase constipation in babies.[72] Check the label on the can of formula, or refer to the formula charts on SproutRight.com, to see whether your formula contains palm olein oil. (Some labels say "or palm olein oil" because they switch between two oils depending on availability.) I came across only two companies that manufacture formula without it. Formula higher in casein than whey can also have constipating results for your baby. Switch to one with a higher level of whey, add in probiotics, and see if that helps. If the problem persists, switch formulas again until your baby is pooing every day. Consult with your doctor as well; an ultrasound or another treatment may be suggested.

WILL STARTING ON SOLIDS RESULT IN CONSTIPATION?

Constipation in babies who are eating solids can be more common when they start on cereal. Any of the cereals has the potential to cause constipation, but I see it more often with rice cereal. One reason for the constipation could be the limited starch-digesting enzymes in babies' digestive systems or the cereal's iron fortification. Although iron in cereal has a low absorption rate (only about 5 to 10 percent is absorbed), the form of iron in cereals is often associated with constipation. If your baby has constipation from eating infant cereals, my recommendation is to remove the cereal until bowel movements are back to normal, giving Meat Broth (see recipe on page 129), fruits, and vegetables. If you'd like to try cereal again (it's really not necessary until you're ready to give homemade brown rice), offer only small quantities and switch to another cereal. I've seen babies do well on oatmeal after they've been constipated with rice cereal. As you progress with solids and introduce new foods, constipation may occur because not enough water was added to the more fibrous vegetable purées. Sweet potato and parsnips, especially, are so fibrous that they need a lot of water to help the fibre move through the digestive tract. An overall lack of fibre, water, or both can lead to constipation in anyone, young or old. Meat is a protein-rich food but is lacking in the fibre of fruits, vegetables, nuts, and grains. If you're giving meat to your baby or toddler for added iron and protein in her diet, remember to serve it with fibre-rich vegetables. I mentioned above that exclusively breastfed babies don't generally suffer from constipation, but this rule changes after solids are introduced. If it's not the food that you're giving to your baby that's causing the constipation, look at mom's diet. Foods that often trigger constipation in baby include dairy, wheat, sugar, chocolate, coffee, and gluten (found in wheat, rye, barley, spelt, and kamut). The only way to find out which food may be causing the constipation is by eliminating some of these possible triggers or any other suspect foods. After avoiding the questionable foods for at least two weeks (four weeks for a more definitive answer), start eating them again. If there's a reaction (remember, it could take three to five days for it to show up), avoid that food and even delay introducing it to your baby.

Wheat, and the gluten it contains, is a very common food sensitivity that's known to cause constipation or harder stools. It's high in gluten and can irritate the lining of the intestines. I caution against giving wheat regularly to babies and even toddlers until closer to one year of age. Wheat is a frequently consumed grain that seems to sneak into just about everything. Parents giving toast, cookies, pasta, bagels, or muffins to their babies or toddlers need to keep in mind that all of these foods contain wheat, and so it can end up being eaten many times throughout the day. The quantity of wheat eaten easily increases as new foods are introduced, especially prepackaged foods of all kinds. Dairy is also associated with constipation, and intake should be evaluated if symptoms appear. Milk, cheese, and yogurt are favourites of both children and adults and, like wheat, make up a large part of our daily food intake. Remove gluten and/or dairy completely for at least two weeks and then reintroduce them to see if the same reaction appears. If it does, then once again keep them out of the diet and go slowly when introducing them directly to your baby. You can replace dairy with other calcium-rich foods, such as the green leafy vegetables included in Green Eggs (page 148), calcium-rich amaranth in Toasted Coconut Amaranth Porridge (page 150) or Amazing Sweet Amaranth (page 168), almonds, sesame seeds and tahini, organic soy, navy beans, and blackstrap molasses.

SIMPLE, EFFECTIVE TREATMENTS

Please don't leave constipation untreated for too long, thinking that it will right itself. Irregular bowel movements can be helped. Having said that, any situation of prolonged constipation should also be investigated by your doctor. A common medical treatment is to give prune juice or puréed prunes, mineral oil, laxatives like lactulose, or suppositories. They're all Band-Aids for what's really going on, so it's still important to determine the root cause. Below are some suggestions to help pass the impacted stool and to make your child more comfortable while you investigate why the constipation is there in the first place.

- Keep a food diary of all foods eaten for three to five days—this should raise some red flags about foods that are eaten regularly and may cause constipation. Remove those foods from mom's diet or baby's diet until the situation resolves.
- Give water to your baby as the diet of solid food increases in complexity and different fibres are introduced. Offering 2 to 4 tablespoons (30 to 60 mL) of water at regular intervals throughout the day should help a constipated baby. Get her to drink as much of it as possible; any water is better than none.
- Give probiotics to your baby daily. They are very helpful in alleviating constipation by normalizing digestive function. Give a human microflora product that contains both

Bifidobacterium and *Lactobacillus* strains of beneficial bacteria. Give ten billion or more CFU bacteria (my *Take This* Bio Boost Baby or Kid is appropriate) daily after "milk" or food.

- Give flax or hemp seed oil as a stool softener. Doctors offer mineral oil to ease constipation, but if you're giving an oil to soften the stool, your baby might as well get some nutritional benefit from it. Flax and hemp seed oil offer both omega-3 and omega-6 essential fatty acids. First offer 1 teaspoon (5 mL), increasing to 2 tablespoons (30 mL) if necessary. But don't become dependent on it—use only as necessary while you figure out the root cause of the constipation.

- Remove food altogether. If your baby has just started on solids and isn't yet eating three regular meals a day, remove the food from his diet and go back to breast milk or formula until you see regular bowel movements. When you start to introduce solids again, start very slowly and only add foods that you know are on the safe list.

- Avoid sugar completely. You may have to look at your diet if you're breastfeeding; if you consume a lot of sugar, avoid it as much as you can. Sugar slows down the muscle movement in the intestines. Try dried fruit as a sweet alternative.

- If you're formula feeding, be sure that your formula isn't "extra iron" fortified or doesn't contain palm olein oil (known to cause constipation and other digestive issues). See SproutRight.com for more suggestions.

- Give your baby dried fruits. Prunes, dried apricots, and raisins all have a laxative effect. But don't rely on prune purée or prune juice for a daily bowel movement—this treats the symptom but doesn't eliminate what's causing the problem.

- Apply castor oil to your baby's abdomen at nap time and bedtime. Rub a loonie-size amount over the abdomen and lower back before bed. Put on the diaper as usual and then older onesies or pyjamas, as the oil may get on them (though it does wash out).

- Consider osteopathy, a hands-on, noninvasive treatment safe for day-old babies and older, which may help by making sure that nerves associated with muscle contraction within the digestive system aren't restricted or constricted. I've seen many babies treated by an osteopath return to normal bowel function.

- I've treated babies and children suffering from constipation with sound therapy in my clinic. It's incredibly balancing and, along with dietary advice, constipation very often gets resolved in less than a month.

All of these recommendations are only meant to help ease the situation. You still need to be a good detective and find the reason why your baby is constipated in the first place. Treating the symptom does not solve the problem and can lead to fear of pooing, even in babies. Hard, compacted stools not only are painful, but can cause tiny fissures in the anus, leading to bleeding and even more pain when trying to poo. That's enough to make any parent willing to do whatever it takes to avoid the problem.

GASSY TUMMY AND BABY TOOTS

Gassiness is a common condition that often causes a lot of pain. Some babies tell you about the pain by crying, and at times they can be inconsolable. It seems that some babies are born gassy, and others develop gassiness with the introduction of solid food. Whatever your baby's age, there could be many reasons for it.

NEWBORN GAS

Gassiness in newborns up to the age of three months is sometimes referred to as colic or fussiness. The persistent crying for, it seems, no particular reason is exhausting for new parents and babies. You might find your baby arching her back or pulling her knees into her chest, trying to alleviate the discomfort. Whether you have a diagnosis of colic or not, the reasons behind gassiness are possibly the same. First, check with a professional to see if your baby has a tongue-tie (see page 51). Then, suspect an imbalance of good and bad bacteria. At birth, baby takes on mom's beneficial bacteria to colonize his gut with billions and billions of good bacteria. If antibiotics were taken by mom while pregnant, during labour and delivery, or postpartum while breastfeeding for whatever reason, that can lead to an imbalance of good and bad bacteria. Bad bacteria cause gas. Babies born by Caesarian section also can have fewer beneficial bacteria. In any of these situations, give a probiotic suitable for a baby that includes both *Bifidobacterium* and *Lactobacillus* strains of beneficial bacteria. Give ten billion or more CFU in a daily dose that's found in my *Take This* Bio Boost Baby.

Your baby may be reacting to something in mom's diet if she's breastfed. Trial-and-error elimination is the only way to find out for sure—dairy, wheat, chocolate, coffee, garlic, spices, cabbage, broccoli, and cauliflower are good places to start. I know, it's quite the list. Dairy is the most common offender, with wheat and chocolate a close second. Eliminate what you suspect for at least two weeks before reintroducing it. Some babies take longer to show an improvement.

If formula fed, your baby may be reacting to his formula. Try to pinpoint when the problem started; if it started with formula or with increased intake, consider changing formulas. Some babies might be fine on 4 ounces (120 mL) of formula, but as that level increases, symptoms appear. See Chapter 3 on formula feeding for suggestions.

The flow of breast milk or formula may be too fast for your baby to keep up with. Swallowing air along with milk causes more air to get into the stomach and either come back up the way it went in or become trapped lower in the digestive tract. Burp your baby throughout her feeding, if possible, to release air. Also, position your baby so that, while nursing, her head is higher than the nipple (hard to imagine, I know, but try a football hold and then lean back into a chair while supporting the back of her head). This should slow down the flow into baby's mouth. Make your baby work for the flow instead of trying to keep up with both gravity and breast milk flow.

In formula-fed babies, buy bottles that help eliminate extra air or have fewer holes in the nipple to reduce the flow. Also, look at the ingredients in your formula and perhaps switch to a formula that isn't sweetened with corn syrup or sucrose. These two sweeteners might be feeding any bad bacteria present, which give off gas and increase discomfort (see Chapter 3 for more detailed information).

Your baby might be getting too much foremilk versus hindmilk. Foremilk is the first breast milk in your baby's meal. It's high in lactose and water, whereas hindmilk supplies fat to sustain your baby. Too much foremilk without the hindmilk can make a baby gassy and fussy. To ensure that baby gets more hindmilk, try to completely drain the milk by compressing your breast once your baby slows down nursing on one side. If you were exposed to antibiotics during pregnancy, labour, or delivery or while breastfeeding, there may be a higher percentage of unfriendly bacteria to good bacteria in her digestive tract. Probiotics are a safe and effective treatment for gassiness and other abdominal symptoms and should be given to baby as soon as possible.

STINKY TOOTS AND POO

Most toots and poo don't smell of roses, but they certainly shouldn't leave a lingering aroma that sends everyone for cover. The smell of your baby's poo will reflect what he's drinking or eating. If that's sweet potato, the poo will have a sweet smell and orange colour. In cases of really stinky toots or poo, you can suspect that less desirable bacteria are present in the digestive tract. Along with the unfriendly bacteria, there may be food that isn't being digested or broken down properly, which increases the nose-holding aroma. You may not realize how sweet smelling your nursery can be until you squash the bad bacteria by having baby's intestines boot it out with good bacteria, or probiotics.

INEFFICIENT BURPING OR TOOTING

Some babies have a hard time dispelling gas from either end. Patiently burping your baby by supporting the front of her body on your chest and slightly over your shoulder and rubbing in an upward motion should help. Some babies do well with the pat style of burping, so try both to see which is more effective. A football hold, with baby's belly down along your forearm, head (or cheek, actually) in your hand, and legs straddling the inside of your elbow, is often a comfortable position. Pressure on the abdominal area from either the forearm or even abdominal massage often helps to alleviate gas.

SUPPORTIVE RELIEF

Osteopathy is a hands-on treatment that aims to release restriction and constriction gently so that normal function can resume.[73] Osteopaths perform craniosacral therapy within their treatments that can help alleviate any tension between the cranium and sacrum and associated nerves or organs. For the treatment of gassiness, colic, constipation—well, anything really—osteopathy can be amazingly effective. Tema Stein, a Toronto-based pediatric osteopath, explains that certain situations in utero or during delivery (the birth itself or use of vacuum or forceps, for example) can lead to health effects later: "If there has been any squeezing of the cranium (skull), you are squeezing on the contents (the nerves and brain). Depending on where the squeezing happens, it can affect different aspects of health, such as gassiness, constipation, colic, ear infections, poor latch, and strong gag reflex, to name a few."[74] Homeopathic remedies also can be very useful in situations of colic. If you're unfamiliar with homeopathy or don't know a homeopath, look for combinations of the most common remedies for colic, such as Boiron's Cocyntal. They're safe to give to mom and baby and are incredibly effective once you find the remedy that best matches the symptoms. They're available at most pharmacies and health food stores. Otherwise, consult with a naturopath or homeopath for specific remedies. Gripe water also helps with gassiness or colic. However, most gripe water is a mixture of sugar and water, and I'd recommend staying away from any product containing sugar for your baby. An herbal, sugar-free gripe water, such as Colic Calm (containing fennel), is a better alternative. Read the label before giving anything to your baby.

Fennel oil has shown great results in reducing colic in babies. In a 2003 study, 121 infants with colic were given either a placebo or an emulsion of fennel seed oil.[75] Colic symptoms decreased by a whopping 45 percent in the infants taking the fennel seed oil formula, compared with only a 5 percent reduction in symptoms in those taking the placebo formula. Fennel seems to "reduce intestinal spasm and to increase the movement (motility) of the small intestines," two factors that often contribute to the development of colic.[76]

Beneficial bacteria may be lacking in the case of any gassiness, not just with colic-type symptoms. Good bacteria do great things like produce vitamins, digest the sugar in milk, and maintain acidity in the intestines to keep bad bacteria under control. When a baby is first born, she has a higher level of *Lactobacillus* bacteria in the intestines, which changes within the first week to primarily *Bifidobacterium*, especially in the breastfed baby. If your baby was born by Caesarean section or has been introduced to formula, that balance can be altered, so give probiotics to your baby daily.

Doctors have begun recommending a pharmaceutical brand of probiotics called BioGaia for the treatment of colic, as research showed positive results. This is a hopeful development for new parents who don't consult a naturopath or nutritionist—the usual way to find out about probiotics.

Probiotics support the development of the digestive system and there are no long-term side effects to giving probiotics.[77] Ensure that your infant probiotics supplement includes *Bifidobacterium* strains as well as *Lactobacillus* strains of bacteria at a level of at least ten billion CFU (found in my *Take This* Bio Boost Baby). The probiotic should be given after nursing or formula feeding one to two times a day, depending on the severity and history of your baby's symptoms of gas, constipation, or diarrhea. A breastfeeding mom can also take an adult probiotic supplement to enhance her own immune system; even though the probiotics that mom takes don't reach breast milk, she'll pass on immune factors that do get into the breast milk and support the baby's immune system further.

5 · ALLERGIES AND THE IMMUNE SYSTEM

The immune system is the backbone of our health. Understanding more about it helps you to navigate all that can affect us, from colds and flus to allergies, pain and inflammation, and even some cancers. Allergies in children are increasing, and parents need help in understanding not only why there's an increase, but also what can be done to support a child with an allergy or friends and family who you may feed, because it really does affect us all.

Fifty percent of all Canadian households are directly or indirectly affected by food allergies. The most recent research, at the time of writing, is that 1 in 3 Canadians is directly affected by allergies. The incidence of food allergies has increased dramatically over the years, affecting 1 to 10 percent of children worldwide.[78] The question that I have, and I'm sure many others do as well, is why? Why are these numbers rising and not looking like they're slowing down?

When I was a kid, allergies existed. Although I wasn't positive to a scratch test, I was sensitive to certain foods that would give me a migraine. For kids and their parents who are allergic, sitting down to eat a meal can be a scary and fear-inducing situation. Whether in the comfort of one's home, out at a restaurant, or over at a friend's house, eating has the potential to cause suffering or put a life at risk.

A 2018 review has listed the most common food allergens as peanuts, tree nuts, fish, shellfish, eggs, milk, wheat, soy, and seeds.[79] The reasons for increased risk of allergy, published in the Canadian Healthy Infant Longitudinal Development (CHILD) Study, include lack of a healthy microbiome or intestinal bacteria, whether there's a pet in the home, where you live and the level of pollution in your area, how your baby was born (Caesarian section or vaginal birth), whether antibiotics were given to mom or baby, and if baby was breastfed or not and for how long.

THE IMMUNE ARMY

This section takes a more in-depth look into how the immune system functions: the workings of specific cells and how they work together as our protective army. If you're more interested in immunity as it relates to your baby specifically, feel free to skip to my practical recommendations starting with The Immature Immune Army on page 87.

The immune system can be thought of as an army made up of generals, soldiers, killers, and a clean-up crew. It's helpful to know how each part of the army acts in our bodies to better understand why an allergic reaction happens.

IMMUNE CELLS

White blood cells (also called leukocytes) are known as the main defenders of the immune system. White blood cells include:

LYMPHOCYTES—THE GENERALS They travel around the blood and lymph system looking for any invaders they don't recognize and mount an attack with the help of others. There are two types of lymphocytes—B and T lymphocytes. Both are developed from stem cells in the liver and bone marrow. T lymphocytes mature and are under the instruction of the thymus gland (part of the immune system), found behind the breastbone. In the family of T lymphocytes there are T helper cells (TH cells), T suppressor cells, and natural killer cells (NK cells). The TH cells help to activate the B lymphocytes to produce antibodies (immunoglobulins, or Igs—see box), whereas the T suppressor cells turn off the activation once the invader has been dealt with and then hold up the victory flag. NK cells are like germ warfare—they produce toxins that can annihilate anything foreign. Both B and T cells leave behind memory cells so that if the same antigen (perceived foreign invader) crosses their path again, they will mount an attack and repeat this process, but more quickly and efficiently next time.

MONOCYTES (FOUND IN BLOOD) AND MACROPHAGES (FOUND IN TISSUES)—THE CLEAN-UP CREW These cells finish off and clean up what the others started by engulfing and digesting the invader through inflammation and signalling other troops that a war is going on. Monocytes present the invader to the T cells so that they can recognize more of their kind in the body and continue the attack. (That's what I call teamwork!)

GRANULOCYTES—THE SOLDIERS These make up the majority of the white blood cells and include neutrophils, eosinophils, and basophils. They also help the clean-up crew and engulf invaders, damaged cells, or debris, supporting the monocytes and macrophages.

MAST CELLS—THE FRONT LINE OF DEFENCE These are mainly residential cells that are found close to entranceways to the body—for example, the mouth and eyes. They produce histamine, which most of us are familiar with. It creates itching, redness, inflammation, and flushing in an allergic response. The main points of entry of any foreign particle can be through the skin (topically or injected), via the mouth or eyes, up the nose, inhaled into the lungs, or even passed upward into the urethra. All of our epithelial cells (or internal skin), at each of these entry points, are coated with mucus to slow down or stop the invader in its tracks. The eyes defend with both mucus and tears, which contain an enzyme called lysozyme that breaks down the cell walls of many bacteria. Saliva is alkaline and antibacterial. The nasal passages and lungs are coated in mucus and trap invaders in the mucus, which are then blown out, sniffed or coughed up, and swallowed (sorry, not a nice picture, but it happens). Mast cells also line the nasal passages, throat, lungs, and skin. Any bacteria or virus that wants to gain entry to your body must first make it past these defences.

> **The Five Classes of Antibodies Called Immunoglobulins (Igs)**
>
> **IgE—involved in type 1 allergic reactions.** The presence of this antibody is a marker for an allergy that your doctor might test for with a scratch test.
>
> **IgG—the most abundant, making up 75 percent of all antibodies in the body.** These antibodies are passed on to the fetus through the placenta and are found in breast milk, along with IgA. IgG attacks bacteria, viruses, and fungi by neutralizing and destroying them. It's also thought to be involved in approximately 60 percent of allergic reactions and is more commonly associated with food sensitivity.
>
> **IgA—found in breast milk, saliva, sweat, tears, blood, the lungs, and intestinal mucosa.** It's also known as secretory IgA, or sIgA. It protects against foreign invaders before they can enter the body. IgA is most abundant in the digestive system. A deficiency of IgA is an indicator of allergy, because IgA is used up while calming the allergic reaction.
>
> **IgM—one of the largest.** This front-liner operating in the bloodstream only comes out strong at the beginning of an infection to disable bacteria. It doesn't cross the placenta.
>
> **IgD—makes up a very small percentage of the immunoglobulin team.** It signals the spleen (another immune organ) that the B cells are ready for action.

THE IMMATURE IMMUNE ARMY

When your baby is born, his immune system is not mature, meaning that it has a lot of learning to do. It can take about two years for your baby's immune system to fully mature and become an effective army of immune cells working together to fight off foreign invaders. In the beginning, your baby relies on the immunity she took from you through the placenta while in utero, on the way out in the birth canal, and in colostrum first and then breast milk, two to three days after birth. This is one important reason for exclusively breastfeeding your baby, even if just for a short while. If possible, avoid supplementing with formula either in the hospital or after you've returned home; formula doesn't provide antibodies or immune support, and it is a potential allergen.

The immune system takes time to mature and strengthen as it practises recognizing what is foreign, or "non-self," while ignoring "self." The more it gets to flex its muscles by mounting an attack and winning the battle, the stronger the immune army becomes. And although it might seem as if your baby has a constantly runny nose (this may also be due to a food intolerance or allergy), his immunoglobulins, neutrophils, mast cells, and lymphocytes are learning what to do with different attackers. However, if the immune system doesn't get the chance to develop in the way it needs to—perhaps a certain aspect isn't challenged and therefore doesn't develop properly—something may go awry. Hyperresponse, or an immune army overreacting to something that's not a foreign invader, such as dairy, might lead to a perpetual runny nose as the immune system keeps on producing mucus to try to capture and eliminate the invader—in this case, dairy.

KEEPING CLEAN—OR NOT?

How do we learn how to do things in life? Something new is presented to us, and through practice we master how to do it. The same thing happens in the immune system. It needs practice dealing with foreign invaders, and if it doesn't get the chance to build itself up through this practice, it may never reach its full potential. The immune system needs exposure to bacteria, viruses, fungi, and other pathogens (foreign invaders) so it can react and become stronger. These are all things that most parents desperately try to keep their babies safe from as they sanitize everything, including hands, toys, floors, and anything that goes near babies' mouths and might lead to sickness. But we actually may be doing more harm than good with this practice. I'm not saying that hygiene isn't important, and especially in recent years, with so many potentially harmful situations from superbugs, crazily named flus, and quarantinable illnesses, we want to keep our children from harm. It's understandable. But what if this constant sanitization is contributing to the increased incidence of allergy? Some dirt, germs, viruses, fungi, and other nasties put the immune army through its paces, increasing its strength each time. The more the immune system is confronted, the stronger it gets. Why does your child get a cold or a cough? If that's all she gets (as opposed to secondary infections such as chest or ear infections), the immune system is doing its job. A compromised immune system or underfunctioning immune army needs to be assessed along with the history of that child to figure out what may have led to the immune system being unable to attack, defend, and kill illness.

IMMUNITY FROM THE BEGINNING

Babies are "sterile" at birth. When they travel through the birth canal, this is, in a sense, their passageway to the big wide world full of bacteria. Mom's vagina is colonized with beneficial bacteria and possibly some fungus (*Candida albicans*) or unfriendly bacteria, such as strep B, which baby takes on before entering either the hospital room or home (in a home birth). No matter where birth takes place, the beneficial bacteria in the vagina help protect your baby from the billions of bacteria in the world she has just entered. Babies born by Caesarean section don't travel through this passageway and, because they miss this important step, might be lacking in immune protection. There may be an association between birth via Caesarean section and a higher risk of allergies. Compared to vaginally delivered babies, C-section babies are also much more at risk for conditions like asthma, allergic rhinitis, celiac disease, type 1 diabetes, and gastroenteritis.[80]

Your baby has taken on your antibodies in utero, including IgE and IgA, for protection as her immune system continues to develop. Nutrients found especially in breast milk supply the immune system with the fuel it needs to function properly. Breast milk contains the antibodies IgE, IgA, and IgM, as well as lactoferrin, which bind to iron in baby's intestines, making it unavailable for bad bacteria to use as fuel. Other immune soldiers are present in breast milk to keep potential bacteria in check. Formula companies have yet to add immunoglobulins or other immune-boosting elements to their products—but one day this might happen.

THE IMMUNE ARMY'S FUEL

Supporting the army is crucial. If it doesn't get adequate nutrition, it's going to be sluggish, fatigued, and unable to rally the troops in defending the body. Nutrients— including vitamins A, C, and E; all the B vitamins, including vitamin B12 and folic acid; and the minerals zinc and copper—allow the army to function by producing lymphocytes as needed, increasing NK cell activity, and producing antibodies. Inadequate nutrition would be like sending troops to war while on a hunger strike!

The wrong fuel also slows the troops down, and sugar is one of the worst. One teaspoon (5 mL) of sugar can stop the immune complexes for up to eight hours. That's a staggering thought. With other possible causes of immune depression, including pesticides, medical drugs, stress, *Candida albicans*, environmental pollution, antibiotic use, trauma, food allergy, and alcohol (not all are applicable to your baby, of course), it's amazing that we fight anything off at all, but somehow we do. However, perhaps our immune system isn't fighting to the best of its ability, which might be the start of a few issues, including allergy.

ANTIBIOTICS: IMMUNE SUPPORT OR NOT?

One of the major medical breakthroughs of our time, antibiotics, has saved countless lives in life-threatening situations. Unfortunately, as they've become more commonplace, antibiotics are also being overused. They're incredibly important in certain situations and may be recommended by your doctor or even your dentist, but they now make up an increasing percentage of prescribed medicines. In my years as a practising nutritionist, I've come across many children who were treated with antibiotics. This is understandable in certain situations; however, so many times I've heard that ear infections, for instance, were treated with three, four, or more courses of antibiotics before tubes were put in a child's ears under general anesthetic. I find this to be a mind-boggling method of treatment.

After the second round of antibiotics, why did no one question why they weren't working? Had a superbug made its way into the ear canal? Doctors are taught to treat the disease, symptom, or illness. Antibiotics are one treatment option they have in their doctor's kit. If one kind doesn't work, maybe another will do the job. I recently heard of a child who was given six different types of antibiotics to treat an ear infection. Unbelievable. I understand the logic, but there must come a point when someone has to say, "STOP!" Take a step back and look at what else might be going on—a food allergy, an immune system not working as it should, or maybe something structural that an osteopath or chiropractor could help with. Furthermore, many researchers are still divided as to whether antibiotics are effective at all in treating ear infections. A *Genome Medicine* article stated about the impact of antibiotics on the microbiome:

> *In addition to the development of resistance, the use of antibiotics heavily disrupts the ecology of the human microbiome (i.e., the collection of cells, genes, and metabolites from the bacteria, eukaryotes, and viruses that inhabit the human body). A dysbiotic microbiome may not perform vital functions such as nutrient supply, vitamin production, and protection from pathogens.*[81]

When antibiotics are taken, about a hundred thousand billion beneficial bacteria are destroyed in the intestines. When the course of antibiotics is over, it can take months for them to be replenished. This is an opportunity for fungi, bacteria, and other antibiotic-resistant organisms to proliferate. It's common to see symptoms of diarrhea, gastritis, and fungal infection after antibiotic use, and there's even the potential for more serious bacteria to take hold, leading to secondary infections (and then more antibiotics). Diarrhea is dangerous for an infant because it can lead to dehydration and fungal infection, or *Candida albicans*, which is an absolute nuisance that can cause many uncomfortable and annoying symptoms of thrush in both mom and baby and also depress immune function. The immune system then becomes so busy trying to keep the *Candida albicans* or bacteria at bay that it's not as available to fight off the next passerby's sneeze, which brings new bacteria to fight off. Antibiotics have their place and are sometimes the only way to deal with an illness. However, if they must be taken, it's essential during and after a course of antibiotics to take probiotics, which have been clinically proven to dramatically reduce negative symptoms, including diarrhea, and lessen the disruption to the beneficial bacterial environment.[82] Broad-spectrum antibiotic use can cause a vitamin K deficiency, as the microbiome is a producer of this vitamin.

Another situation that occurs with antibiotic use is that white blood cell (the general) production is turned off. The antibiotics are doing the job of the immune system, but only up to a point. When the general can't rally his soldiers and clean-up crew, the infection may never be dealt with completely.

OVERUSE OF ANTIBIOTICS AND SUPERBUGS

Superbug is a word that the father of penicillin, Sir Alexander Fleming, may not have considered when he discovered the first antibiotic. He would have known after further testing that some micro-organisms were resistant to his new find. But since that time, micro-organisms that were killed by antibiotics have mutated into superbugs that can't be treated with antibiotics. On the rise now are serious illnesses from antibiotic-resistant bugs such as *Clostridium difficile* (*C. difficile*), a diarrhea-causing pathogen; *Staphylococcus aureus*, a bacteria found on the skin and mucous membranes; and many others. The mention of a superbug brings a feeling of dread, as even the strongest antibiotics are of no use. Studies show that one of the most effective treatments for *C. difficile* is probiotics of a strain called *Saccharomyces boulardii*; recolonizing the digestive tract with good bacteria has brought improved health to very sick patients.

HEATING THINGS UP: FEVER

A fever is an increase in body temperature above the normal 37°C (98.6°F). Fever usually comes on as the body's response to a bacterial or viral invasion—viruses usually involve a low-grade fever hovering around 38°C to 39°C (100.4°F to 102.2°F), and bacterial infections are accompanied by fevers of 39°C (102.2°F) and higher. Many viruses and bacteria don't survive in a body with an elevated temperature, and the heating up of the body increases the production, speed, and effectiveness of all white blood cells.

Complications of a fever may include dehydration and febrile seizures—a convulsion in young children, usually lasting a minute or so, that's caused by a sudden spike in their temperature. Keeping a child with a fever hydrated is extremely important. Febrile seizures may be genetic and occur in a very small percentage of children, usually without long-term negative effects. Medical attention is necessary if your child suffers a seizure.

It's most common to treat a fever with acetaminophen or ibuprofen, to make the child more comfortable and to bring down the fever (note that ibuprofen is not advised for babies under 6 months of age). However, allowing the immune system and its army to deal with this challenge is preferable, if possible. Remember that it's in training and needs to flex its muscles to try to win this assault and raise the victory flag. It's important to consult your doctor if a fever persists, if your child seems listless, or if you're worried about serious illness.

When the body's temperature is on the rise, let it learn to do what it needs to do to fight it off. Offering water to sip is important to prevent dehydration, but keep in mind that although you would like your child to eat something, appetite is usually suppressed in times of illness and fever.

Supporting the immune system with vitamin C is a simple yet powerful strategy: put some vitamin C powder into your child's water and let him sip it while resting. Lukewarm baths, cold water compresses, or my favourite, cold, wet cotton socks covered by wool or woolly socks (usually adult size) to draw the heat away from the head and toward the feet, are all effective ways to treat a fever with hydrotherapy (water therapy).

HOLES IN A GARDEN HOSE: LEAKY GUT

Leaky gut may sound like a strange term, but it encompasses the porous state of the intestines perfectly. Ideally, our intestines are a complete entity, with strength in the mucosa, or internal skin, of the intestinal wall. Like a garden hose, cell structure is strong all the way along the length of the small intestine, allowing chewed food particles to enter and stay put while enzymes break them down into smaller molecules, which are transported across the intestinal wall into the bloodstream for use elsewhere in the body. In a large portion of the population, it's as if the garden hose (the intestine) has been attacked by a hole punch, allowing the water that you want to reach your planter to leak out all over the driveway. This, essentially, is what leaky gut looks like. Within the intestines, there are tiny holes (not that you'd be able to see them with the naked eye) that allow some food particles that haven't been digested or broken down yet, as well as bacteria and toxins, to cross into the bloodstream. The circulating immune army is then alerted to these foreign invaders, the food particles. The immune army doesn't differentiate between a nut or dairy particle and bacteria or a virus and attacks by producing antibodies. So, in the situation of leaky gut, the immune army is always hard at work defending you against your last meal.

Leaky gut is essential in babies—it's how they survive. The description of an immature digestive system takes into account this leaky gut that all babies are born with. The holes in their intestines allow the minerals, vitamins, antibodies, proteins, carbohydrates, and fats found in breast milk to be easily absorbed and transported into the bloodstream. Formula is partially broken down or "digested" already to ease the digestion of its ingredients, and formula companies are always doing research to come up with improved absorption and digestion with minimal reactions. Perhaps you can now see why some babies commonly react to a dairy formula that hasn't been hydrolyzed, or broken down, as the larger milk protein molecules leak from the intestines into the bloodstream, where they shouldn't be. Then, the immune system comes along, producing antibodies, and an allergy begins. Dairy is one of the most common allergies in infants and children, and this is why. As your baby gets older, the holes are patched up and her digestive system becomes stronger; with less leaky gut, there's less potential for allergies.

> **Symptoms of Leaky Gut**
>
> Just about any symptom can be attributed to leaky gut, but here's a list so you can fully understand the extent to which leaky gut can affect the body: asthma, abdominal pain, indigestion, chronic joint pain, chronic muscle pain, poor immunity, foggy thinking, confusion, gas, mood swings, and nervousness. Leaky gut also gives rise to poor memory, anxiety, fatigue, recurrent vaginal infections, skin rashes, diarrhea, bedwetting, recurrent bladder infections, constipation, shortness of breath, bloating, aggressive behaviour, and the digestive diseases of ulcerative colitis, food allergy and intolerance, and irritable bowel syndrome. Most of the items on these lists won't be relevant to your baby, but they illustrate the far-reaching effects of having holes that aren't supposed to be there in the intestines.

CLASSIC OR TYPE 1 ALLERGY

The term *allergy* refers to a misguided reaction by the immune system to what it perceives as a foreign invader. A nonallergic individual can be challenged by the same "foreign invader," such as a food particle, and not produce a reaction. Allergy was first defined in the mid-1920s to describe an adverse reaction to food in which the immune system is involved by producing IgE antibodies. This definition is still in use within the medical community, but reactions to foods are far more commonplace today and so the symptomatology of allergies may need to be extended from this original definition.

Classical symptoms of allergies can range from a slightly runny nose to anaphylaxis. Other allergic symptoms include coughing; wheezing; itching; swelling of the lips, eyes, and/or tongue (anaphylaxis); shortness of breath; itchy mouth; vomiting; diarrhea; headache; and hives and other skin reactions. Allergies also show in situations of autism, celiac disease, colitis and Crohn's disease, eczema, asthma, and migraines. Any swelling of the throat or airway needs immediate medical attention.

The immune system can react to dust, mould, pollen, animal hair, insect venom, drugs (such as penicillin and tetracycline), metals (most commonly nickel), food additives, chemicals found in household cleaners, pesticides, and even modern adulterations in genetically modified organisms (GMOs). It seems as if the immune system is confused in its reactions. But why, and how? These are literally million-dollar questions that parents of allergic children would give their right arms to have answered. Reacting to peanuts, for instance, seems like such a strange thing. A peanut isn't a bacteria, parasite, or virus that can cause illness in the body, so why does the immune system react in this way? And why do some people tolerate peanuts while others can die from ingesting microscopic amounts? It all comes back to the individual's immune system.

Researchers are trying desperately to understand the mechanisms of allergy with the hope of eliminating it altogether. Years ago, I attended a conference titled "The Development Origins of Disease" given by microbiologist Dr. Nigel Plummer, who's known internationally for his work with both fish oils and probiotics. He had an enlightening way of describing some contributing factors to allergies. Armed with numerous studies to illustrate his point, Dr. Plummer explained how a lack of beneficial microflora (or good bacteria) in a newborn's digestive system doesn't allow for the normal development of a balanced immune system. Both mom and babys' immune systems are downregulated during pregnancy, so that the two immune armies aren't fighting against each other while in utero. This ensures that mom's body and immune army don't reject the fetus.

Because of this, baby is born with an immature immune system. The cell-mediated (or TH1) side of his immune system is downregulated, and his antibody response (antibody-mediated or TH2 side) is dominant. This imbalance means that your baby is born biased toward allergy as his antibodies react to perceived foreign invaders. Balancing these two aspects of the immune system by stimulating the TH1 side starts when your baby takes on your beneficial bacteria during delivery through the nose, mouth, and mucous membranes as he travels through the birth canal. Unfortunately, this important step is missed when babies are born by Caesarean section or antibiotics are given to mom during delivery and even while breastfeeding. But the good news is that you can stimulate and mature the nonallergic TH1 side of baby's immune system with infant probiotics, which will help to rebalance or steer the immune system away from the TH2 allergic response. I highly recommend supplementing newborn babies with human microflora varied strains of *Bifidobacterium* and *Lactobacillus acidophilus*. This will help to replace any missed or lessened beneficial bacteria and, ideally, reduce allergic reactions and symptoms such as eczema and asthma. The key here seems to be that both mom and baby take probiotics—mom while pregnant and while breastfeeding and baby as soon as she is born. Dr. Plummer published a large double-blind, placebo-controlled trial (a long name for a trial where the researchers and patients don't know who is given the real treatment and who is given a placebo) in South Wales, where he and his team discovered that probiotics can prevent child-onset type 1 allergy (IgE) by 50 percent. They used an HMF product including *Bifidobacterium* and *Lactobacillus* strains of good bacteria. Called the Swansea Study, this was certainly one study I was eagerly awaiting the results of. For more information from Dr. Plummer, go to https://youtu.be/aFN1MnmzaAs

Eczema is a first symptom of a potential allergy. In my own practice, I tell parents that any rash or eczema indicates that something's going on internally, not just on the surface of the skin. Using cortisone or steroid cream clears the skin reaction on the surface (suppressing the symptoms) but doesn't deal with why the rash was there in the first place. Often, the rash will disappear for a while (even years) and then reappear in another place on the body. Some children with asthma first had eczema and were treated with cortisone cream, which got rid of the rash but sent the problem to another organ to try to get rid of it—in the case of asthma, the problem was sent to the lungs. The inflammation first seen on the skin is the body's way of trying to excrete something through one organ, the skin; when that's unsuccessful, the body tries to eliminate it using the lungs and inflammation known as asthma. In my years of consulting, I've seen this progression first-hand in children with asthma. Eczema is multicausal and usually involves several factors, including *Candida*, food allergies and sensitivities, vaccines, poor digestion, too much bad bacteria in the gut, an unhealthy diet, and nutritional deficiencies. I see eczema a lot in my practice, and most often it's the direct result of food allergy or sensitivity, the biggest culprits being wheat, dairy, soy, corn, peanuts, eggs, and sugar. In addition to other recommendations, I often advise removing these allergenic foods and supplementing with probiotics to help support the immune system. It's best to see a nutritionist and/or a naturopath to assess your baby's individual situation and treat the problem. I've seen improvement using probiotics without diet modifications, but eczema can come back with a cold, flu, or teething.

Genetically Modified Foods

Genetically modified (GM) foods have been created by large companies trying to feed our growing population (and make a buck or two in the process). There are four major GM food crops: soybeans, corn, canola, and cotton. All are used to make vegetable oils, and soy and corn components are used in many processed foods. GM seeds are resistant to herbicides, allowing the crops to be sprayed without the plant dying from the chemicals. Some see genetic modification of the seed as revolutionizing food. For most, though, this is considered tampering with nature and an unpredictable practice. GM foods have expanded to include salmon, milk (growth hormones), sugar, aspartame, zucchini, yellow squash, and papaya.[83] It's advisable to avoid as many GM foods as possible because of the potential link to an increase in food allergies and to disorders such as autism, reproductive disorders, and digestive problems that have all increased dramatically since GM foods were introduced. Between 1996 and 2008, U.S. farmers sprayed an extra 383 million pounds of herbicide on GM crops.

THE MOST COMMON FOOD ALLERGIES

There are many possible food allergies, but the most common ones, as listed in a 2018 review, are peanut, tree nuts (for example, hazelnuts, walnuts, pecans), fish, shellfish, egg, milk, wheat, soy, and seeds.[84] Other common allergies include corn and beef. It's the protein within these foods that the immune system reacts to.

The beta-lactoglobulin milk protein, found in whey, is the most common protein that infants and children react to. Casein is also an allergen for some, more so in the case of autism. The father of Pablum (fortified cereal), Dr. Alan Brown, was physician-in-chief at the Hospital for Sick Children in Toronto from 1919 to 1951. He was convinced that feeding babies cow's milk was harmful and stated that "cow's milk is for calves."[85] He was completely right—cows produce milk that's meant for their calves, just as women produce breast milk that's perfectly suited for their infants.

INTRODUCING ALLERGENIC FOODS TOO SOON?

The old recommendation followed in North America, the United Kingdom, and Australia advised avoiding peanuts until age three. That has been changed, and the new recommendation advises introducing peanuts and all allergens at six months of age, and most certainly before baby's first birthday.

This change was supported by a study in Israel that looked at Jewish primary school–age children in both Israel and the United Kingdom. More than eight thousand children were included in this study, which was carried out by questionnaire. The study found that children in the United Kingdom were ten times more at risk for peanut allergy than children in Israel. Israeli infants are exposed to peanuts from an average age of eight months, whereas UK infants avoid peanuts until closer to age three.[86] Other studies question why, in countries such as China, peanuts are consumed regularly without the greater incidence of peanut allergy seen in North America. One study suggested that it was because peanuts are boiled in China, perhaps taking away some of their allergenic potential, whereas roasting peanuts may increase the allergic potential.[87] A 2017 study shows that delaying the introduction of common allergens (cow's milk, eggs, and peanuts) until after the first year may increase the risk of developing an allergy to these foods.[88] More research is now showing that early introduction, before six months of age, of common allergen foods may prevent allergy to those specific foods.[89]

In the case of cow's milk allergy, a study looked at the introduction of cow's milk formula to babies born via Caesarean section and vaginally who were given supplementary formula directly after birth. In this study, 92.5 percent of babies delivered by C-section were exposed to cow's milk protein in the first few days of life, compared to only 50 percent of those delivered vaginally. The study suggested that the use of hydrolyzed-protein formula may reduce this very high risk of allergy to cow's milk.[90] It would have been interesting to have continued the questioning in this study to see if mom was given antibiotics during labour or took probiotics toward the end of her pregnancy, as the Swansea Study showed a 44 percent reduction of allergy in pregnant mothers and babies who took ten billion CFU of *Bifidobacteria* and *Lactobacillus* strains of probiotics. Currently, the standard recommendation made by Health Canada is to give allergenic foods earlier, from six months of age. Before that age, have peanut butter in the house and after a parent has eaten some, give baby a kiss to share a trace amount of the protein.

ALLERGY TESTING

The most common test for allergy is the skin prick or scratch test, in which a drop of the potential allergen in solution is put on your skin and a scratch is made through the solution with a needle. If you're allergic, inflammation, redness, and itchiness show up. This test is useful for certain types of allergies, mainly inhalant allergies. It doesn't do well testing for foods, as the IgE antibody is not found in the skin, but in other areas of the body—the intestines, for instance. The scratch test fails to detect 50 percent of food allergies.[91] Allergists use the results, along with the patient's history and family potential for allergies, to decide whether there's an allergy. The RAST, or radioallergosorbent, test also measures IgE, but in the blood. This is a good test for airborne allergies, such as seasonal allergies or hay fever. ELISA testing is a method used to test mainly delayed reactions, but IgE reactions (instant allergic responses) as well as IgA and IgM reactions do show up. The ELISA test uses components of the immune system and chemicals in the patient's blood to detect immune responses in the body.

FOOD INTOLERANCE OR SENSITIVITY

What's the difference between a food allergy and sensitivity? The distinction is in the way the immune system reacts. Allergy involves IgE antibody production, whereas intolerance or sensitivity most commonly involves IgG antibody production or could be from a lack of a particular enzyme, leaky gut, and chemical sensitivities.

The term *sensitivity* is often used as a catch-all for both allergy and intolerance, so to avoid confusion I'll use the term *intolerance* for all IgG reactions. Doctors are not so quick to accept that the IgG reactions that millions of people suffer with are real. Food intolerance doesn't show up with medical testing and therefore often isn't recognized as a problem. Intolerance reactions are not life threatening, but they can reduce quality of life. Symptoms are generally delayed, unlike with allergies, sometimes taking up to seventy-two hours to present. By that time, you've forgotten what you ate three days ago, making it hard to pinpoint the offending food.

INTOLERANCE SYMPTOMS

Food intolerance is different from allergy in having not only delayed symptoms but also less severe ones. Some symptoms of intolerance are similar to those of allergy, making it that much more confusing to diagnose. Food intolerance symptoms in babies and children can include colic; persistent diarrhea; recurrent ear infections; asthma; stomach aches; rash on the body, bum, or face; dark circles under the eyes; runny nose or what seems like a constant cold; eczema; hives; infant insomnia; bedwetting; headache or migraine; fatigue; hyperactivity; depression; anxiety; recurrent mouth ulcers or canker sores; aching muscles; vomiting; nausea; and stomach and duodenal ulcers.

As you can see from this list, just about any symptom can be attributed to a food intolerance. Although there are tests for intolerance, the gold standard is to remove a suspected food for at least four weeks and then reintroduce it with a large serving. If symptoms return, there's a good chance you've found the culprit. However, you may have realized already that you felt better while not eating that food. Or, if you're avoiding a suspected food while breastfeeding and your baby improves, I would suggest keeping it out of your diet. Once you are ready to give that food to your baby, start slowly and watch for similar symptoms.

Quite often, foods that are not tolerated are the ones that become food cravings. The reaction in the body actually provides a natural high, usually leading to food cravings and therefore increased consumption.

COMMON FOOD INTOLERANCES

The most common, well-known food intolerance is to lactose found in milk. The deficiency of the lactase enzyme leads to an inability to digest lactose, the milk sugar, resulting in a wide variety of symptoms that often differ between individuals. Although lactose is naturally present in breast milk, most of the population stops manufacturing the lactase enzyme between age two (when most babies are weaned) and adolescence. Carolee Bateson-Koch comments, "This is why 70% of the world population is lactase deficient."[92] When you think about it, cow's milk is produced for nursing calves (which weigh about 36 to 45 kg/80 to 100 pounds at birth), not adult humans.

Other potentially intolerated foods include wheat, dairy products, soy, corn, nuts, yeast, alcohol, sugar, red meat, eggs, and caffeine. Another complication with food intolerance is that it may take eating a lot of a particular food before you show symptoms.

The most commonly intolerated foods, wheat and dairy, are eaten many times a day, sometimes every day. Our bodies were not meant to eat the same foods on a regular basis. I commonly see problems with dairy in infants or toddlers at age one as they move on to milk as a replacement for formula. The slow introduction of cow's milk may not produce a reaction straight away, giving a false sense of security. As milk intake increases, symptoms start to show, but because no reaction occurred when it was first given, milk is not suspected as the problem. Any food can be a problem, especially when you consider the health of the digestive system, the potential for leaky gut from taking antibiotics, or the early introduction of solid food.

WHAT CAN BE DONE ABOUT FOOD ALLERGIES AND INTOLERANCE?

The only way to "cure" an allergy is to re-establish tolerance or prevent loss of tolerance in the first place. These are big words for a big problem. See below for some possible strategies.

• Be proactive—give probiotics. There is a 57 percent chance that the potential for allergy may be reduced with probiotics. Remember that the colony of good bacteria in the digestive system pushes the developing immune system to respond normally. Give your baby an infant probiotic with at least ten billion CFU in a daily dose. For toddlers and children, give at least fifteen billion CFU each day. Take a potent probiotic with at least twenty-five billion CFU while you're pregnant to ensure that a strong colony is present before baby is born (see chart in Chapter 1, page 43).
• Don't be too clean—put away the sanitizer and antibacterial products. The immune system needs to be challenged with some unsavoury "dirt." Washing hands, floors, and toys is important, but don't go overboard.

- Stay away from sugar—even in small quantities and especially in small bodies, sugar reduces the strength of the immune system for up to eight hours.
- Offer common allergens at around six months of age—delaying the introduction of common allergens (cow's milk, eggs, and peanuts) until after the first birthday may increase the risk of developing an allergy.[93] Identify any potential allergies. If symptoms show up in baby as a breastfeeding mom drinks or eats dairy, it's a sign and dairy should be avoided. Follow the starting solids recommendation of meat broth and give probiotics before baby is given any dairy directly. Although it's good to expose baby early to prevent allergies, giving a food that is not well tolerated, like dairy, on an ongoing basis isn't recommended.
- Allow the leaky gut to heal—babies are born with a leaky gut and need time for it to mature. Give meat broth as recommended in Chapter 7 (page 104). Start offering food at six months of age, no later. It's a myth that solid food before six months helps your baby to sleep better.
- If eczema appears, figure it out—it may be a sign of greater risk of allergy. So, if you see it, adjust your diet if you're breastfeeding to eliminate common allergenic foods such as dairy, or investigate what the cause might be if your baby's on formula or solid food. Note when the eczema started and whether it correlates with an immunization or medication.
- Avoid antibiotics unless there's no alternative—antibiotics annihilate the good bacteria in the intestines, leaving them exposed to foreign invaders and bad bacteria. Find a good naturopath, homeopath, or nutritionist who can teach you what to do to treat different types of sicknesses.
- Eat organic—pesticides and herbicides weaken the immune system and increase the toxicity in your baby. Also, when any plant grows in soil that is fertilized using natural methods—for example, compost in organic farming—naturally occurring beneficial bacteria are present. Pesticides kill off these beneficial bacteria.
- Take immune-boosting vitamins—vitamins A, C, and E; all of the B vitamins, including vitamin B12 and folic acid; and the minerals zinc and copper allow the immune army to function at full strength. Take these as part of a multinutrient if breastfeeding or offer some vitamin C powder mixed with water or food to your baby. Vitamin C shouldn't be given directly to newborns.

POSSIBLE TREATMENTS

For the treatment of allergies, neutralization or desensitization treatment looks promising. Researchers are still conducting trials on small groups of children. Oral immunotherapy[94] has successfully treated a small group of children with peanut allergy in the United Kingdom; these children were able to tolerate up to ten peanuts without any adverse consequence. This approach requires medical treatment and should never be tried at home.

I've come across another very accessible treatment that seems to help both allergies and intolerance. The results of the treatment depend on the individual, and success should be discussed with your practitioner. It's known as bioenergetic intolerance elimination, or BIE. I got the lowdown from Janet Neilson, a homeopath who uses it in her practice: It's essentially electro-acupuncture—no needles—used to clear symptoms of allergies or sensitivities to substances (food, pollens, chemicals, etc.). Using a small probe, the device carries energetic frequency information about various allergens or sensitivities to the immune system via acupuncture points. These points are like little doorways into the body, and stimulating them (for 20 seconds) presents the immune system with information to counter or cancel out its typical response to a food or substance it's normally sensitive to. For example, cat hair cancels out a cat hair reaction, and wheat cancels out a wheat reaction.[95] Check out the Institute of Natural Health Technologies at www.inht.ca for more information and know that there are many new methods similar to BIE available every year.

ALLERGY DIAGNOSIS: NOW WHAT?

Your child has been diagnosed with an allergy and you need to clear out your kitchen and reconfigure what you're going to feed them. This is an incredibly overwhelming time, but it will get easier as you find your groove. Reach out to friends with kids who have allergies and find a nutritionist who can help you create meal plans and navigate the healthy options, taking into consideration what you will have to avoid. Here are some ways to find your new groove.

1. Take the time to read all labels and know what various terms mean and the differences between them. Certain allergens can sneak their way foods that you would never think would carry them, so make sure you know what you're looking for.

2. Watch out for extras on food labels. Things like nitrates and nitrites, sulphites, artificial flavours, and food dyes are not good for your children, especially if they have one or more allergies.

3. An excellent resource for substitutions and alternatives to common food allergens is the Stanford Children's Health website (www.stanfordchildrens.org). Lists, charts, and substitutions are all there for eggs,[96] wheat,[97] and soy.[98] Note: Not all of the suggested alternatives and substitutions are healthy or ideal options. It will take a bit of time and effort to navigate avoiding allergenic foods and maintaining a healthy diet. A consultation with a nutritionist will help you navigate resources like this one.

4. Download a food allergy app to help you with your food choices. When I went to Apple's app store, the free app Yummly looked most helpful. New apps are being launched all the time. They can serve as useful tools for those looking for easy recipes and for an easy way to generate grocery lists.

5. Exploring healthier and allergen-free options may be challenging. My recommendation of eating a rainbow of colourful fruits and vegetables every day is the perfect place to start (see page 4). Foods that come in fun shapes and a variety of colours keep mealtime more interesting and much more fun. Try out vegetable cutter shapes and let the fun begin!

Friends with Allergies

Your kids likely will have friends with allergies, and having them visit your home can be a scary thought for both you and your kids' friend. Don't take it personally if it takes a while for an allergic child to eat your food. They've been taught to be very careful, and they know that food from home is the safest. A great friend of mine, whose son has many allergies, once said to me when I offered to feed him, "I don't think you want to be responsible for my kid having a reaction and ending up in hospital, so I'll give you food to feed him." I fully understood what she meant, and I gladly took the meals for her son until we all became confident enough that I could cook butter chicken (of all things) made with safe ingredients. Soon, he started coming for dinner every week, and I was thrilled to be able to feed him safely! Here are some tips to help you navigate this uncomfortable situation.

TIP 1

Get in the know. Kids know about their allergies and may wear a MedicAlert bracelet, but always discuss the issue with the child's parents to get the whole story. What is the child allergic to? How severe is the allergy? If the child is a little older, does he carry medication like an EpiPen with him, or do you need to have Benadryl on hand? By having this conversation, parents are better equipped if their own child ever develops an allergy, and they will serve as a stronger support system for the child with the allergy.

TIP 2

If you are planning to offer food to your child's friend, check with the parents first. Offer a safe list of foods and even suggest that the child bring a meal with her. If you're hosting a birthday party, save the boxes or wrappers of packaged foods, including cake mixes and decorations, so that you can answer questions about the ingredients.

TIP 3

Ask the parent for safe meal or snack suggestions, or ask the child to bring his own snacks. There's no need to feel badly about it. It really is better to be safe than sorry.

TIP 4

Look through the recipes in Chapter 10 to identify what's gluten-, dairy-, egg-, nut-, and wheat-free, vegan (dairy- and egg-free), or vegetarian.

6 · MAKING HOMEMADE BABY FOOD

Making your own baby food is simple and rewarding. Knowing what goes into your baby's food and feeding nutrient-packed foods with intense flavours is crucial for expanding a baby's palate. I've seen it time and time again: when babies eat homemade foods, their taste buds have a dance party as they explore the food you're offering.

If you're not confident about making homemade food, don't worry—you've got all the recipes you need here, and you'll also find a tremendous community of parents in the same situation as you in my New Eaters Club online. The club teaches you to make food, with more than fourteen step-by-step videos, and features an online program all based on the Mommy Chef cooking classes I taught for years. I believe that with detailed and expert instruction that builds a strong base of knowledge, anyone can make food for their precious baby that will give baby the best possible start. You'll find more information on SproutRight.com under New Eaters Club.

Unlike setting up baby's nursery, setting up your kitchen to make baby food is easy, and a lot fewer decisions need to be made! First, make sure you have knives, utensils, and small appliances that you love to work with. You won't be motivated to cook a batch of butternut squash if your peeler doesn't work well. I've listed the essentials you'll need on page 16–17.

LET'S GET COOKING!

Making your own baby food is fast, easy, and economical. For some reason, there's a misconception that homemade baby food is a lot of work, but it's really so easy and worth the time it takes for all the great benefits it gives your baby. Preparing your own food allows you to choose exactly what goes into your baby's tummy and to customize it to suit your baby's tastes. You can even adjust the food to create chunkier textures as your baby gets older.

The taste and texture of food made at home expose your baby to real food that will eventually be served at family meals. When was the last time you saw cilantro, parsley, garlic, or ginger in a jar or pouch? Most store-bought baby foods in jars or pouches are combined foods that don't have a strong taste of any particular food, so the vibrant taste of blueberries, for instance, doesn't ever become understood by the palate. Remember that it can take eight to twelve tries before your baby takes to a particular flavour or food, so don't think that your homemade meals aren't a hit because you've done something wrong. Just keep trying!

A HEALING START: MEAT BROTH

The ingredients of Meat Broth (page 129) are meant to heal and nourish your baby with minerals, gelatin (and collagen), and fat. The fat is incredibly important to transport the nutrients needed to help heal leaky gut, a normal situation in babies. Salt can put a strain on maintaining water balance and stress the kidneys, so an unsalted broth is best.

Meat broth differs from bone broth: meat broth is made from a lot of meat with a few bones, cooked for a short period of time. Bone broth is made from a lot of bones with a small amount of meat, cooked for a long period of time. Drawing out nutrients and protein from the meat is crucial for your baby. Bone broth offers slightly different nutrients and is perfect for later, when the gut is healed. It's still a nutritious offering, just not in the early stages. The recipe in this book cannot be replaced by store-bought tetra packs, stock cubes, or even butcher-made broth that contains salt. These products aren't made with the same ingredients that offer the needed nutrition, and they contain flavour enhancers and salt, neither of which is suitable for baby.

A few days before you start your baby on solid foods, give meat broth to him as a drink from a spoon or bottle and then add it to any purée or recipe in this book instead of water. As a vegetarian alternative, try Vegetable Broth (see recipe on page 130). It doesn't contain the healing properties of gelatin and collagen, but it's still a great addition to many recipes.

COOKING FIRST FOODS

I recommend starting with butternut squash and then, three to four days later, pear as baby's first puréed foods—they have the perfect taste and texture for new palates. Add in Meat Broth (page 129) to smooth the squash (pear doesn't need any added liquid) and to increase the iron and nutrient content. After squash and pear, you can follow the list below in no particular order, alternating different-coloured vegetables and fruits and adding in steamed or soft pieces of fruit or vegetable to incorporate my Hybrid Feeding Method (see page 115). Mix it up!

VEGETABLES

- Asparagus
- Beets
- Broccoli
- Butternut squash
- Carrots
- Cauliflower
- Green beans
- Green peas
- Parsnip,
- Sweet potato
- Turnip
- Zucchini

FRUITS

- Apples
- Apricots
- Avocado
- Banana
- Blueberries
- Cherries
- Dried apricots
- Mango
- Papaya
- Pears
- Plums
- Prunes

HOW TO PREPARE FIRST FOODS

1. Peel, core, and chop the fruit or vegetable into small cubes. The smaller you chop them, the faster they'll cook. Adjust the steaming time depending on the size of the cubes.

2. Fill your saucepan with enough water so that it won't boil away, keeping in mind that harder vegetables such as carrots and beets take longer to steam. Put the pot on the stove over high heat and bring to a boil with the lid on to heat it up faster.

3. Put your cubed food in the steamer basket and place it on top of the boiling water. Reduce the heat to medium so that the water doesn't boil over.

4. Steam with the lid on until tender. You'll know it's cooked when a knife can slide through the food or it can be mashed easily without any resistance.

5. Empty the contents of the steamer into a bowl suitable for puréeing.

6. Purée using a hand (immersion) blender, high-speed blender, or food processor before adding any broth or water.

7. Add water or broth, ¼ cup (60 mL) at a time. As you make more food for your baby, you'll learn roughly how much water you need, but at first, add it slowly (see the recipes in Chapter 7 for approximate amounts).

8. Continue to purée until you achieve the texture of a smooth, thick soup for first meals. As your baby gets older, add a bit less water to your purée and leave a few lumps or bumps in it.

Some vegetables, including sweet potatoes and parsnips, are more fibrous than others and will need more broth or water to achieve the right consistency. Add ¼ to ½ cup (60 to 125 mL) water or broth, and expect to add about 1 to 2 cups (250 to 500 mL) for a large batch. Each fruit and vegetable will need a different amount of water or broth, so be sure to mash it first to get a sense of the consistency if you haven't made it before. The added water or broth not only creates a texture that your baby can swallow, but also with some of the more fibrous vegetables, helps to move the fibre through baby's digestive system easily, lessening the chance of constipation. Don't be put off by the combination of broth and food you're making. Your baby doesn't know that apples with a chicken taste isn't normal. Using the broth provides more fat, highly absorbable minerals like iron and magnesium, calcium, gelatin, and collagen, making it a more nutrient-dense and filling food.

Note: Dried fruit such as apricots or prunes should be boiled in a saucepan with enough water to cover them until they become plump. Add the water from the saucepan to the purée when blending, and use extra if you plan on freezing it.

MASH AND SERVE

Ripe banana, avocado, and papaya can be mashed with a fork or the back of a spoon and served. They're great foods for when you're on the go. As your baby gets older and more accustomed to texture, purée pear and blueberry without steaming them first.

TO PEEL OR NOT TO PEEL

- Peel the first foods for your baby—the skin adds texture that might not be well received. As she gets older, leave the skin on pear, apple, and sweet potato, being sure to wash it well.
- Always peel the skin of butternut squash after washing it.
- Scrub or peel carrots, beets, parsnips, and turnips.
- Peel the stalk of broccoli and chop it to yield more food.
- Don't peel zucchini, plums, apricots, nectarines, blueberries, and green beans or take the skin off peas.
- Chop cauliflower and remove the stalk.
- Take the peel off avocado, banana, mango, and papaya.
- Any of the above can be used frozen, if applicable. Frozen wild blueberries, for example, are available all year and are usually cheaper than fresh.

WATER AND BROTH

We usually take a lot of care when choosing the types and quality of food for our babies, but we often don't give water as high a priority. I highly recommend using filtered water to drink or add to baby's food—both when adding water to purées and when making broth. Depending on the filter, it can remove contaminants of bacteria, spores, lead, chlorine, and other pollutants, including medication. Filters range from Brita to reverse osmosis water filtration systems. There are also whole house water filters for those with skin conditions and sensitive skin.

PREPARING CHUNKY MEALS WITH TEXTURE

My general guideline is to introduce textured and chunky meals at seven to eight months of age, although your baby may be ready for lumpier food earlier. Try introducing it to your baby. If she "gags," she's not ready; simply try it again in a week or two. When you see that gag reflex ease, leave some chunks and lumps in the foods you've been making smooth and start to prepare more meals with texture. At this stage, the method of cooking changes from steaming most purées to cooking in a saucepan to make more of a thick and chunky soup or stew-like meal. Foods can still be puréed to the texture your baby likes, and little by little you can purée them a bit less, leaving a few lumps or bumps, or reduce the amount of water or broth to create a thicker purée and textured meal. If you've been using mostly store-bought food, you might find that you need to wean your baby onto the flavourful recipes in Chapter 7. Start with a bit of what he knows and likes, adding in a teaspoon (5 mL) of the new food at a time to let him get used to it. If your baby isn't quite sure about what you're making now, it could have a more intense texture or flavour than she's used to.

At this stage, you will slowly add more texture to baby's food each week or so. This is where the versatility of making your own baby food comes into play. Start slowly and give your baby time to adjust to the new texture in his mouth.

The meals you make in this progression of texture and taste will include a wider variety of fruits and vegetables, all cooked in the same saucepan. You'll also start giving legumes (beans, peas, and lentils), brown rice, and gluten-free grains and seeds, which are high in fibre, protein, iron, and many other vitamins and minerals.

HOW TO PREPARE CHUNKY MEALS

1. Peel or scrub, core, and chop fruit or vegetables into small cubes.

2. Add these to a saucepan with water or homemade meat broth and a choice of legumes (beans, peas, and lentils), brown rice, or gluten-free grains.

3. Simmer until the fruits or vegetables are tender and the grain, bean, or legume is well cooked.

4. Empty into a bowl suitable for puréeing and mash with your hand blender. If the mixture is too thick, add water or broth to thin it.

5. Remember that you can always add more water (or even breast milk or formula) upon serving if it's too thick.

6. As your baby gets older, you can adjust the texture by "pulsing" the hand blender to create a little more texture with lumps and bumps. When she's close to toddler age, you might not even have to purée her food at all.

You can find recipes for chunky meals in Chapter 8. See Chapter 8 for a full list of finger foods (other than fruits and vegetables) as well as dips.

STORAGE

To store baby's food, let it cool and then spoon it into bisphenol A–free baby food trays, cubes, or silicone trays and freeze for at least twenty-four hours. Once frozen, pop out the cubes into a storage freezer bag, and label the bag with the contents and date. Prepared food will keep in the refrigerator for three days and in the freezer for up to three months. You can also store it in glass containers or jars.

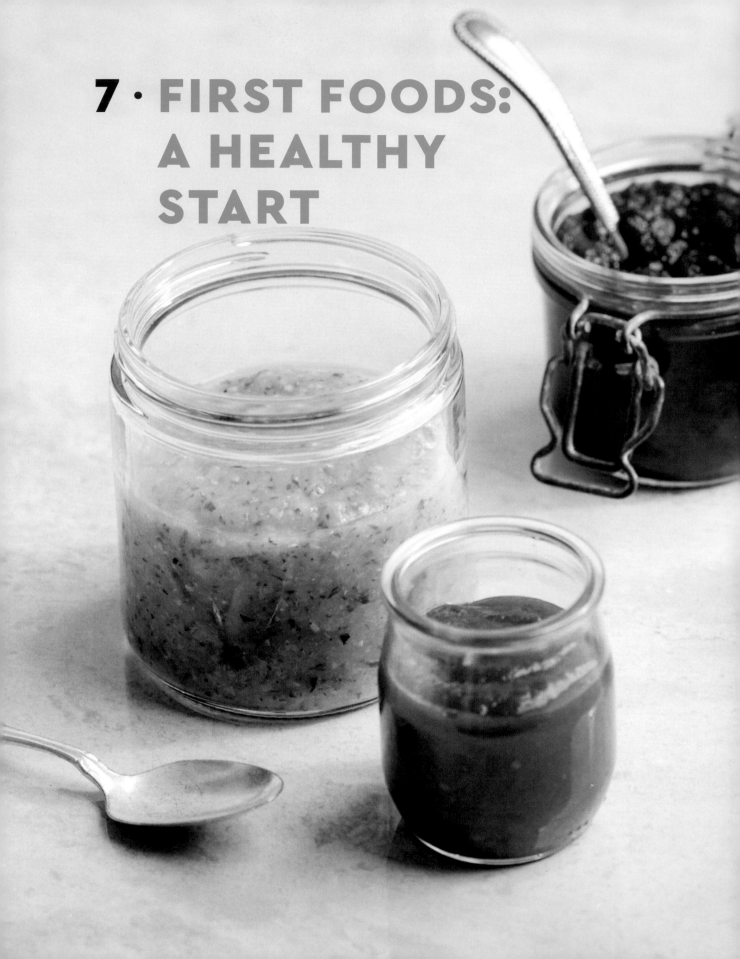

7 · FIRST FOODS: A HEALTHY START

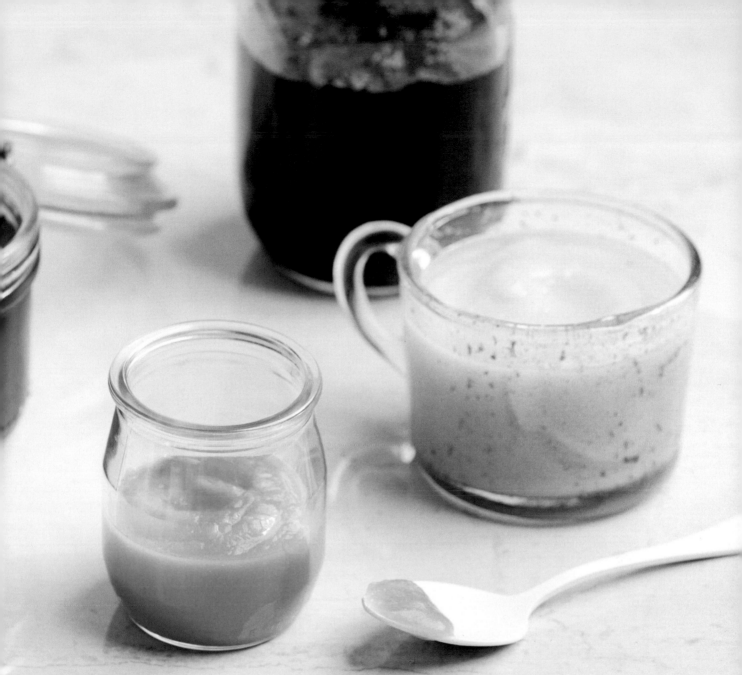

Starting your baby on solids can be a daunting yet exciting time. There's a lot of conflicting advice out there, not to mention the opinions of others: moms, your mother-in-law, friends, the internet, and, of course, your doctor. Here, I break down weaning to solid foods into easy steps, including baby-led weaning and my Hybrid Feeding Method, and explain why you should introduce certain foods at different times, taking into account the most recent recommendations from Health Canada and what foods are best to offer to decrease the chance of allergy.

STARTING SOLIDS

Both Health Canada and the World Health Organization recommend exclusively breastfeeding or formula feeding for the first six months of your baby's life. Around the world, the same recommendation stands. The United States, United Kingdom, and Australia all recommend starting solids at six months of age to give enough time for the digestive system to become ready for solid food in addition to breast milk and formula. I still hear from clients that their doctor recommends starting solids at four months of age; however, all research and recommendations by international health bodies support starting solids at six months of age.

Breast milk and formula provide all the nutrition your baby needs and will continue to do so as solid food is introduced and slowly increased over time. It's best if you can continue breastfeeding or formula feeding along with solid food until at least one year of age. The longer you breastfeed, the more your baby will gain the benefits of your own immune antibodies and super-absorbable vitamins, minerals, and enzymes that help her digest the essential fats in breast milk. The long list of benefits of breastfeeding extend into later life and include protecting from necrotizing enterocolitis and diarrhea during the early period of life and a lower incidence of inflammatory bowel diseases, types 1 and 2 diabetes, and obesity later in life. Breastfeeding is also associated with a reduction in the risk of acute otitis media (ear infections), nonspecific gastroenteritis, severe lower respiratory tract infections, atopic dermatitis, asthma (young children), childhood leukemia, and sudden infant death syndrome. Breast milk becomes more concentrated in some minerals and proteins as your baby starts to breastfeed less (around the time when solids increase) to ensure that she's still getting everything she needs.[99] Formula-fed babies should also be fed formula exclusively, without solid food, until six months of age, and formula should remain the main source of nutrition until age one.

"I want food" Signs
- Baby shows interest in your plate, tries to grab your food or cutlery, or shows new interest in what's happening at the table.
- She mimics your eating or mouth motions.
- She can sit up on her own.
- Her tongue's sucking reflex has relaxed and food can pass into the throat.

READ THIS FIRST

Before you set up the high chair and choose a bib and bowl with a matching spoon, sit down and read and absorb this first: *starting solids is a daily experiment of introducing and trying out new foods, tastes, and textures and getting feedback from your baby's taste buds and body.* Now, take a deep breath and lower your expectations. Do not assume that the transition to solids is going to be a breeze and that all will go according to plan (you may have already learned that lesson once or twice in the first six months of your child's life). The whole feeding process is new—the food coming toward him on a spoon, learning to self-feed rather than accepting food from the breast or bottle—and there are so many new tastes and textures, too. Then there's the need for his digestive system to work on something other than "milk" (breast or formula). It's all new, from the inside out. The amount of food your baby eats as she starts could be literally a thimbleful. You're not alone if you think it's hardly worth the time and effort to peel, chop, cook, and purée or give pieces of carrot, but remember that she'll eat it eventually. If not on the first or second try, maybe on the fifth or tenth. If you've come across a strict schedule of how introducing solids should happen, with times of day and how much she should be eating, throw it out. It's too much pressure for you and your baby to live up to those expectations, and feeding often doesn't happen on schedule in the beginning. Guidelines are helpful, but remember that you're the expert on your baby and it will take time to hone the skill of eating. You need to learn what your baby wants and needs, likes and dislikes. If my recommendations about when to start and progress with solids aren't working well, change them to make them work for you and your baby and call it a success.

Your baby may show signs that he's ready to start on solids at four or five months; however, it's best to wait until he's six months old because the digestive system will continue to mature. This maturity may reduce the risk of allergies, and you're not starving your baby if you wait. Every baby is different in his eagerness to start, so assess your own situation, but don't be fooled into starting too early.

Reaction Confusion

Be sure to start food on a day when your baby is healthy and free from any immune challenges like colds or viruses, teething episodes, or recent vaccinations. This is especially important when introducing allergenic foods like peanuts, other nuts, seeds, dairy, and eggs. Immune challenges can complicate the smooth introduction to solids, as your baby may suffer symptoms that include rash, fever, or out-of-sorts behaviour.

When introducing potentially allergenic foods, be sure to allow at least five hours between the time you give the food and bedtime so you can be sure baby doesn't experience an adverse reaction to it.

ADDING CEREAL TO THE BOTTLE: A BAD IDEA

There's some old thinking that mixing rice cereal in your baby's bottle before he's four months old will help him sleep. It's not true. If you offer any food other than breast milk or formula before four months of age, you run the risk of increasing the potential for allergies, digestive complaints, and skin rashes and slowing down the maturation of the digestive tract. Don't do it—that tiny digestive system isn't ready yet.

Contrary to the myth, introducing solids too early actually may cause sleep problems for your child because his digestive system isn't ready for them—gassiness, constipation, or colic-like symptoms of wailing for hours may result. In an online poll of moms that I conducted, 24 percent of moms tried giving their baby solids to help improve sleeping patterns, but 60 percent said it didn't work, and 7 percent said it made sleep worse.[100] All too often, I see new moms starting their baby on solids out of desperation, in the hope that it will help baby sleep. If this actually worked, there would be a lot of very well-rested new moms, full of energy and not mentioning how much they dread nighttime. In my years of listening to the conversations of new moms, I've learned that sleepless nights are the norm. We're all exhausted most of the time and pray for the miracle of a good night's sleep. A great friend and colleague, Tracey Devine, also known as "The Sleep Doula" (sleepdoula.com), says:

> One of the most common suggestions my clients are given by medical professionals is "Just wait till they start solids—they'll start sleeping through the night." But to their surprise, after solids are introduced, there is still no change or improvement. A baby or toddler isn't going to eat well during the day if they know they can eat or nurse all night long. I liken it to an all-night buffet, and why would they give up the service? For sleep? Probably not. At around four months they get a new awareness of what's around them, become distracted, maybe nibble during the day as opposed to a full feeding. At night you see them start waking every two to three hours. Whatever is given to put them to sleep—breast, bottle, or something else—they will need that same tool to go back to sleep again in the middle of the night. A very high percentage of sleep problems are due to habit, not hunger.[101]

TIME OF DAY TO START

I suggest that you first start solids around lunchtime. That could be anytime between 11:00 am and 3:00 pm. Breakfast seems to be the least successful meal to start with; in fact, it may end up being the last meal of the three that you introduce. Once you've offered a food and there's been no reaction like a rash, digestive discomfort, constipation, or diarrhea, move that food to dinner and keep introducing new foods at lunchtime. It's better to be able to see if a food produces a reaction, and if you give a new food at dinner, it's too close to bedtime, and a reaction could appear overnight and you won't see it.

Give Potentially Allergenic Foods Early

Health Canada suggests giving foods like peanuts, egg yolk, fish, dairy, and wheat as you start solids at six months. Studies show that offering allergenic foods earlier lessens the chance of allergy. Even before your baby starts eating solids, if you eat any of these foods, give your baby a kiss. The transfer of allergenic proteins through that kiss desensitizes the immune system and can reduce reactions. When you're ready to give a potential allergenic food, take a small amount in your finger and wipe it on the inside of your baby's bottom lip. This provides a small introduction as the first try. Watch for anything different in your baby's skin, digestive system, or mood.

MILK FIRST, THEN FOOD

Because breast milk or formula is your baby's main source of nutrition, I recommend continuing with your routine milk feeding and offering food afterwards. Remember that starting on solids is about trying out food as opposed to relying on nutrients from it, and you don't want to take away from the broad nutrition that comes from milk. So, nurse or bottle-feed your baby as usual, be sure she has had a nap and isn't tired, and within a half-hour or so of the milk feeding, give her a meal of solids. The solids will offer extra calories and nutrients on top of the usual daily nutrition she receives from milk. Adjust the time between nursing and food depending on your baby and her schedule. If your baby isn't interested in solids after milk, it may not be because she's already full. Some babies are slow to start when introducing food. You could try a different time of day and see if that's any more successful. As his food intake increases, you may notice that your baby starts to nurse less or leave an ounce or two of milk or formula in his bottle. This is his way of weaning himself off milk as his food intake increases. Let him be in charge of this unless he refuses milk altogether. Making the transition is a balancing act that you can manage as his food intake increases. Moving too quickly away from milk might leave him deficient in certain nutrients, as it provides him with protein, fat, carbohydrates, vitamins, minerals, and antibodies (in breast milk). You won't find all of that in 2 tablespoons (30 mL) of butternut squash!

The following sections will help you create a plan of how much food to start with, when to start solids, and what to do if you see a reaction. Having a plan makes it easier to work through the first couple of weeks and can ease the transition to solids.

HOW MUCH TO START WITH

Remember, giving solid foods is more about the experience than about nourishment in the first weeks. Your baby may start with something between a fingertip of food and a tablespoon (15 mL) of food—really, that's all you can expect at the beginning. Whatever she chooses to accept, start slowly. If your baby takes to this like a duck to water, you have to be in charge of the amount; otherwise, you might see what you've just served her come right back up. That small stomach will only hold so much, so if after 2 tablespoons (30 mL) your baby is still keen, I suggest managing the pace. If 1 teaspoon (5 mL) is taken in and swallowed, you're off to a great start. You may see complete love or rejection of a food, and at other times you might see a funny face or two.

Expect some of the food to end up on your baby's face or hands, and remember that it's about the experience more than the quantity swallowed. If you consistently see his tongue pushing the food out of his mouth, your baby's tongue thrust reflex may not have relaxed yet, so try again in another week or so. If there are concerns over your baby's lack of weight gain (see Tipping the Scale: Solids and Weight Gain, page 124), still take your time. Although you want more food to go in for a higher calorie intake, your baby may not be able to handle as much food as you want him to.

To progress, increase the amount of food until you see your baby taking in a consistent amount, whatever that may be—about 2 to 4 tablespoons (30 to 60 mL).

Then you can add another meal; if you started with lunch, add dinner. If dinner was the first meal, give lunch. Breakfast is usually the last meal added. It may take a number of weeks before you offer a second and then third meal. For instance, offer one meal for two to three weeks; if that's going well, introduce the next meal. The third meal may not start until well into the second month of solids, around the time that baby is eight or even nine months old. Some babies go slowly, but in general I suggest trying to have your baby on three meals a day by the time she's nine months old.

Some babies do well with one meal and then the second meal also goes down easily; others can take it or leave it. If another meal isn't going well, leave it for a week or two and try again. There is no set amount that your baby should be eating; although you might come across some recommendations, I usually suggest following your baby's cues. Keep up the same milk intake until she starts to want less. Your baby will let you know.

The amount of food your baby eats on any given day can change dramatically. During a growth spurt, expect the intake to increase; later, it may go back to what it was previously. If a cold or any sickness is coming on or you detect a teething episode, expect a decrease in appetite. You can't force-feed your baby, so try not to worry. Whatever the reason, it usually passes, and although it can take some time to get back to where you once were, you will get there.

PURÉE VERSUS BABY-LED WEANING

Puréed fruits, vegetables, grains, and meat are the usual foods used to begin your baby's food adventure. In recent years, baby-led weaning (BLW), the practice of offering your baby only pieces of food that are of a size and shape he can easily handle for self-feeding, rather than spoon feeding, became a different way of introducing solids.

BLW started to gain momentum in early 2000 and now presents itself as an alternative to starting with smooth purée. In a recent update by Health Canada, the recommendation to offer pieces of food, such as a broccoli floret, was included along with fruits, vegetables, meat, and cereal. BLW allows baby to explore food, whether anything is eaten or not. Just like crawling, walking, rolling, and all other development milestones, eating pieces of food can take time. This leaves how quickly she expands the type, texture, and kind of food she wants to consume up to her. From a nutrition standpoint, one study found that BLW eaters ate more saturated fat and consumed less iron, zinc, and vitamin B12.[102] At a time when iron is a concern, my recommendation is to follow my Hybrid Feeding Method, discussed next. Concerns about babies choking are a rational fear. While she's learning how to manage the pieces of food in her mouth, her reactions may look very similar to gagging and choking. Gagging is a safety reflex where the throat stops something questionable from going down the windpipe. The sound and physical motion of the gag reflex is enough to make a parent's heart stop until they see and hear their child inhale. This is when choking first aid training is absolutely essential. However, a study showed that the rate of choking was no higher in BLW eaters.[103]

HYBRID FEEDING METHOD

As I learned about BLW after the first edition of this book was published, I realized that introducing purées and then chunky meals and finger foods, as I had taught for years, could be combined. The adventure of eating expanded to include exploration with pieces of food in a broader way. Some babies take to it and others aren't too sure and don't quite get it until nine months of age. I have adapted how I recommend starting food to keep purée as the foundation of a meal offering taste, vitamins and minerals, antioxidants, fibre, and energy, *and then* to give pieces of the same food used in the purée at the same meal. It's a great structure for a meal. Remember, starting on solids is really an adventure in food, and offering pieces of food for baby to independently feed himself is part of that adventure.

TEXTURE CONFUSION?

In speaking with some parents, I've heard concerns about giving both purée and pieces of food for fear of baby not chewing and being confused. Baby needs to learn to switch from just swallowing food (a light chew with purée) to chewing pieces of food. Learning to deal with both is another part of the adventure. Sit in front of your baby and show her when and how to chew. She can chew purée for practice. I don't feel that this is enough of a concern to avoid both nutrient-dense purée and the experience of pieces of food. Watch how your baby does with this and adjust accordingly.

VARIETY, TASTE, AND NUTRIENTS

The variety of ingredients you can include in a purée provides important nutrition. From meat broth to garlic, onions, kale, other leafy greens, and tasty herbs like cilantro, parsley, and dill, food combinations can expand the palate further. When foods like avocado aren't favourites, they can be combined with pear, blueberry, and banana in the Fabulous Fresh Fruit Purée (page 177). Cinnamon, ginger, and nutmeg in the Spiced-Up Apples (page 177) make new taste sensations that explode on those wee tastebuds. Both of these combinations can be self-fed; however, if given as single pieces of food, the taste won't be the same.

STARTING WITH THE HYBRID FEEDING METHOD

Ideally, start with Meat Broth (page 129)—if you are a vegetarian or vegan family, offer Vegetable Broth (page 130)—followed by purée for the first couple of weeks. You can allow your child to self-feed and assist with a few spoonfuls here and there. I promise, he will sit at a table and self-feed, one day in the future. Next, add in some pieces of food like steamed broccoli trees, soft cauliflower, or whatever food you're offering as a purée. Do not leave your baby unattended with pieces of food. You should also stick to the recommendation of offering one food for four days in a row to see if there's a reaction to it. No matter what method you choose to introduce solids—BLW, Hybrid Feeding Method, or purée only—take a slow and steady approach to weaning onto solid food.

FINGER FOODS AND SELF-FEEDING SUGGESTIONS

• Aim for as much organic food as possible without any added refined sugar.

• Small pieces of ripe pear (no skin) is a soft fruit to start with. Progress to kiwi, avocado, melon, plum, peach, mango, papaya, raspberries, banana, apricots, and apples (no skin).

• Small pieces of grapes (I peeled some of the skin off with my teeth the first few times, as it made my daughter gag) or champagne grapes (these are very small and available in summer).

• Frozen organic wild blueberries (smaller than non-wild blueberries) are flavourful and packed with antioxidants. They are one of nature's superfoods. Keep them frozen so they're not quite as messy; frozen berries also feel great on sore gums.

• Steamed and sliced veggies: green beans, sweet potato, asparagus, broccoli, carrots, beets, peas, cauliflower, corn, and parsnips.

See more suggestions in Chapter 8 on chunky meals and finger foods.

MEAL IDEAS FOR HYBRID METHOD FEEDING

• Zucchini Purée (page 138) with avocado wedges and pear slices on the side

• Cauliflower Purée (page 135) or pieces mashed with diced mango

• Peach, banana, and apple purée with a dash of ground cinnamon and wild blueberries

• Lentil, Sweet Potato, and Red Pepper Purée (page 153) with steamed cauliflower pieces

• Egg yolk mixed with pear purée and steamed green beans

• Beany Green Dip (page 181) with steamed carrot, beet, and parsnip sticks

• Toasted Coconut Amaranth Porridge (page 150) with steamed or ripe peach on the side

• Immune-Boosting Purée (page 169) and Parsnip Chips with Paprika (page 151)

Offer purée first and add in finger foods as you and baby feel comfortable.

PURÉE ONLY

For some parents and babies, purée is the preferred way forward. Parents who are too scared or babies who have an overly sensitive gag reflex may take more time to become comfortable with texture, so purée is the way to start. It's important to offer pieces of food by nine months of age and more texture to see if the gag reflex has relaxed. Be guided by your baby, deal with your fears, and keep nudging him along.

START FROM THE BEGINNING

For the first two weeks, give your baby three or four foods so you can set a foundation and see how the foods go down, how much is eaten, and if there's a reaction. Start with meat broth a few days before solid food. Whether fed from a bottle, spoon, or cup, it's the perfect nutrient-dense food to begin with (unless you've found an allergy to chicken). After that, whichever food comes next with—butternut squash, banana, or pear—offer the same food for three to five consecutive days before moving on to a new one. You'll have heard that it's recommended to wait three days before trying a new food, but I prefer four or five days for more sensitive babies. Especially if your baby has a history of eczema, you had to change your diet while breastfeeding, or you had to change the formula milk offered, I suggest waiting an extra day or two before moving on to a new food. If your baby does have a reaction—and there's no reason to assume she will—it's easier to figure out what caused it when there's a bit more time to let the body show you. Say that you start with banana on a Monday, giving it each day until Wednesday. On Thursday morning you start on apple, and a rash appears. It could be caused by the apple that was just eaten or by the banana from yesterday. Feeding one food for at least four days gives your baby's system time to show a reaction, or not. Use the Baby Feeding Calendar on page 127 to make note of what your baby is drinking and eating and any symptoms that might emerge.

WHAT IS A REACTION?

For a clear outline of symptoms of allergic reaction and food intolerance or sensitivity, read Chapter 5 on allergies and the immune system. But for quick reference, you're looking for anything new or different in your baby. Allergic symptoms include digestive problems like diarrhea, hives, or swelling of the face, eyes, or airway. In some people, a food allergy can cause severe symptoms or even a life-threatening reaction known as anaphylaxis. Common symptoms of food sensitivity appear more slowly and include a rash on the bum, face, torso, arms—well, just about anywhere—a change in bowel habits (diarrhea or constipation), gassiness, discomfort, and throwing up or spitting up, but your baby could show different symptoms.

Generally, food allergies show up faster than food intolerances. Allergic reactions involve an immune system reaction that can occur within minutes to an hour of eating a certain food. On the first introduction of an allergenic food, a lesser reaction may take place, but subsequent exposure could lead to stronger reactions.[104] For instance, the first time I gave my daughter egg yolk, at nine months of age, she broke out in hives all over her body. A month later I tried again, and she violently threw up. I knew it was a problem for her and kept it out of her diet until she was over one year old; then, I found that because she was older, she could tolerate it. Although an allergy didn't show up in a scratch test, eggs clearly didn't sit well with her. I did eat a lot of eggs during my pregnancy, and I've seen in countless other situations that what mom eats a lot of during pregnancy can show up as a food allergy or sensitivity in baby. She now eats eggs regularly without reaction.

In children, food allergies are commonly triggered by proteins in peanuts, tree nuts, eggs, cow's milk, wheat, fish, and soy. Some allergies can weaken with age, but be sure to check with your doctor before offering any food that has shown a reaction in the past. Skin reactions such as eczema can appear for the first time, or existing patches may flare up. For instance, a bum rash may appear or worsen with the introduction of a sugary food—or sometimes dairy. Be sure to read the label of the food you're about to introduce if you haven't made it yourself.

Food intolerance or sensitivity can sometimes take up to seventy-two hours, which is why feeding solids may involve some detective work. You also may have noticed that many of the reaction symptoms mentioned above are very similar to symptoms of teething, so it can be tough to keep things straight. When I speak with parents about food reactions in a consultation, we always look back to the days leading up to the symptoms—the answer is usually there somewhere. For example, if your baby has constipation, look back at what she ate over the previous three days. Was there an increased amount of a cereal? Did you just start on formula or mix cereal with formula? Either situation could be the cause. The Baby Feeding Calendar on page 127 can help you keep track of the foods you've introduced and any new reactions. Relying on memory at this point may not be your best strategy (mommy brain is real!).

If you do suspect a reaction to a food, remove it, make a note with a red flag, and wait at least three weeks before trying it again. When you give that food again, make sure there's nothing else going on—recent vaccination, teething, a cold, or other sickness. Look for the same or other symptoms. If they return, wait three months before reintroducing the food. Discuss your findings with your doctor for her records and advice (although doctors don't always recognize food intolerance reactions).

THE CEREAL DEBATE

Doctors are under the impression that baby's iron stores run out at six months of age, but that may not be the case. A medical student once told me she was taught that breast milk contains no iron, and therefore the potential for iron deficiency in babies is a concern. Yet it's been proven again and again that breast milk does in fact contain iron, and in the most absorbable form. This is a disconnect in what doctors are learning at medical school and leads to confusion when it comes to advice around food for babies. In fact, breast milk contains proteins called lactoferrin and transferrin that transport iron so it can be easily and effectively absorbed by baby. Bad bacteria that commonly live in the digestive tract can feed on iron from cereals and formula, leaving baby iron deficient. Iron levels can be lower in formula-fed babies without the supplementation of probiotics. So, those iron-fortified cereals (which contain no lactoferrin or transferrin) don't seem to do what the doctors want them to, especially with the common situation of high bad bacteria and low good bacteria levels, particularly after antibiotic use in either mom or baby and with babies born by Caesarian section.

Infant cereals have been recommended for years because they're fortified with iron and the thinking is that it's a suitable iron source for babies. Cereal is a processed food and far from its original state in being an iron-rich food. The processing of rice cereal, for instance, removes the bran and outer shell, where most of the nutrients, including iron, are. Because of this loss, during processing all cereals are fortified with iron in the form of ferrum sulphate. Ferrum sulphate has a low absorption rate of about 5 percent of what's ingested; however, it's known for digestive aggravation, leading to constipation. I've seen countless babies unnecessarily suffer with constipation after introduction of cereal.

Despite the link with constipation and the low iron absorption rate, the pressure from some doctors to feed cereals is real and over time can lead to chronic constipation in babies who are not yet one year old. In addition to the problems that fortified iron may cause, the grains in most infant cereals, including rice, oats, and barley, contain starch and need to be broken down by enzymes. When babies are born, they haven't yet developed their full spectrum of enzymes, including the carbohydrate (starch)–digesting enzymes ptyalin and amylase. Ptyalin, found in saliva in the mouth (also known as salivary amylase), and amylase are specifically needed to digest starches found in cereals. Around six months of age, amylase slowly increases to digest carbohydrate or starchy foods, but possibly not enough is produced to handle the quantity of cereals given. Prune or other juices are commonly recommended to ease this common complaint; if that doesn't help, mineral oil or lactulose ingestion is the next step. Why the first suggestion isn't to stop cereal intake until the problem corrects itself still baffles me. If constipation correlates with the start of cereals and could be the cause, why not remove cereals and see what happens? In most cases I see, digestion improves and constipation eases.

When my first daughter was four months old, I began researching which food to start her on. I was hesitant about starting with the usual cereal, having known other babies who became constipated with cereal, so I was cautious and wanted an alternative for her. My naturopath recommended that I start her on fruits and vegetables instead. Since then, introducing fruits and vegetables first has become more common, so my recommendation to start with fruits and vegetables is no longer out of the ordinary. Those babies I know who've followed this method are growing up healthy and without iron deficiency anemia.

A Concern: Rice and Arsenic

Trying to understand all aspects of health can sometimes be overwhelming. For example, maybe you thought you were making a healthy choice by buying brown rice, and then heard about arsenic being found in rice.

A 2017 investigation by Healthy Babies Bright Futures reported that there is six times more arsenic in infant rice cereals than in other types of infant cereals (including oatmeal and multigrain). Brands tested that had arsenic in them included Gerber, Earth's Best, Beech-Nut, Bio-Kinetics, Happy Baby, and Healthy Times (which is organic). However, the non-rice and multigrain cereals made by the same brands had much lower levels of arsenic.[105]

As it turns out, where rice is grown has an impact on the amount of arsenic found in the grain. Avoid buying white rice grown in the southeastern United States. Rice grown in Arkansas, Louisiana, Missouri, and Texas had higher levels of total arsenic. Rice grown in California and imported basmati and jasmine rices (from Pakistan and India) are better options, and they may have lower arsenic levels.[106]

To reduce the amount of arsenic in your rice, rinse it thoroughly with filtered water before cooking to eliminate some contaminants. Rinse it up to six times. When cooking rice, use a ratio of 6 cups (1.5 L) of water to 1 cup (250 mL) of rice and, once cooked, drain the excess water. Some of the nutritional value could be lost, but this method will reduce the arsenic level.

PROGRESSING FROM A BOTTLE TO A CUP

The UK, Australia, and Canada all recommend introducing baby to a cup when introducing solid foods, and there's research to back up the idea that changing the vessel your baby drinks from is worth considering as he starts on solids. Offering water in a cup or a free-flowing sippy cup without a valve helps your baby learn to sip. Also, several health reasons are cited for transitioning from a bottle to a cup that contains water (please don't give juice, as it's high in sugar and so a concentrated source of sweetness and not good for teeth) and eventually breast milk or formula:

1. Sucking can change the position of adult teeth down the line and affect the development of facial muscles and the palate.

2. Drinking while lying down (such as lying in bed) increases the chance of ear infections.

3. Bottles boost tooth decay—both from milk and especially from juice.

4. Prolonged use of a bottle is linked to obesity.

It can take time to get the hang of using a sippy cup with a spout or straw, so persevere until baby gets it.

FIRST FOODS

This is where it all starts: your baby's food adventure. I will guide you through the most nutritious, colourful, tasty, and nourishing options with recipes so you can make your baby homemade food with ease. Having her taste buds jump for joy as the food adventure begins is so important for fostering a healthy and lifelong love of nutritious food. Start with iron-rich meat broth (or vegetarian broth) and move on to purées and combined dishes that will encourage your new eater to become a food adventurer in no time.

MEAT BROTH

Broth is a very traditional food that's become "trendy" in the health market once again. None of its great benefits went away, but the way we make and consume it did. Stock cubes, cans, and tetra packs of store-bought broth made it a quick and tasty option to add to recipes. Sadly, the store-bought varieties contain a lot of flavour enhancers and have fewer actual nutrients and health benefits. Those amazing benefits are why I'm recommending broth as a first food for your baby, so taking the time to make this homemade classic is worth it. As with most things, it's super-easy to make once you've done it once or twice, so don't be put off, as this truly is a throw-it-all-in-a-pot recipe that involves lengthy cooking time but very quick prep.

Benefits of Meat Broth

- Gelatin, one of the key nutrients that I'm most interested in, is abundant in meat broth, both in the liquid and captured in the fat. It helps to heal the gut lining, or "leaky gut," as your baby starts on solids (most of us have a degree of leaky gut, and babies much more so). Improving gut integrity by healing leaky gut helps to reduce the chance of food sensitivities and allergies. It's also a key component of bone growth and improves the growth of beneficial bacteria, as it is a prebiotic that feeds the good bacteria in your baby's intestines.
- Meat broth contains the minerals calcium, magnesium, phosphorus, silicon, and sulphur in forms that the body can easily absorb. These minerals are used to build strong and healthy bones and teeth.
- Electrolytes found in meat broth can help to improve hydration, which is why it's recommended during or after sickness of any kind.
- Chondroitin sulphate and glucosamine found in meat broth are components of healthy joints. It may not seem important right now as your baby is growing, but what you put in now will benefit him both now and later.
- Meat broth is packed with amino acids (the building blocks of protein) that help to improve digestion, support the building of muscle tissue, and boost immunity. With those benefits, it's worthy of being called a "superfood"! One of the amino acids in meat broth called glycine may also help to improve sleep.
- Meat broth is the best source of natural collagen, which is important for cartilage and joint health, skin health and integrity, and healing.

Meat broth can be started as baby begins solid foods and can be offered in addition to breast milk or formula and solid foods. Use meat broth as a drink or in place of water when making purées and other foods like any of the soup and stew-type recipes for older babies. I've also included a vegetable broth recipe for vegetarian and vegan families. It doesn't have the same gut-healing and iron-rich benefits, but it does offer more nutrients and taste than just water. Start with around 1 tablespoon (15 mL) and work up to 3 tablespoons (45 mL) or so. Give the broth by syringe, bottle, or spoon, or in a cup or mug. Broth can be frozen in mason jars of various sizes (the safest way to store it) or in safe plastic ice cube trays, then gently warmed in a saucepan (not in the microwave) as needed.

FRUITS AND VEGGIES

After meat broth, I suggest starting with banana, apple, pear, avocado, carrots, yams or sweet potato, butternut squash, or parsnips—not necessarily in that order. My favourites to start with are butternut squash as the first vegetable and pear as the first fruit during the first two weeks of solids. It's a common misconception that starting with fruits will predispose your baby to a sweet tooth. However, if you want to be on the safe side, start with butternut squash, a sweeter vegetable than broccoli, for instance. In case you haven't tasted breast milk or formula, it's much sweeter than most fruits and vegetables, so starting with a not-so-sweet vegetable such as broccoli may or may not be the success you hope it to be.

ALLERGENIC FOODS

After two weeks of meat broth, fruits, and veggies, it's time to introduce egg yolk and allergenic nuts like peanuts and almonds. I suggest starting with egg yolk before whole egg, as Health Canada recommends, because I see more reactions to egg white than I do to the yolk. Egg yolk is a very nutritious food that's a great source of iron, so if your baby isn't eating a whole lot as you start solids, giving egg yolk will provide more nutrition in each bite.

The ever-increasing research on reducing allergies continues. As it stands right now, those who avoided peanuts, milk, or egg in the first year were nearly twice as likely to be sensitized to those foods compared to infants who consumed them before twelve months of age.[107, 108] While it's a scary situation to give your baby the most allergenic foods in the first month of introducing food, it's a very important leap to take for two reasons. First, it's done on your watch. You know the health of your baby in the previous weeks and can use that knowledge to assess any reaction. You are also in control of the amount given. Second, because you know that a potential allergic food has been given and there's no cross-contamination from another food you don't know about, if a reaction shows up, you will know it's directly correlated to the food that has just been consumed.

Here's a rundown of what you're looking for, according to BabyCentre.ca:[109]

- Hives around your child's mouth, nose, and eyes, which can spread across his body
- Mild swelling of his lips, eyes, and face
- A runny or blocked nose, sneezing, and watery eyes
- An itchy mouth and irritated throat that will likely show as irritation and rubbing
- Nausea, vomiting, and diarrhea
- Eczema rash

However, delayed allergic reactions are more common, and symptoms include:

- Reflux
- Colic
- Diarrhea
- Constipation
- Eczema, which is common in babies with a milk allergy

As mentioned before, do not introduce an allergenic food when your baby is experiencing an immune challenge. That means any kind of sickness, virus, eczema flare-up, teething episode, or vaccine. These challenges all require help from immune reserves and if a potentially allergenic food is given, the immune system is more likely to overreact. Find a window of calm, if possible, then give a small amount of one of the following: egg, peanut butter (natural, without extra ingredients), almonds, sesame seeds in the form of a paste called tahini, dairy, yogurt, cheese, milk, or fish. Give that same food again on the following two days and watch for a reaction. If none appears, then carry on to the next food.

The Lipstick Swipe

When giving any allergenic food, a whopping spoonful of the food is not needed. A small amount, on the end of your finger, wiped just inside your baby's bottom lip—as you would apply lipstick—is enough of an introduction. An allergy can show with even the smallest trace of a food. Giving a smaller amount can also have more of a desensitizing effect, so be sure to go slowly with allergenic foods. Give a small amount once in the morning and no more for the rest of the day. Give a bit more on the following day and again watch for a reaction. Discuss any reaction with your doctor and stop offering a concerning food immediately.

MEAT

Meat is a good source of heme iron (with about 40 percent heme iron and the rest non-heme), a more absorbable form of iron from food that's good for your baby. After you introduce fruits, vegetables, and allergenic foods, it's time to introduce meat—after about a month of solid foods is an ideal time. The good bacteria or acidophilus cultures that live in your baby's digestive system become unbalanced with the introduction of meat, more so than with fruits and vegetables. The ratio of good to not-so-good bacteria in babies eating fruits and vegetables is fifty-fifty. When meat is introduced, it changes to closer to 90 percent unfavourable bacteria and 10 percent good guys. As you may remember from previous chapters, the benefits of good bacteria for your baby include keeping his immune system strong, helping to digest food, synthesizing B vitamins and vitamin K, and helping to reduce the incidence of allergies. It's important to maintain this healthy balance or microbiome for overall health.

Introducing meat is a good idea, as it's a rich source of iron. The effect it has on the microbiome means that giving probiotics is even more important. When giving meat, be sure to provide it in balance with high-fibre and antioxidant-rich fruits and veggies. High levels of protein in anyone's diet lead to greater acidity in the body, but our bodies need to be more alkaline to maintain overall balance. To keep this balance, the body calls on calcium to buffer the acid and maintain its alkalinity. When your baby's body is building bone strength by depositing calcium into bones, a balance of protein and iron from meat with alkaline fruits and vegetables, while giving a daily probiotic, is key.

INTRODUCING DAIRY

Dairy is the number one allergenic food, even over peanuts. Symptoms to look out for in a dairy allergy include inconsolable crying, colic, skin rashes, vomiting, diarrhea, blood in the stool, and constipation. Your baby may have had issues with mom consuming dairy while breastfeeding or with a particular formula. Those are possible signs that dairy given directly to your baby may cause further problems.

Offering cow's milk is not recommended before about nine months of age, but other dairy products can be offered before milk: yogurt, cheese, and cottage cheese. Ease into dairy, though; offer it slowly after a month of broth, fruits and vegetables, and other allergenic foods mentioned above. Because the symptoms of dairy allergy aren't as severe as most reactions to peanuts, for example, I find that it's not addressed as quickly as other allergies.

While it's thought that dairy is the best source of calcium for us, it isn't. I've mentioned better sources of dairy on page 37, so if your baby does have an allergy, don't fret! Finding other calcium-rich foods isn't difficult.

FOODS TO AVOID COMPLETELY

There's only one food that should be completely avoided until age one: honey. Honey may be contaminated with botulism, which your baby's digestive system can't fight off until around eight months, so it's recommended to avoid it completely until age one.

OTHER POTENTIAL ALLERGY CONCERNS

Other foods to be aware of, though not necessarily avoided include:

• Tomatoes, which may cause rash on the face or bum.
• Citrus fruits—including oranges and grapefruit, in particular, as they're usually eaten in larger quantity—and limes and lemons are acidic and potentially cause rashes. A bit of lemon or lime juice in water or food shouldn't cause any problems.

TIPPING THE SCALE: SOLIDS AND WEIGHT GAIN

Sometimes a baby's weight doesn't increase as quickly as your doctor might like according to the growth chart you see at each visit. However, most of these charts are based on formula-fed babies, so if you're breastfeeding, your baby may be in the lower percentiles for growth. It's more important that your baby follow her own trajectory, whether breastfed or formula fed. Some babies are on the leaner side and some on the more robust side.

These charts can cause stress for many parents. Following growth and weight provides great information and can be important, but at the same time, thinking that your baby is healthier or growing better because he's closer to the 100th percentile is incorrect. The chart shows the trajectory of his growth and highlights spurts and plateaus. Use it as overall information, but if your baby drops in percentile, don't panic. Look at other reasons why this might be the case. Genetics play a part in the size and weight of your baby, and development also should be taken into account. If you have an early crawler who's tearing around the house (okay, maybe this is a slight exaggeration), calories are being used up faster than in a baby who hasn't started moving yet. Maybe he's just had a growth spurt and shot up a centimetre or two, so the ratio of height to weight has changed. There are many factors to consider.

To give an example of how weight can fluctuate, I know an almost six-year-old girl who now weighs about 45 pounds (20 kg), an average weight for her age. She was born weighing 8 pounds, 9 ounces (about 4 kg) and at four months had just about doubled her weight to 18 pounds, 9 ounces (8.5 kg). By six months, she weighed 20 pounds (9 kg), and by nine months, 20 pounds, 9 ounces (9.3 kg)—yes, weight can plateau around nine to twelve months). For most of her life, up until today, her weight was off the growth charts. She was breastfed exclusively until seven months, when she started on solids. No one was worried except her mom, who had to dress her in clothes for eighteen-month-olds at age nine months and carry her around all day long. At one year, she weighed 23 pounds, 5 ounces (10.5 kg); at 18 months, 25 pounds (11 kg); and at five years, 40 pounds (18 kg). Now, she is a completely average weight for her age. She levelled out and is doing just fine.

Sometimes low weight can be a concern, more so if the weight gain increases slowly. If your baby genuinely needs to put on a few extra pounds, be sure to include some higher-fat foods, which provide 9 calories per gram as opposed to the 4 calories per gram provided by protein and carbohydrate foods. Avocado, egg yolk, olive oil, and flaxseed oil are all healthy higher-fat foods. Coconut milk can be added to purées to provide extra fat (coconut is not considered a tree nut, by the way).[110] I've heard butter and cream suggested as fatty foods to introduce, which is fine but not as healthy as the suggestions above. Also, consider that dairy has higher allergic or sensitizing potential, so it may not be the right choice for your baby. Feeding more regularly—at least three times a day—while incorporating the higher-fat foods listed above can quickly increase weight. If your baby was light at birth, he'll most likely catch up with his weight before you get to the point of starting solids, so it may not be necessary to keep up the higher calorie intake if his weight increases within his own growth chart. Your doctor will be monitoring your baby's weight and will know if there's a concern outside a routine weight plateau. If you feel that your baby is losing weight, discuss it with your doctor and seek help from a nutritionist and naturopath, too, as minerals like tissue salts can help to increase appetite.

SCHEDULE FOR INTRODUCTION OF SOLIDS

Here is a general guideline to follow from the introduction of solids to the time when your baby's eating three meals a day, usually by nine months of age. But don't worry if your baby isn't following this order exactly—every baby is different, and this table is intended simply to give you an example of how to introduce solids and progress. Start with either lunch or dinner (this table shows lunch), and continue to give baby either breast milk or formula upon rising, at bedtime, and before naps.

INTRODUCTION OF SOLIDS	BREAKFAST	LUNCH	DINNER
First 2 weeks	Milk	Milk, then half an hour to 1 hour later, solid food. To progress, increase the number of teaspoons in a feeding.	Milk
Next 2 to 4 weeks	Milk	Milk and solids, including allergenic foods like egg yolk, peanut butter, almond butter, tahini, fish, and dairy over the next 2 to 4 weeks.	Milk, then half an hour to 1 hour later, introduce the second meal. To progress, increase the number of cubes in a feeding.
From about age 7 to 9 months onward	Milk, then half an hour to 1 hour later, introduce the third meal. To progress, increase the number of cubes in a feeding.	Milk and solids	Milk and solids

"Milk" is either breast milk or formula.

FIRST FOOD CHECKLIST

Use a chart like the following sample checklist when introducing fruits and vegetables to your baby. You'll find a complete downloadable chart on SproutRight.com, or you can make one yourself. I recommend starting with butternut squash and then pear, as they have the perfect texture and flavour. After that, you can alternate between other recommended first foods (see page 120), testing each new food for five days before moving on to the next one.

FOOD	DATE FIRST GIVEN (PURÉE/PIECE)	LIKED	PREFERENCE (PURÉE/PIECE)	DISLIKED	TRIED AGAIN
VEGETABLES					
Butternut squash					
FRUITS					
Pear					

BABY FEEDING CALENDAR

Here's another chart you might find helpful to keep track of the introduction of solids; overall food, breast milk, or formula intake; reactions; and digestive output. Fill in a chart like this one each week to keep a record of the details.

	MON	TUES	WED	THURS	FRI	SAT	SUN
Milk (ML/TIME)							
Food							
Reactions							
Poo							
Other (TEETHING/ VACCINA- TIONS/ SICKNESS)							

MILK: How many mL of formula, or length of time if breastfed?

FOOD: What did baby eat, how much, and at what time?

REACTIONS: Any rashes anywhere on the body, runny nose, constipation, diarrhea, gassiness, bloating, etc.?

POO: How many? Describe.

OTHER (TEETHING/VACCINATIONS/SICKNESS): Is anything else going on that may contribute to symptoms?

RECEIPES

MEAT BROTH MAKES ABOUT 8½ CUPS (2 L)

DAIRY-FREE • EGG-FREE • GLUTEN-FREE • NUT-FREE • WHEAT-FREE

This recipe cannot be replaced by store-bought tetra packs, stock cubes, or even butcher-made broth that contains salt. Store-bought broths are made with flavour enhancers and high in sodium. The purpose of this broth is to nourish your baby with minerals (including iron), gelatin, collagen, and fat. The gelatin and fat is incredibly important to heal leaky gut, a normal situation in babies. Do *not* add salt to this recipe. Salt upsets the body's fluid balance and affects the kidneys. Ideally, use organic or naturally raised poultry only.

4 to 6 chicken thighs and/or legs, bone in, skin on
2 celery stalks, roughly chopped
1 onion, cut in half
2 to 3 carrots, scrubbed and roughly chopped
2 cloves garlic, smashed (optional)
1-inch (2.5 cm) piece fresh ginger (optional)
4 quarts (4 L) filtered water

1. Add all ingredients to a large pot. Bring to a boil on high heat, then reduce the heat and simmer, partly covered, for up to 4 hours. By then, the vegetables should be very soft, the chicken should be cooked thoroughly, and the broth should be a rich, deep yellow colour.
2. Remove the chicken and vegetables by straining the broth through a colander. Save the chicken for another dish or to add to a purée or soup.
3. Store the broth in mason jars with 1 inch (2.5 cm) of room at the top to allow for expansion during freezing or in BPA-free plastic ice cube trays. Keep in the fridge with the lid on for up to 4 days or in the freezer for up to a month.

TIP: **1.** You can make the broth using a Crock-Pot or slow cooker. Add the ingredients to the Crock-Pot or slow cooker and cook on high for 1 hour, then reduce heat to low and cook for an additional 6 hours. When done, strain and store as above. **2.** You can also make the broth using an Instant Pot or any electric pressure cooker. Add the ingredients to the Instant Pot to the max line. Put the lid on and adjust the valve to seal. Set to manual for 30 minutes. Let it turn off on its own and allow the pressure to release naturally. This can take up to 30 minutes. Remove the lid and let cool before straining and storing as above.

NUTRITIONAL INFORMATION This nutrient-dense broth is a great source of minerals, especially calcium, and proteins like collagen.

VEGETABLE BROTH MAKES AROUND 12 CUPS (3 L)

DAIRY-FREE • EGG-FREE • GLUTEN-FREE • NUT-FREE • VEGAN • VEGETARIAN • WHEAT-FREE

For a different flavour or for vegetarians, vegans, or those following a plant-based diet, use this recipe. Vegetable broth doesn't have the same benefits as meat broth, so if you can use chicken or other meat, it's preferable.

1 onion, roughly chopped

1 carrot, scrubbed and roughly chopped

1 tomato, sliced into quarters

1 cup (250 mL) button or cremini
   mushrooms, cleaned

1 bunch parsley stems

6 cloves garlic, smashed

1½-inch (4 cm) piece fresh ginger, chopped
   into 3 pieces

1 bay leaf

5 whole black peppercorns

4 quarts (4 L) filtered water

1. Add all ingredients to a large pot and bring to a boil.

2. Reduce the heat and simmer for 1 hour. Strain the stock through a sieve (a colander will also work, but more fibrous parts will fall through).

3. Store the broth in ice cube trays or mason jars with an airtight seal, being sure to leave 1 inch (2.5 cm) of room at the top of the jar to allow for expansion during freezing. Keep in the fridge for up to 4 days or in the freezer for up to a month.

BUTTERNUT SQUASH PURÉE

MAKES ABOUT 3 CUPS (750 ML)

DAIRY-FREE • EGG-FREE • GLUTEN-FREE •

NUT-FREE • VEGAN • VEGETARIAN • WHEAT-FREE

I recommend this as a first food. Babies love the smooth texture and flavour, and it's sweet and smooth—but not too sweet.

1 pound (450 g) butternut squash
½ to 1 cup (125 to 250 mL) filtered water

1. Peel, seed, and chop the squash into small cubes.
2. Steam until tender, about 15 to 20 minutes.
3. Purée the squash, adding water until it reaches the texture of a smooth, thick soup.
4. Store the purée in an airtight container in the fridge for up to 3 days or in the freezer in ice cube trays or baby-safe food containers for up to 3 months.

TIP: **1.** Squash tends to be a little watery after defrosting, so make this purée slightly thicker if you're going to freeze it. **2.** Substitute Meat Broth (page 129) or Vegetable Broth (page 130) for the water for more nutrients and taste.

NUTRITIONAL INFORMATION Butternut squash is a good source of vitamin A (in the form of beta carotene); vitamin C; potassium; fibre; manganese; folic acid; vitamins B1, B3, and B6; copper; and pantothenic acid.

PEAR PURÉE

MAKES ABOUT 3 CUPS (750 ML)

DAIRY-FREE • EGG-FREE • GLUTEN-FREE •

NUT-FREE • VEGAN • VEGETARIAN • WHEAT-FREE

Pear is a lovely second food to introduce. Smooth and sweet, it's a common favourite!

8 pears (D'Anjou, Bartlett, or Bosc)

1. Peel, core, and chop pears into medium-size cubes.
2. Steam until tender, about 7 to 10 minutes.
3. Purée until smooth (no added water needed).
4. Store the purée in an airtight container in the fridge for up to 3 days or in the freezer in ice cube trays or baby-safe food containers for up to 3 months.

TIP: After the first couple of times you make this recipe, skip peeling the pears and steam with the skin on.

NUTRITIONAL INFORMATION Pears are a good source of vitamin C and fibre.

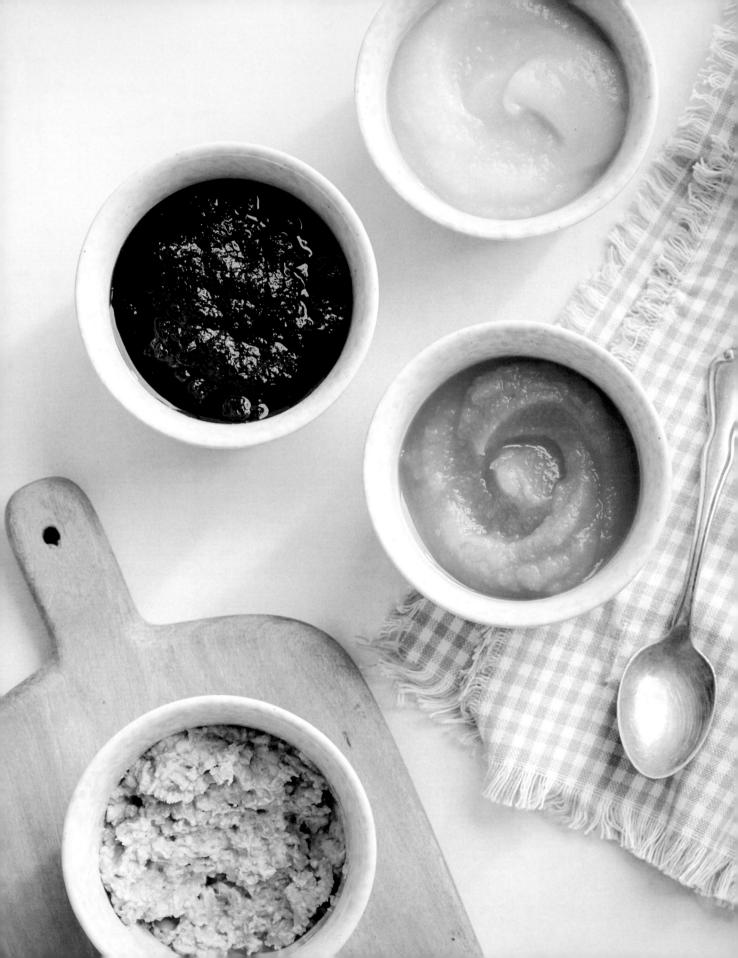

BLUEBERRY PURÉE

MAKES ABOUT 2½ CUPS (625 ML)

DAIRY-FREE • EGG-FREE • GLUTEN-FREE •

NUT-FREE • VEGAN • VEGETARIAN • WHEAT-FREE

Don't be afraid to serve your baby this purée, even though it can be messy! Keep in mind that the blueberry skins will give it more texture than other purées, so it might be best to wait until four or more foods have been introduced before serving this one. Expect blueberry poo to be a dark colour.

2½ cups (625 mL) frozen or fresh wild
  blueberries
¼ to ½ cup (60 to 125 mL) filtered water

1. Steam blueberries until just heated through, about 5 to 7 minutes.
2. Purée until smooth, about 5 minutes, adding ¼ to ½ cup (60 to 125 mL) water, depending on how much liquid the blueberries lost during steaming.
3. Store the purée in an airtight container in the fridge for up to 3 days or in the freezer in ice cube trays or baby-safe food containers for up to 3 months.

TIP: Substitute Meat Broth (page 129) or Vegetable Broth (page 130) for the water for more nutrients and taste.

NUTRITIONAL INFORMATION Blueberries are high in antioxidants and a good source of vitamin C, manganese, fibre, and vitamin E.

AVOCADO PURÉE

MAKES 2 TO 4 TABLESPOONS (30 TO 60 ML)

DAIRY-FREE • EGG-FREE • GLUTEN-FREE •

NUT-FREE • VEGAN • VEGETARIAN • WHEAT-FREE

Avocado is a powerhouse of nutrients and monounsaturated fat. It's an amazing food for putting on extra weight if your baby needs it, but don't shy away from it if she doesn't.

¼ to ½ ripe avocado
2 tablespoons (30 mL) meat or vegetable broth
  (if needed)

1. Remove the pit from the avocado and scoop out the flesh with a spoon. Mash with a fork or the back of a spoon until smooth, and serve immediately. This purée is not suitable for freezing.

TIP: Add 1 or 2 tablespoons (15 or 30 mL) of Meat Broth (page 129), Vegetable Broth (page 130), breast milk, or formula, if necessary, to thin out the avocado purée.

NUTRITIONAL INFORMATION Avocados are a good source of vitamin K, fibre, vitamin B6, vitamin C, folate, copper, and potassium.

BANANA PURÉE

MAKES ABOUT ½ CUP (125 ML)

DAIRY-FREE • EGG-FREE • GLUTEN-FREE •
NUT-FREE • VEGAN • VEGETARIAN • WHEAT-FREE

Banana is a well-loved fruit and so easy to prepare. When you're out and about and stuck for something to feed your baby, find a banana, mash, and serve.

1 ripe banana

1. Peel and mash the banana with a fork or the back of a spoon. Stir in breast milk or formula to desired consistency.
2. Store the purée in an airtight container in the fridge for up to 2 days. This purée is not suitable for freezing.

NUTRITIONAL INFORMATION Bananas are a good source of vitamin B6, vitamin C, potassium, dietary fibre, and manganese.

APPLE PURÉE

MAKES ABOUT 3 CUPS (750 ML)

DAIRY-FREE • EGG-FREE • GLUTEN-FREE •
NUT-FREE • VEGAN • VEGETARIAN • WHEAT-FREE

Apple purée, or applesauce, is one dish you'll be making for a long time! It's a firm favourite from the baby stage well into adulthood.

8 apples (Fuji, Gala, or Pink Lady)
¼ to ½ cup (60 to 125 mL) filtered water

1. Peel, core, and chop the apples into small cubes.
2. Steam until tender, about 10 minutes.
3. Purée, adding water until it reaches the texture of a smooth, thick soup.
4. Store the purée in an airtight container in the fridge for up to 3 days or in the freezer in ice cube trays or baby-safe food containers for up to 3 months.

TIP: Substitute Meat Broth (page 129) or Vegetable Broth (page 130) for the water for more nutrients and taste.

NUTRITIONAL INFORMATION Apples are a good source of fibre, vitamin C, and flavonoids.

BROCCOLI PURÉE

MAKES ABOUT 3 CUPS (750 ML)

DAIRY-FREE • EGG-FREE • GLUTEN-FREE •
NUT-FREE • VEGAN • VEGETARIAN • WHEAT-FREE

Many parents worry that broccoli will give their babies gas, but that's not necessarily the case. As with any other food, try it and watch for a reaction.

1 head broccoli
¼ to ½ cup (60 to 125 mL) filtered water

1. Peel the broccoli stem to remove the fibrous outer layer and cut about 1 inch (2.5 cm) off the bottom and discard. Chop broccoli florets and stem into small pieces.
2. Steam until tender, about 10 to 15 minutes.
3. Purée, adding water until it reaches the texture of a smooth, thick soup.
4. Store the purée in an airtight container in the fridge for up to 3 days or in the freezer in ice cube trays or baby-safe food containers for up to 3 months.

TIP: Substitute Meat Broth (page 129) or Vegetable Broth (page 130) for the water for more nutrients and taste.

NUTRITIONAL INFORMATION Broccoli is a good source of calcium, magnesium, beta carotene, folic acid, potassium, and vitamin C.

CAULIFLOWER PURÉE

MAKES ABOUT 3 CUPS (750 ML)

DAIRY-FREE • EGG-FREE • GLUTEN-FREE •
NUT-FREE • VEGAN • VEGETARIAN • WHEAT-FREE

Cauliflower's delicate, creamy taste lends itself to many combinations of purée. I've occasionally seen babies become gassy with cauliflower, but not as often as you might think!

1 head cauliflower
¼ to ½ cup (60 to 125 mL) filtered water

1. Remove the core and stem from the cauliflower and chop the florets into small pieces.
2. Steam until tender, about 15 minutes.
3. Purée, adding water until it reaches the texture of a smooth, thick soup.
4. Store the purée in an airtight container in the fridge for up to 3 days or in the freezer in ice cube trays or baby-safe food containers for up to 3 months.

TIP: Substitute Meat Broth (page 129) or Vegetable Broth (page 130) for the water for more nutrients and taste.

NUTRITIONAL INFORMATION Steamed cauliflower is a good source of vitamin C, folate, fibre, vitamin B5, vitamin B6, and manganese.

DRIED APRICOT PURÉE

MAKES ABOUT 3 CUPS (750 ML)

DAIRY-FREE • EGG-FREE • GLUTEN-FREE •
NUT-FREE • VEGAN • VEGETARIAN • WHEAT-FREE

Dried apricots have a laxative effect, so they're great for treating constipation. Buy organic brown and unsulphured dried apricots—they're brown because they don't contain sulphites, which can trigger asthma and gas.

1 cup (250 mL) unsulphured dried apricots

1. Put the apricots in a saucepan and cover with filtered water. Simmer until the apricots are plump and softened, about 10 minutes.
2. Transfer all contents, including any remaining water, to a bowl; purée until it reaches the texture of a smooth, thick soup. If you're freezing the purée, you may need to add an extra ¼ cup (60 mL) of water so it will freeze solid.
3. Serve alone or combine with pears, papaya, avocado, or any other favourite fruit or vegetable.
4. Store the purée in an airtight container in the fridge for up to 3 days or in the freezer in ice cube trays or baby-safe food containers for up to 3 months.

TIP: Substitute Meat Broth (page 129) or Vegetable Broth (page 130) for the water for more nutrients and taste.

NUTRITIONAL INFORMATION Apricots are a good source of beta carotene, potassium, iron, calcium, silicon, phosphorus, and vitamin C. The copper and cobalt in apricots is beneficial in treating anemia. In some animal studies, dried apricots were just as effective as liver, kidney, or eggs in treating iron deficiency anemia. Ounce for ounce compared to fresh apricots, dried apricots contain 12 times as much iron, 7 times as much fibre, and 5 times as much vitamin A!

SWEET POTATO PURÉE

MAKES ABOUT 4 CUPS (1 L)

DAIRY-FREE • EGG-FREE • GLUTEN-FREE •
NUT-FREE • VEGAN • VEGETARIAN • WHEAT-FREE

Babies seem to love orange vegetables, and this one's definitely a favourite. Sweet potatoes are high in fibre, so you'll need to add a lot of liquid to thin this purée and help that fibre move through baby's digestive system. Try adding 1 tablespoon (15 mL) ground cinnamon the next time you make a batch.

2 medium sweet potatoes or yams
1¾ to 2½ cups (425 to 625 mL) filtered water

1. Peel and chop the sweet potato into small cubes.
2. Steam until tender, about 15 to 20 minutes.
3. Purée, adding ½ to ¾ cup (125 to 175 mL) water until it reaches the texture of a smooth, thick soup.
4. Store the purée in an airtight container in the fridge for up to 3 days or in the freezer in ice cube trays or baby-safe food containers for up to 3 months.

TIP: 1. Sweet potato tends to be a little watery after defrosting, so make this purée slightly thicker if you're going to freeze it. 2. Substitute Meat Broth (page 129) or Vegetable Broth (page 130) for the water for more nutrients and taste.

NUTRITIONAL INFORMATION Sweet potatoes are a good source of beta carotene, fibre, potassium, and vitamins C and E.

CARROT PURÉE

MAKES ABOUT 3 CUPS (750 ML)

DAIRY-FREE • EGG-FREE • GLUTEN-FREE •
NUT-FREE • VEGAN • VEGETARIAN • WHEAT-FREE

Carrots are well liked for their sweet flavour and pack a powerful antioxidant punch. They can also be used to introduce a slightly more earthy flavour, especially if you use organic carrots.

10 medium carrots
½ to 1 cup (125 to 250 mL) filtered water

1. Peel and chop the carrots into small cubes.
2. Steam until tender, about 20 minutes.
3. Purée, adding ½ cup (125 mL) of water at a time, until it reaches the texture of a smooth, thick soup.
4. Store the purée in an airtight container in the fridge for up to 3 days or in the freezer in ice cube trays or baby-safe food containers for up to 3 months.

TIP: Substitute Meat Broth (page 129) or Vegetable Broth (page 130) for the water for more nutrients and taste.

NUTRITIONAL INFORMATION Carrots are a good source of beta carotene and fibre.

PARSNIP PURÉE

MAKES ABOUT 3 CUPS (750 ML)

DAIRY-FREE • EGG-FREE • GLUTEN-FREE •
NUT-FREE • VEGAN • VEGETARIAN • WHEAT-FREE

Babies love this smooth, creamy purée.
I constantly hear, "I've never tried parsnip before," from the moms in my cooking classes. Now's your chance!

5 to 6 medium parsnips
1½ to 2 cups (375 to 500 mL) filtered water

1. Peel and chop the parsnips into small cubes.
2. Steam until tender, about 10 to 15 minutes.
3. Purée to desired consistency, adding water until it reaches the texture of a smooth, thick soup.
4. Store the purée in an airtight container in the fridge for up to 3 days or in the freezer in ice cube trays or baby-safe food containers for up to 3 months.

TIP: Substitute Meat Broth (page 129) or Vegetable Broth (page 130) for the water for more nutrients and taste.

NUTRITIONAL INFORMATION Parsnips are a good source of fibre, calcium, iron, potassium, some B vitamins, and vitamin C.

ZUCCHINI PURÉE

MAKES ABOUT 3 CUPS (750 ML)

DAIRY-FREE • EGG-FREE • GLUTEN-FREE •

NUT-FREE • VEGAN • VEGETARIAN • WHEAT-FREE

A simple yet delectable purée that's fast to make! Zucchini is quite watery, so no extra water is needed. It's an easy taste to add to other purées if you're looking to incorporate more nutrients from a green vegetable.

2 large zucchini, washed

1. Trim the ends off the zucchini and chop into small cubes.
2. Steam gently until tender, about 5 to 10 minutes.
3. Purée until smooth (no water needed).
4. Store the purée in an airtight container in the fridge for up to 3 days or in the freezer in ice cube trays or baby-safe food containers for up to 3 months.

NUTRITIONAL INFORMATION Zucchini is a good source of manganese, vitamin C, magnesium, vitamin A, fibre, potassium, copper, folate, and phosphorus.

BEETROOT PURÉE

MAKES ABOUT 3 CUPS (750 ML)

DAIRY-FREE • EGG-FREE • GLUTEN-FREE •

NUT-FREE • VEGAN • VEGETARIAN • WHEAT-FREE

A good source of iron, beets have a lovely sweet but earthy flavour. If your baby isn't sure about the taste, try beets as a finger food.

2 large fresh red beets

½ to 1 cup (125 to 250 mL) filtered water

1. Peel and chop beets into very small pieces.
2. Steam until tender, about 45 minutes.
3. Purée, adding water until it reaches the texture of a smooth, thick soup.
4. Store the purée in an airtight container in the fridge for up to 3 days or in the freezer in ice cube trays or baby-safe food containers for up to 3 months.

TIP: Substitute Meat Broth (page 129) or Vegetable Broth (page 130) for the water for more nutrients and taste.

NUTRITIONAL INFORMATION Beets are a good source of folic acid, manganese, potassium, fibre, vitamin C, magnesium, iron, copper, and phosphorus.

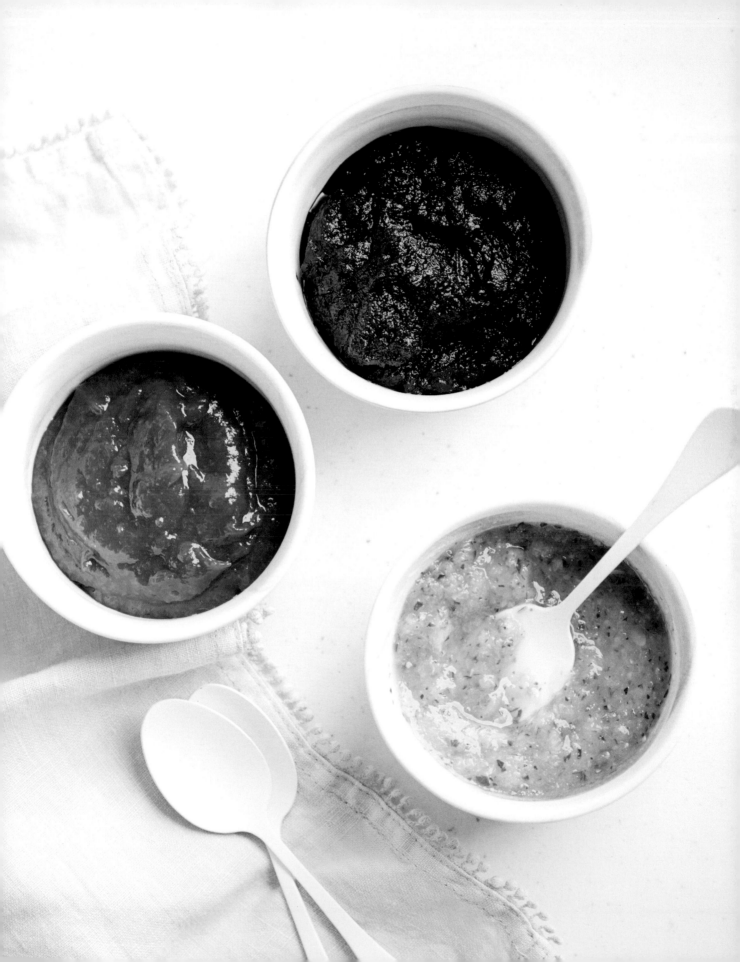

PLUM PURÉE

MAKES ABOUT 3 CUPS (750 ML)

DAIRY-FREE • EGG-FREE • GLUTEN-FREE •
NUT-FREE • VEGAN • VEGETARIAN • WHEAT-FREE

The dark pigment of plums lets you know that they're high in antioxidants. This luscious purée is a treat for anyone. If the plums are too tart, stir in some apple or pear purée.

10 ripe plums

1. Slice the plums in half vertically, and twist to reveal and remove the pits (no peeling required). Cut into quarters.
2. Steam until tender, about 10 minutes.
3. Purée, adding water if needed, until it reaches the texture of a smooth, thick soup.
4. Store the purée in an airtight container in the fridge for up to 3 days or in the freezer in ice cube trays or baby-safe food containers for up to 3 months.

TIP: Substitute Meat Broth (page 129) or Vegetable Broth (page 130) for the water for more nutrients and taste.

NUTRITIONAL INFORMATION Plums are a good source of vitamin C, vitamin A, vitamin B2, potassium, and fibre.

FRESH APRICOT PURÉE

MAKES ABOUT 3 CUPS (750 ML)

DAIRY-FREE • EGG-FREE • GLUTEN-FREE •
NUT-FREE • VEGAN • VEGETARIAN • WHEAT-FREE

A treat in the summer when apricots are fresh. Apricots are on the list of fruits to buy organic. It may not be necessary to add filtered water or broth, so check the texture before you add extra.

10 ripe apricots

1. Slice the apricots in half vertically, and twist to reveal and remove the pits. Cut into quarters.
2. Steam until tender, about 10 minutes.
3. Purée, adding water if necessary, until it reaches the texture of a smooth, thick soup.
4. Store the purée in an airtight container in the fridge for up to 3 days or in the freezer in ice cube trays or baby-safe food containers for up to 3 months.

TIP: Substitute Meat Broth (page 129) or Vegetable Broth (page 130) for the water for more nutrients and taste.

NUTRITIONAL INFORMATION Apricots are an excellent source of vitamin A, vitamin C, fibre, and potassium.

GREEN BEAN PURÉE

MAKES 3 CUPS (750 ML)

DAIRY-FREE • EGG-FREE • GLUTEN-FREE •
NUT-FREE • VEGAN • VEGETARIAN • WHEAT-FREE

You can make this with both green and yellow beans. The recipe can also be made with frozen beans if you're making it out of season. This is a beautiful sweet green purée that's surprisingly loved.

1½ pounds (675 g) fresh or frozen green beans
¼ to ½ cup (60 to 125 mL) filtered water

1. Trim the stem ends and chop the beans into ¾-inch (2 cm) pieces.
2. Steam until tender, about 5 to 10 minutes.
3. Purée, adding water until it reaches the texture of a smooth, thick soup.
4. Store the purée in an airtight container in the fridge for up to 3 days or in the freezer in ice cube trays or baby-safe food containers for up to 3 months.

TIP: Substitute Meat Broth (page 129) or Vegetable Broth (page 130) for the water for more nutrients and taste.

NUTRITIONAL INFORMATION Green beans are a good source of vitamin C, vitamin K, manganese, vitamin A, fibre, potassium, folate, and iron.

ASPARAGUS PURÉE

MAKES 3 CUPS (750 ML)

DAIRY-FREE • EGG-FREE • GLUTEN-FREE •
NUT-FREE • VEGAN • VEGETARIAN • WHEAT-FREE

Asparagus is a nutritious spring vegetable that can be purchased conventional (not organic). Bugs don't like them, so they don't need to be sprayed with pesticides much, if at all.

12 asparagus spears
2 to 3 tablespoons (30 to 45 mL) filtered water

1. Chop ¾ inch (2 cm) off the bottom of each asparagus spear, or snap off the woody ends, and discard.
2. Chop asparagus into ¾-inch (2 cm) pieces.
3. Steam until tender, about 5 to 7 minutes.
4. Purée, adding water until it reaches the texture of a smooth, thick soup.
5. Store the purée in an airtight container in the fridge for up to 3 days or in the freezer in ice cube trays or baby-safe food containers for up to 3 months.

TIP: Substitute Meat Broth (page 129) or Vegetable Broth (page 130) for the water for more nutrients and taste.

NUTRITIONAL INFORMATION Asparagus is a good source of vitamin A, vitamin C, potassium, folic acid, zinc, and fibre.

OAT CEREAL   MAKES ABOUT 2 TABLESPOONS (30 ML) CEREAL (WITHOUT THE FRUIT PURÉE)

DAIRY-FREE • EGG-FREE • GLUTEN-FREE (IF USING GLUTEN-FREE OATS) • NUT-FREE • VEGAN • VEGETARIAN • WHEAT-FREE

If you choose to give your baby cereal, I recommend oats, as they're the least allergenic and are naturally high in both soluble and insoluble fibre as well as iron. Double the recipe and freeze some for later!

1 cup (250 mL) steel cut oats

¼ cup (60 mL) filtered water

1 to 2 tablespoons (15 to 30 mL) fruit purée (like Pear Purée, page 131; Apple Purée, page 134; or Fresh Apricot Purée, page 140)

1. Grind the oats to a fine powder using a coffee grinder, food processor, or high-speed blender. Store in an airtight container.

2. To make the cereal, pour the water into a small saucepan and bring to a boil.

3. Slowly add 1 tablespoon (15 mL) ground oats while whisking vigorously. Reduce the heat and simmer for about 10 minutes.

4. Set aside to cool, then stir in your baby's favourite fruit purée for natural sweetness and a nutrient boost. You can also thin the cereal with breast milk, formula, meat or vegetable broth, or water. Serve immediately.

5. Store the cereal in an airtight container in the fridge for up to 3 days.

TIP: Substitute Meat Broth (page 129) or Vegetable Broth (page 130) for the water for more nutrients and taste.

NUTRITIONAL INFORMATION Oats are a good source of manganese, selenium, iron, vitamin B1, fibre, magnesium, protein, and phosphorus.

PEA AND MINT PURÉE

MAKES ABOUT 1½ CUPS (375 ML)

DAIRY-FREE • EGG-FREE • GLUTEN-FREE •
NUT-FREE • VEGAN • VEGETARIAN • WHEAT-FREE

Mint perfectly complements the peas and adds unexpected zip.

1 medium carrot
1½ cups (375 mL) fresh or frozen peas
¼ teaspoon (1 mL) chopped fresh mint
2 to 4 tablespoons (30 to 60 mL) filtered water

1. Peel and chop the carrot into small cubes and steam for about 15 minutes. Add peas and steam until tender, about 5 to 10 minutes longer.
2. Purée, adding mint and enough water to reach the texture of a smooth, thick soup.
3. Store the purée in an airtight container in the fridge for up to 3 days or in the freezer in ice cube trays or baby-safe food containers for up to 3 months.

TIP: Substitute Meat Broth (page 129) or Vegetable Broth (page 130) for the water for more nutrients and taste.

NUTRITIONAL INFORMATION Green peas are a good source of vitamin C, vitamin K, manganese, fibre, folate, thiamine (vitamin B1), and iron.

PEAR AND APPLE PURÉE

MAKES ABOUT 3 CUPS (750 ML)

DAIRY-FREE • EGG-FREE • GLUTEN-FREE •
NUT-FREE • VEGAN • VEGETARIAN • WHEAT-FREE

A scrumptious purée with loads of extra fibre and minerals! Combining two of the most loved fruits introduces a new flavour to expand your baby's palate further. Add in ground cinnamon, curry powder, or sage the next time you make it.

4 medium apples (Gala, Fuji, or Pink Lady)
4 medium pears (D'Anjou, Bartlett, or Bosc)
1 tablespoon (15 mL) chia seeds
2 to 4 tablespoons (30 to 60 mL) filtered water

1. Peel, core, and chop the apples and pears into small cubes.
2. Steam until tender, about 15 minutes.
3. Add chia seeds and purée, adding water until it reaches the texture of a smooth, thick soup.
4. Store the purée in an airtight container in the fridge for up to 3 days or in the freezer in ice cube trays or baby-safe food containers for up to 3 months.

TIP: Substitute Meat Broth (page 129) or Vegetable Broth (page 130) for the water for more nutrients and taste.

NUTRITIONAL INFORMATION This purée is a good source of fibre, vitamin C, and flavonoids.

AVOCADO AND PEAR PURÉE

MAKES ABOUT 1 CUP (250 ML)

DAIRY-FREE • EGG-FREE • GLUTEN-FREE •

NUT-FREE • VEGAN • VEGETARIAN • WHEAT-FREE

Creamy and delicious, avocado is a good source of nutritious fat to add to any purée. You can add some raw garlic before mashing if baby is getting sick—it's a great way to boost the immune system.

½ ripe avocado
½ ripe pear

1. Remove the pit from the avocado and scoop out the flesh with a spoon. Peel the pear.
2. Mash together or use your hand blender or chopper until the desired consistency is achieved. Serve immediately.
3. Store the purée in an airtight container in the fridge for up to 3 days. This purée is not suitable for freezing.

TIP: Papaya or banana can be used in addition to or instead of pear. Next time, add some blueberries as well.

NUTRITIONAL INFORMATION Avocados are a good source of vitamin K, fibre, vitamin B6, vitamin C, folate, copper, and potassium.

CARROT, APPLE, AND SPINACH PURÉE

MAKES ABOUT 3 CUPS (750 ML)

DAIRY-FREE • EGG-FREE • GLUTEN-FREE •

NUT-FREE • VEGAN • VEGETARIAN • WHEAT-FREE

This is a simple dish that's high in antioxidants. Spinach doesn't have much taste, so it's a well-liked addition.

4 medium carrots
4 apples (Gala, Fuji, or Pink Lady)
Handful of baby spinach
2 to 4 tablespoons (30 to 60 mL) filtered water

1. Peel and chop the carrots into small cubes. Steam for about 15 minutes.
2. Peel, core, and chop the apples into 1-inch (2.5 cm) chunks and add to the carrots. Steam until tender, about 10 minutes longer. Just at the end, add in the spinach and let it wilt for a couple of minutes.
3. Purée, adding enough water to achieve the texture of a smooth, thick soup, or leave chunky.
4. Store the purée in an airtight container in the fridge for up to 3 days or in the freezer in ice cube trays or baby-safe food containers for up to 3 months.

TIP: Substitute Meat Broth (page 129) or Vegetable Broth (page 130) for the water for more nutrients and taste.

NUTRITIONAL INFORMATION This purée is a good source of vitamin A, vitamin C, vitamin K, fibre, and potassium.

BUTTERNUT SQUASH AND PEAR PURÉE

MAKES ABOUT 3 CUPS (750 ML)

DAIRY-FREE • EGG-FREE • GLUTEN-FREE •
NUT-FREE • VEGAN • VEGETARIAN • WHEAT-FREE

Your baby will love this wonderful combination. Try sprinkling it with a bit of ground cinnamon, too. For an added boost of protein and fibre, you can add hemp or sesame seeds and purée.

1 pound (450 g) butternut squash

1 very ripe pear

1 tablespoon (15 mL) hemp seeds or sesame seeds (optional)

2 to 4 tablespoons (30 to 60 mL) filtered water

1. Peel, seed, and chop the butternut squash into small cubes. Steam for about 10 minutes.
2. Peel, core, and chop the pear into small cubes and add to the steamer. Steam until tender, about 5 minutes longer.
3. Mash or purée, adding hemp seeds (if using) and water if necessary to achieve the texture of a smooth, thick soup.
4. Store the purée in an airtight container in the fridge for up to 3 days or in the freezer in ice cube trays or baby-safe food containers for up to 3 months.

TIP: Substitute Meat Broth (page 129) or Vegetable Broth (page 130) for the water for more nutrients and taste.

NUTRITIONAL INFORMATION This purée is a good source of beta carotene, vitamin C, potassium, fibre, and manganese.

PLUM AND PEAR PURÉE

MAKES 3 CUPS (750 ML)

DAIRY-FREE • EGG-FREE • GLUTEN-FREE •
NUT-FREE • VEGAN • VEGETARIAN • WHEAT-FREE

This fast, fresh purée is packed with vitamins, antioxidants, and fibre. Tart plums and sweet pears combine wonderfully.

4 ripe plums

2 ripe pears

1 tablespoon (15 mL) filtered water

1. Cut the plums in half and remove the pits. Peel and core the pears. Cut all fruit into small pieces.
2. Steam until tender, about 5 minutes.
3. Purée, adding only a small amount of water if needed to reach the texture of a smooth, thick soup.
4. Store the purée in an airtight container in the fridge for up to 3 days or in the freezer in ice cube trays or baby-safe food containers for up to 3 months.

TIP: Substitute Meat Broth (page 129) or Vegetable Broth (page 130) for the water for more nutrients and taste.

NUTRITIONAL INFORMATION This purée is a good source of vitamin C, vitamin A, vitamin B2, potassium, and fibre.

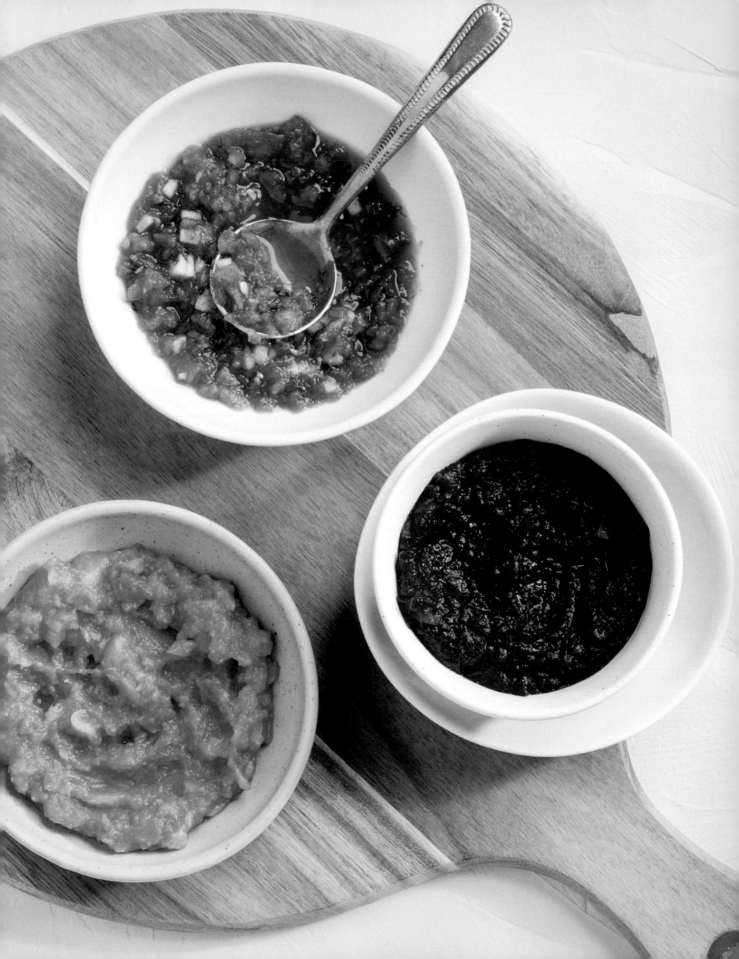

BEET AND APPLE PURÉE

MAKES 3 CUPS (750 ML)

DAIRY-FREE • EGG-FREE • GLUTEN-FREE •

NUT-FREE • VEGAN • VEGETARIAN • WHEAT-FREE

You can substitute two medium parsnips for the apples to make a lovely smooth, pink purée!

1 large fresh red beet
4 apples (Gala, Fuji, or Pink Lady)
2 to 4 tablespoons (30 to 60 mL) filtered water

1. Peel and chop the beets into very small cubes. Steam for about 40 minutes.
2. Peel, core, and chop the apples and add to the steamer. Steam until tender, about 10 minutes longer.
3. Purée, adding enough water to reach the texture of a smooth, thick soup.
4. Store the purée in an airtight container in the fridge for up to 3 days or in the freezer in ice cube trays or baby-safe food containers for up to 3 months.

TIP: Substitute Meat Broth (page 129) or Vegetable Broth (page 130) for the water for more nutrients and taste.

NUTRITIONAL INFORMATION This purée is a good source of vitamin C, folic acid, manganese, potassium, magnesium, iron, copper, and phosphorus.

CARROT AND PARSNIP PURÉE

MAKES ABOUT 3 CUPS (750 ML)

DAIRY-FREE • EGG-FREE • GLUTEN-FREE •

NUT-FREE • VEGAN • VEGETARIAN • WHEAT-FREE

Carrots and parsnips are a wonderful combination that your baby is sure to enjoy.

5 medium carrots
2 medium parsnips
½ cup (125 mL) filtered water

1. Peel and chop the carrots into small cubes. Steam for about 10 minutes.
2. Peel and chop the parsnips and add to the steamer. Steam until tender, about 15 minutes longer.
3. Purée, adding enough water to reach the texture of a smooth, thick soup.
4. Store the purée in an airtight container in the fridge for up to 3 days or in the freezer in ice cube trays or baby-safe food containers for up to 3 months.

TIP: Substitute Meat Broth (page 129) or Vegetable Broth (page 130) for the water for more nutrients and taste.

NUTRITIONAL INFORMATION This purée is a good source of vitamin A, vitamin C, vitamin K, fibre, calcium, iron, potassium, and some B vitamins.

WATERMELON, PEACH, AND BASIL PURÉE

MAKES ABOUT 5 CUPS (1.25 L)

DAIRY-FREE • EGG-FREE • GLUTEN-FREE •

NUT-FREE • VEGAN • VEGETARIAN • WHEAT-FREE

This refreshing "raw" purée is packed with enzymes and nutrients.

2½ cups (625 mL) diced seedless watermelon

2 cups (500 mL) diced peaches

1 teaspoon (5 mL) chopped fresh basil or mint

1. Purée the watermelon and peaches with the basil in a food processor or with a hand blender until smooth.

2. Store the purée in an airtight container in the fridge for up to 3 days or in the freezer in ice cube trays or baby-safe food containers for up to 3 months.

NUTRITIONAL INFORMATION This purée is a good source of vitamin C, vitamin A, vitamin B6, thiamine, potassium, and magnesium.

GREEN EGGS

MAKES 1 SERVING

DAIRY-FREE • GLUTEN-FREE • NUT-FREE •

VEGETARIAN • WHEAT-FREE

This is a great way to green up eggs for your baby with a different texture and broader nutrients. Egg yolk seems to cause less reaction than a whole egg and is also a better source of iron than egg white. This is a vibrant and delicious meal on its own or a nice addition to some fruit purée. The spinach wilts beautifully and can add a little texture to the egg yolk.

½ tablespoon (7 mL) virgin coconut oil

1 egg yolk

¼ cup (60 mL) spinach, finely chopped or puréed

1. Heat the coconut oil in a small skillet over medium heat.

2. Add the egg yolk and spinach to the skillet and scramble until fully cooked. Let cool a bit and serve immediately.

NUTRITIONAL INFORMATION These eggs are a good source of vitamin A, vitamin B5, vitamin D, folate, phosphorus, potassium, selenium, choline, and iron.

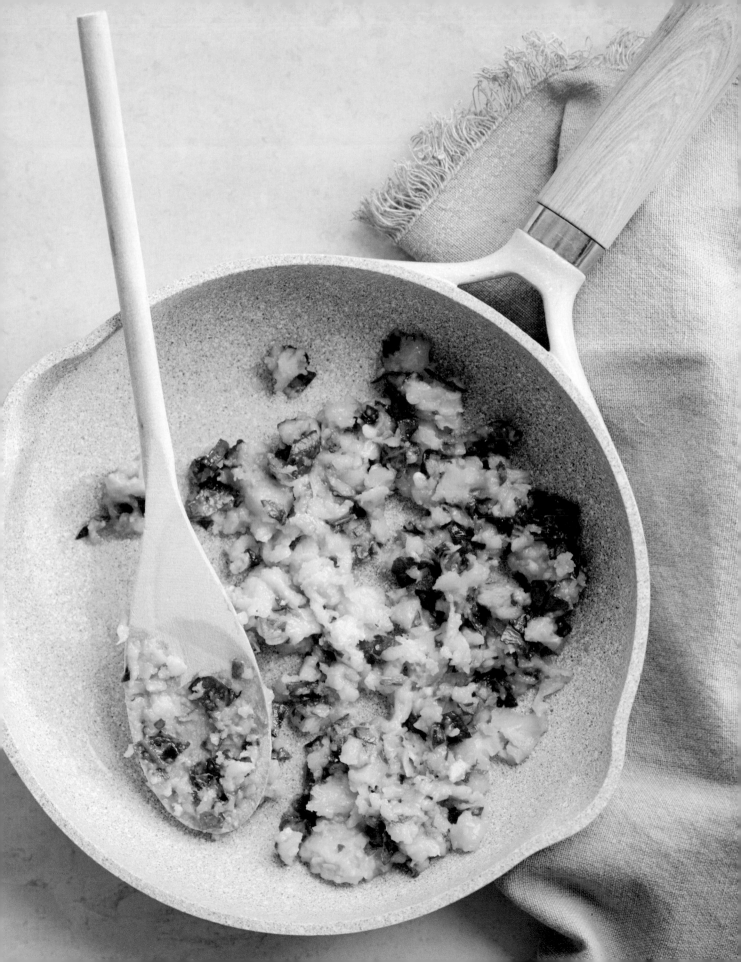

TOASTED COCONUT AMARANTH PORRIDGE MAKES 1½ CUPS (375 ML)

DAIRY-FREE • EGG-FREE • GLUTEN-FREE • NUT-FREE • VEGAN • VEGETARIAN • WHEAT-FREE

Amaranth is a very small gluten-free grain that's packed with nutrition and taste. Feel free to add any fruit purée to this porridge and create a whole new taste.

¼ cup (60 mL) unsweetened coconut flakes

1½ cups (375 mL) filtered water

½ cup (125 mL) organic amaranth

1 teaspoon (5 mL) ground cinnamon

½ cup (125 mL) full-fat canned coconut milk

1. Preheat the oven to 350°F (180°C). Line a rimmed baking sheet with parchment paper.

2. Spread the coconut flakes evenly on the baking sheet. Toast for 5 minutes or until the coconut is fragrant and golden brown.

3. Cool, and then grind the toasted coconut flakes to a coarse texture using a coffee grinder, small food processor, or blender (or skip this step if your baby loves texture).

4. In a small saucepan with a tight-fitting lid, bring the water to a boil. Add the amaranth and cinnamon. Reduce the heat to low and cover, simmering for 20 minutes or until the water is absorbed.

5. Remove the pan from the heat and stir in the coconut milk and toasted ground coconut flakes. Serve with 1 or 2 tablespoons (15 to 30 mL) of fruit purée, if desired.

TIP: Substitute Meat Broth (page 129) or Vegetable Broth (page 130) for the water for more nutrients and taste.

NUTRITIONAL INFORMATION This porridge is a good source of calcium, folate, iron, and fibre.

KALE, ONION, GARLIC, AND APPLE PURÉE

MAKES ABOUT 1 CUP (250 ML)

DAIRY-FREE • EGG-FREE • GLUTEN-FREE •
NUT-FREE • VEGAN • VEGETARIAN • WHEAT-FREE

The superfood kale packs a mineral punch that is swiftly followed by the immune-boosting garlic and onion and vitamin C–rich apple.

1 tablespoon (15 mL) virgin coconut oil
¼ cup (60 mL) red onion, finely chopped
1 clove garlic, minced
1 medium apple, peeled and chopped (Fuji, Gala, or Pink Lady)
Large handful of kale, stems removed and roughly chopped

1. Heat the coconut oil in a medium skillet over medium heat. Add the onion and cook until soft and translucent.
2. Add the garlic and apple and sauté for 5 minutes.
3. Top the mixture with the kale and continue to cook, covered, until the kale is soft and wilted.
4. Purée until the desired texture is achieved. Serve immediately.
5. Store in an airtight container in the fridge for up to 3 days or in the freezer in ice cube trays or baby-safe food containers for up to 3 months.

NUTRITIONAL INFORMATION This purée is a good source of vitamin C, vitamin K, calcium, potassium, magnesium, and phosphorus.

PARSNIP CHIPS WITH PAPRIKA

MAKES ABOUT 1 CUP (250 ML)

DAIRY-FREE • EGG-FREE • GLUTEN-FREE •
NUT-FREE • VEGAN • VEGETARIAN • WHEAT-FREE

These chips are perfect to introduce something crunchy to your baby. They're great for the rest of the family, too.

1 medium to large parsnip
½ cup (125 mL) virgin coconut oil
Sweet paprika

1. Peel the skin from the parsnip using a vegetable peeler and discard. Using the peeler, peel the rest of the parsnip into long, thin strips.
2. Heat the coconut oil in a small skillet over medium heat. Add the parsnip strips in small handfuls (be careful not to crowd them) and cook until golden brown and crisp.
3. Transfer the parsnip chips to a plate lined with a few layers of paper towel to drain. Sprinkle with paprika and serve once they've cooled slightly.
4. Store the chips in an airtight container in the fridge for up to 2 days.

NUTRITIONAL INFORMATION These chips are a good source of vitamin C, magnesium, phosphorus, calcium, choline, and folate.

CHICKEN PURÉE MAKES ABOUT 3 CUPS (750 ML)

DAIRY-FREE • EGG-FREE • GLUTEN-FREE • NUT-FREE • WHEAT-FREE

This is the perfect recipe for baby's first introduction to chicken. It includes a mix of protein and iron, along with fibre and great taste. Make sure you use dark meat, as it's higher in iron.

1 tablespoon (15 mL) extra virgin olive oil

1 small yellow onion, chopped

½ cup (125 mL) organic chicken (dark meat), cut into chunks

1 medium carrot, peeled and chopped into small cubes

1¼ cups (300 mL) sweet potato, peeled and chopped

1¼ cups (300 mL) filtered water

1. Heat the olive oil in a medium saucepan over medium heat. Add onion and sauté for 3 to 5 minutes until soft and transparent. Add the chicken and sauté for 3 to 5 minutes longer. Stir in the carrot, sweet potato, and water and bring to a boil.

2. Turn down the heat to low. Simmer, covered, for about 30 minutes or until chicken is cooked through and vegetables are fork-tender. Purée to the desired consistency.

3. Store the purée in an airtight container in the fridge for up to 3 days or in the freezer in ice cube trays or baby-safe food containers for up to 3 months.

TIP: **1.** You can substitute dark-meat turkey for the chicken. **2.** Substitute Meat Broth (page 129) or Vegetable Broth (page 130) for the water for more nutrients and taste.

NUTRITIONAL INFORMATION This purée is a good source of protein, fibre, niacin, phosphorus, calcium, iron, zinc, and vitamins B6, B12, C, and D.

BABY'S FIRST FISH

MAKES ABOUT 3 CUPS (750 ML)

DAIRY-FREE • EGG-FREE • GLUTEN-FREE •

NUT-FREE • WHEAT-FREE

I suggest introducing protein slowly. Fish is a potential allergen, so go especially slow with this one. For a tasty dish the whole family will enjoy, serve this fish before you purée it.

1 tablespoon (15 mL) extra virgin olive oil

1 medium yellow onion, chopped

2½ cups (625 mL) filtered water

1 cup (250 mL) brown rice, rinsed

¾ cup (175 mL) peas, fresh or frozen

1 medium carrot, peeled and chopped

¼ cup (60 mL) fresh flat-leaf or curly parsley or cilantro, chopped

1 clove garlic, minced

½ pound (225 g) cod, skinned, filleted, and cut into cubes

1. Heat the olive oil in a medium saucepan over medium heat. Add the onion and cook for 3 to 5 minutes until soft and translucent.
2. Stir in the water, rice, peas, carrot, parsley, and garlic. Bring to a simmer. After 15 minutes, add the cod. Simmer for an additional 15 minutes, or until the rice is tender.
3. Purée to the desired consistency.

TIP: **1.** Substitute haddock or sole for the cod for more nutrients and taste. **2.** Substitute Meat Broth (page 129) or Vegetable Broth (page 130) for the water for more nutrients and taste.

NUTRITIONAL INFORMATION This meal is a good source of protein, fibre, selenium, manganese, magnesium, B vitamins, omega-3 fatty acids, and vitamin D.

LENTIL, SWEET POTATO, AND RED PEPPER PURÉE

MAKES ABOUT 3 CUPS (750 ML)

DAIRY-FREE • EGG-FREE • GLUTEN-FREE •

NUT-FREE • VEGAN • VEGETARIAN • WHEAT-FREE

Lentils are a good source of protein and fibre. Try this recipe, before you purée it, for the rest of the family.

¼ cup (60 mL) virgin coconut oil

1 small leek, white part only, finely sliced

½ small sweet red pepper, chopped

½ medium sweet potato, peeled and diced

1 medium tomato, chopped

1 cup (250 mL) dry red lentils

1 cup (250 ml) filtered water

1. Heat the coconut oil in a large saucepan over medium-high heat. Add the leek and red pepper to the pan and cook until softened, about 5 to 7 minutes.
2. Add the sweet potato, tomato, lentils, and water, and bring to a boil. Reduce the heat to low, cover, and let simmer for 10 or 15 minutes, until the sweet potato is soft and the liquid has been absorbed by the lentils.
3. Using a hand blender or food processor, blend to desired consistency. Serve immediately.
4. Store the purée in an airtight container in the fridge for up to 3 days or in the freezer in ice cube trays or baby-safe food containers for up to 3 months.

TIP: Substitute Meat Broth (page 129) or Vegetable Broth (page 130) for the water for more nutrients and taste.

NUTRITIONAL INFORMATION This purée is a good source of vitamin A, vitamin C, calcium, potassium, phosphorus, and folate.

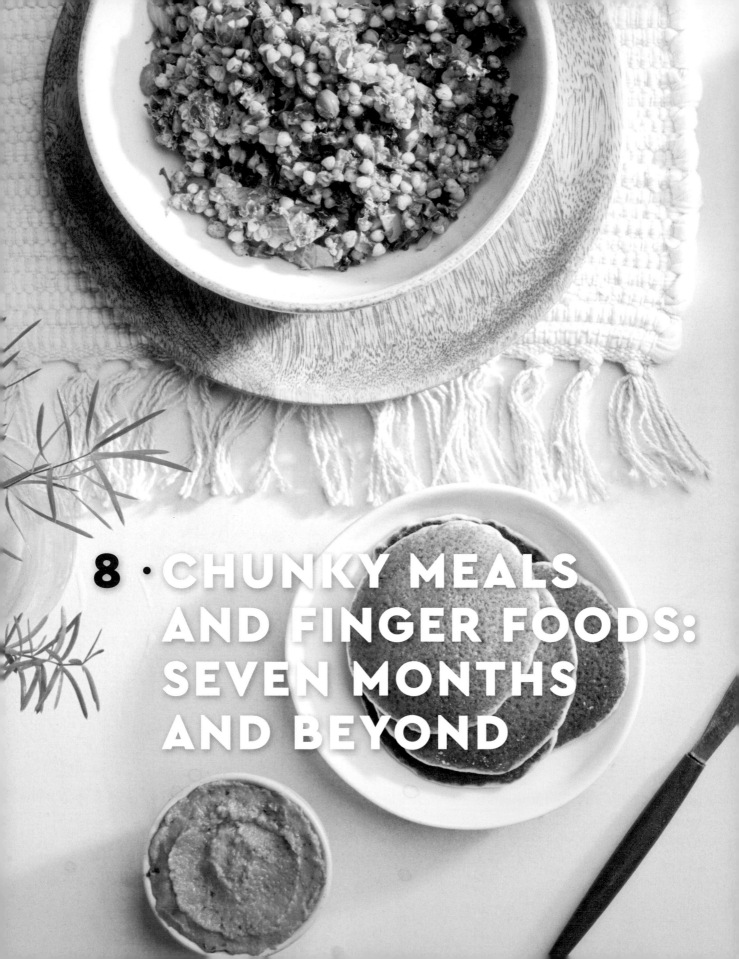

8 · CHUNKY MEALS AND FINGER FOODS: SEVEN MONTHS AND BEYOND

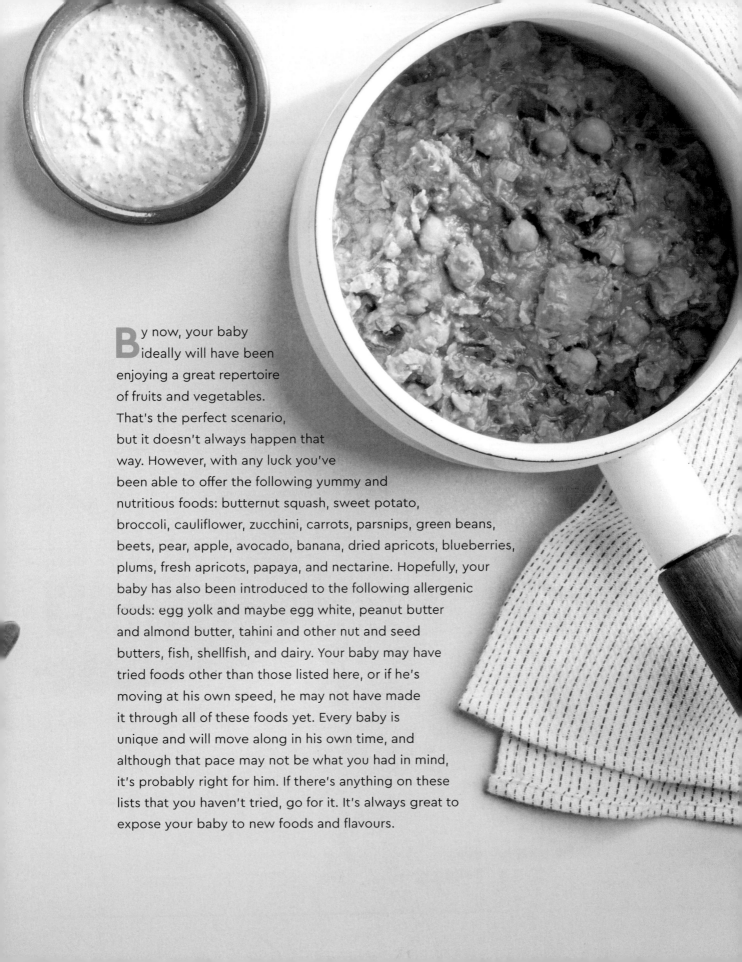

By now, your baby ideally will have been enjoying a great repertoire of fruits and vegetables. That's the perfect scenario, but it doesn't always happen that way. However, with any luck you've been able to offer the following yummy and nutritious foods: butternut squash, sweet potato, broccoli, cauliflower, zucchini, carrots, parsnips, green beans, beets, pear, apple, avocado, banana, dried apricots, blueberries, plums, fresh apricots, papaya, and nectarine. Hopefully, your baby has also been introduced to the following allergenic foods: egg yolk and maybe egg white, peanut butter and almond butter, tahini and other nut and seed butters, fish, shellfish, and dairy. Your baby may have tried foods other than those listed here, or if he's moving at his own speed, he may not have made it through all of these foods yet. Every baby is unique and will move along in his own time, and although that pace may not be what you had in mind, it's probably right for him. If there's anything on these lists that you haven't tried, go for it. It's always great to expose your baby to new foods and flavours.

WHAT TO DO AFTER PURÉE

If you've stuck with simple purées and some pieces of food using my Hybrid Feeding Method, chunkier meals with more texture and a wider variety of herbs and spices is the next step. You could start to purée the food you're making a bit less, leaving some chunks, lumps, or bumps in your scrumptious creation. If feeding then goes well, less puréeing of some foods is the new way forward. But you can continue to offer smooth purées as well, to vary the textures for baby. If your baby still gags with the slightest chunk, try again in another week, as the gag reflex needs to relax before lumpier food can pass.

Around eight to nine months of age or even earlier, new independence and skills bring a whole new meaning to mealtimes. You may see the pincer grip (first finger and thumb coming together) in action, with baby picking up small pieces of food, small objects, or even the smallest bit of fluff on the floor that you need a magnifying glass to see. Offering small pieces of food as well as larger, easy-to-hold pieces or spears helps your baby practise her hand–eye coordination. The pincer grip is a lot of fun but can lead to a great big mess. However, baby needs practice to master this new skill. Not all babies start with the pincer grip at nine months—some begin at eight months, others closer to ten months. Some babies start with the full-hand pickup, where they grab at some food on their plate or tray and try to get it into their mouths, with or without opening their hands (it's good for a laugh, that's for sure!). As baby gets older and these skills become more precise, she learns how to open her hand to grasp the food in a full-hand pickup—an important new understanding.

Most parents worry about their baby choking on chunky meals and finger foods, to the point where they might put off offering them. Choking is rare and not to be confused with gagging, which is very normal. Usually, this is when parents think about signing up for first aid training, which includes what to do in the case of choking— essential information for every parent. Now that you know what to do, you can offer new foods with more confidence if you're just starting.

There are certain foods I would suggest staying away from until your baby is much older, including small, round foods such as whole grapes (cut them into small pieces until baby is twelve to eighteen months old, and then just be mindful), but don't let fear stop you from allowing your baby to move toward chunkier foods and finger foods. Everyone needs to gain confidence when it comes to starting on finger foods, both parents and baby.

Gagging, the thrusting of food from the back of the throat forward into the mouth, is an important reflex to keep your baby from harm. And it works well in most circumstances, protecting your baby from a food she's not ready for.

The recipes for Super-Chunky Meals and Mashes in this chapter are suitable for babies who are ready for family meals, even if puréed. They are perfect for everyone to eat, including toddlers. All recipes can be puréed or mashed until baby is ready, and although it's scary to give more texture to your baby, it's an important step in her development.

HELP FOR GAGGING

Osteopathy can help with a premature or hyperactive gag reflex, which interestingly may have something to do with a forceps birth. If your baby has a really hard time swallowing lumps or bumps without gagging, find your nearest osteopath, ask if she treats babies and children, and make an appointment. Although offering purées (though not always smooth) for a long time can get a wider variety of nutrients into your child, having a strong reflex that leads to throwing up the whole meal isn't to his benefit. Osteopathy is a gentle, hands-on treatment that aims to release restriction and constriction so that normal function can resume.

FINGER FOODS—IF YOU'RE JUST STARTING

If you haven't offered any finger foods to your baby by nine months, get going, but start slowly. Putting finger foods on the high chair tray after a meal is a great way to start. Try placing a ¼-inch (5 mm) well-steamed piece of carrot, halved or quartered, in baby's mouth and see what happens. Steamed cauliflower pieces melt in the mouth (try it first yourself), so this is another good food to try. Some parents get very excited about self-feeding. Your baby independently feeding herself is excellent, alongside some mashed or puréed foods that offer a variety of ingredients. Some babies are more independent and want to feed themselves but can't self-feed with a spoon just yet. Keep practising. A problem arises when baby's food consumption drops because there's only so much she can feed herself at one sitting. You can also get a better variety of foods into a purée than onto the high chair tray. I commonly see a drop in baby's weight and a change in overall eating habits in this scenario, usually not for the better. Parents sometimes worry that their baby isn't getting what he needs because of the limited number of foods that can be offered safely in small pieces or as spear finger foods. That can lead to all sorts of new foods, including toast and cheese, becoming a staple because they're quick and easy. It's very difficult to get leafy greens into anything other than a purée at this stage. So, do what you can to keep purée a part of most meals for as long as you can—offer his main meal of purée first, then a few pieces of finger food to play with afterwards. Although there seems to be a mysterious pressure to steer your baby away from purée toward table foods, I'd rather see one-year-olds eating textured purées or soft foods, such as noodles mixed with a rainbow of coloured vegetables puréed as a sauce. Purée is also the perfect place to hide those fruits or vegetables that offer fantastic nutrition but are not well loved.

Another aspect of finger feeding is that it can be messy—food ends up all over baby, on the floor, or all over you, and you might feel that you're the one who needs the bib. Try to get over the need to be clean while eating. Feeling what happens to a handful of steamed broccoli when it's scooped up into a little hand and squished is good for the tactile senses. Clean your baby up at the end or have the bath ready for a full body wash.

This is the stage when avoiding cereals and grains becomes trickier, with peer pressure to give off-the-shelf foods that a friend's baby loves. But toast, bread, and other refined starches fill your baby up with less nutrient-dense foods that can be hard to digest because he may not yet be producing the digestive enzyme amylase at full strength.

My best tip at this stage is to stay out of the baby aisles at the supermarket. Foods that are marketed for babies are not necessarily the healthiest. Even the organic ones. One of the oldest baby cookies, Farley's Rusks, were first made in the United Kingdom by Heinz and are well known in other countries. An article published in *The Times* newspaper in England commented that the original biscuit "contains more sugar than McVitie's dark chocolate digestives," a cookie coated on one side with chocolate.[111] Baby Mum-Mums are another popular, well-marketed baby cracker available in Canada. The original rice rusk (read about arsenic and rice on page 119) was made of japonica rice, sugar, skim milk powder, and salt. Pause and think about those ingredients for a moment: *white rice, sugar, milk, and salt.* Whoever advised that these foods were appropriate for a baby? I believe that any doctor or dentist would agree that these ingredients are not beneficial for anyone—let alone your baby!

Other teething biscuits found in the baby aisle have attempted to use other sweeteners like fruit juice, syrup, or honey. If you must buy something packaged, do read all labels and assess the nutrition chart. Just as adults are quite partial to cookies and bars, your baby could get used to having Goldfish crackers or teething cookies as snacks and miss out on the good stuff. Your baby's stomach is only so big, and you want to fill it with nutritious food that will support her development and growth, not slow it down.

So, if you're going to stay out of the baby aisle in the supermarket, which finger foods are nutritious and safe? I've listed some suggestions below, with explanations so you'll know which foods are nutritious and which may be more useful for giving baby practice with his new self-feeding skills. Remember, when you're introducing a new food, try to wait four days before offering another new one if your baby has been sensitive in the past. Maintaining this practice can get complicated, but if you don't, it might be the one time that you'll see a reaction and won't know where it came from.

Sugar and the Immune System

Sugar slows down the body's ability to fight off infections, so it's best to avoid it when your baby has a cold or is teething, if not all the time as a preventive measure. When white blood cells are exposed to high levels of sugar in the bloodstream, they are less able to engulf bacteria and have weakened systemic resistance to all infections.

MORE CHALLENGING FINGER FOOD AND SELF-FEEDING SUGGESTIONS

Aim for as much organic food as possible, without any added refined sugar.

• Cut-up dried fruit: apple, apricots, and raisins. Dried fruit is very high in iron and makes an excellent snack. It has some texture and encourages chewing even if baby doesn't have teeth yet (the gums are quite powerful). Dried fruit also needs to be broken down with the gums or teeth to get the nutritional benefit. If you find that your raisins are too hard, soak them in boiling water for a few minutes to soften, and cool before serving. As your baby gets more teeth, be sure to give them a wipe or brush after eating dried fruit, as the fruit can stick between or in premolars or molars and cause cavities.

- Peas and beans: chickpeas (garbanzo beans); black-eyed peas; and adzuki, cannellini, kidney, black, navy, pinto, mung, and borlotti beans. Start slowly with these, as they pose a choking hazard, and remove the skin from chickpeas so baby doesn't choke on it. Squish with your fingers or mash with a fork to serve, offering small pieces to start. Eventually your baby will get the hang of round foods like green peas and enjoy them whole without any help.

The following recommendations are for cereal products that are gluten-free, sugar-free, and dairy-free.

- Rice Puffs cereal (Nature's Path): not rice crisps but puffs (organic, whole grain, and sugar-free). I call this the novice picker-upper food. These puffs melt in the mouth easily and are big enough to practise the pincer grip with. Nutritional value is limited, but they're a great practice tool.
- Millet Puffs cereal (Nature's Path): excellent for giving purée more texture, so add it to any purée you make. The puffs don't lose their shape when added to food, either. They're a bit too small to pick up with the fingers, but useful to keep your little one busy practising his pincer grip while you make dinner.
- Rice cakes (brown rice, salt-free, and organic): start by breaking off small pieces to eat. Then, as confidence grows, give half and then whole cakes. Try to find thin rice cakes at health food stores. Spread them with hummus or almond butter or even make a rice cake sandwich with apple butter or fruit juice–sweetened fruit spread, a healthier jam.
- Short-grain brown organic rice: there's a lot of texture here, so start by mixing it with a vegetable-rich purée. The rice alone can be put on baby's tray. It provides great nutrients, including B vitamins, iron, and fibre. Short-grain rice tends to be a bit stickier than long-grain rice, so it's easier for little fingers to pick up. Do read about rice and arsenic on page 119 if the few rice products listed here become fast favourites.
- Noodles made from brown rice, quinoa, beans, lentils, or amaranth. Start with penne or elbow macaroni and cut the tubes into smaller pieces. These can be added to a purée (my favourite is Lovely Lentils on page 165) or served plain as a finger food.

NEW FOODS ON THE MENU

As your baby grows, his digestive system continues to mature. You may feel a bit bored with your menu options of simpler fruits and vegetables, so here are a few new foods to jazz up mealtime if you haven't already given them a try.

- Legumes and beans such as chickpeas, kidney, adzuki, cannellini, and mung; split peas; and lentils open up a whole new world of possibilities. Red lentils are fantastic when added to any purée or soup at this stage. Cooking vegetables in a saucepan (as opposed to steaming them) with adequate water and a handful of rinsed red lentils increases the fibre, protein, and beta carotene content of any dish. Red lentils add a great texture because they don't maintain their shape as green lentils (also known as French or du Puy lentils) do.

- Chickpeas cook well in purées and can be mashed to make hummus. Once chickpeas have been offered in purée, you can start to give them as a finger food with care (they are a good size for choking).
- Whole egg is an excellent source of nutrients, including iron; zinc; calcium; magnesium; potassium; selenium; folic acid; vitamin B12; fat-soluble vitamins A, D, E, and K; essential fatty acids (from chickens fed with essential fatty acid–rich seeds); and cholesterol. The yolk has an exceptionally absorbable form of protein, second only to that found in breast milk, according to Dr. Sears.[112]

Eggs have been unfairly stigmatized as being high in cholesterol and possibly contributing to heart disease. This isn't completely true. The egg scare came about because of a study in the 1930s in which people consumed large quantities of dried egg powder. This was shown to raise cholesterol. But dried egg powder contains oxidized fat, which is rancid fat, and that is what raised the cholesterol levels. In subsequent studies, some people have been able to eat three fresh hardboiled eggs a day for thirty days without their cholesterol levels going up![113] So, giving eggs offers your baby a nutrient-packed food that's low in saturated fat. Choose organic eggs for your baby. Conventional chickens are usually given genetically modified (GM) feed (containing corn), which can pass into the egg and is then eaten by you or your baby. GM foods are a concern and continue to crop up in our food chain. Keep up to date with information from the Institute for Responsible Technology (www.responsibletechnology.org).

If you haven't yet introduced allergenic foods, start with egg yolk. Boil an egg for seven to eight minutes (add it to already boiling water) until it's completely cooked but not dried out and chalky. Cool, separate the white from the yolk, mash the yolk, and serve (see page 123 for the lipstick swipe introduction). You can also try mixing the yolk with a favourite purée, as in the Green Eggs recipe (page 148). Once you're sure there's no reaction, you can do an egg yolk scramble or omelette to vary the texture. If your baby has had a reaction to her vaccinations, offer a very small amount of egg yolk at first, as she may already have developed antibodies that will produce a reaction. Avoid egg white to start, as I've seen more reactions to the white than to the yolk. If you mix the two as in a scrambled egg and an issue arises, you'll have to avoid the whole egg.

Next are the nut and seed butters; peanut butter, almond butter, sesame seed butter (tahini), and sunflower seed butter are powerhouses of essential fatty acids; minerals such as calcium, magnesium, manganese, and zinc; and fibre and protein. In the form of raw butters, they offer a full spectrum of beneficial fats, whereas roasted or toasted butters have been heated, denaturing these good fats. Use them as a spread or add to purées to increase nutritional content and protein.

As with eggs, nuts and seeds have a higher allergic potential. Assess your own situation—if you have a family history of allergies or if your baby has eczema, for instance, proceed slowly. On first introduction, give a small amount of these butters without any other new food. Giving a small quantity allows the body the chance to react to a lesser degree, while ideally having a more desensitizing effect. If you introduce almond, sesame seed, or sunflower seed butter in a controlled situation, you'll be better able to assess the reaction than if your baby is exposed to it without your knowledge and you have no idea where the resulting rash has come from. The next ingestion might also cause more serious symptoms. See Chapter 5 for more on allergies.

Iron- and zinc-rich foods are important in the chunkier meals to continue to support the growth and maturation of tissues. Fibre, found in all fruits and vegetables, is encouraged to promote intestinal health and the colonization of good bacteria in the intestines. Daily bowel movements are essential for your baby's good health. Both herbs and spices boast a wide variety of important nutrients, not just extra flavour. If you haven't already, start adding some fresh or dried herbs to your baby's food for a new taste experience; try basil, oregano, rosemary, thyme, tarragon, cilantro, parsley, dill, and sage. Spice up simple purées or combined purées with cinnamon, coriander, cumin, curry powder, ginger, turmeric, paprika, and even saffron strands.

Iron-Rich Foods
- Beef, lamb, pork, chicken, and turkey (especially dark meat)
- Beans, chickpeas
- Potatoes (with skin)
- Pumpkin
- Peas, lentils
- Sweet potatoes
- Pasta
- Whole-grain bread
- Quinoa
- Dried apricots, dried peaches, figs, raisins
- Prunes and prune juice
- Nuts
- Tofu
- Blackstrap molasses
- Sunflower and pumpkin seeds

Zinc-Rich Foods
- Beef, lamb, poultry, pork, liver
- Egg yolks
- Milk products
- Fish and seafood
- Whole grains
- Beans
- Nuts
- Pumpkin seeds
- Peas, carrots, beets, cabbage (contain some zinc)

DRINK UP: MOVING ON TO A SIPPY CUP

I wrote about changing to a cup as your baby starts solids in Chapter 7 on first foods. Again, if you haven't made the switch yet, it's time to move to a sippy with or without a valve or a cup with a straw. Some sippy cups have a soft, chewy top, and others have a hard one. It really doesn't matter which you offer, though your baby might find one easier than the other. If the lid has a valve you can remove, put a small amount of water or broth in the cup, replace the lid without the valve, and demonstrate the cause and effect of tipping up the cup to get the water. Once you've tried that a couple of times, put the valve back in and let your baby practise. Not only is the suck required for a sippy cup different than that required for a bottle, but tipping up the cup takes some getting used to. If your baby already takes a bottle with formula or breast milk in it, think about transitioning to one of these cups. Some moms prefer to keep one type of vessel for specific fluids—a bottle for breast milk or formula and a sippy cup for water. It's a better idea for the reasons I outline on page 120. You don't want to take away from the quantity your baby's drinking of either breast milk or formula, as it's still the main source of nutrition, even on an expanded diet offering a wide variety of foods.

THE WATER DEBATE

Water is such a simple thing, or it should be. But H2O has become as confusing as what food to start feeding your baby. Bottled, tap, distilled, spring, reverse osmosis, oxygenated, carbonated, and vitaminized water are all available to choose from. With so many options, how on earth do you decide what's best to serve your baby?

Most tap water is under strict scrutiny for any contaminants that may harm us, and local water authorities boast about how clean and safe it is. In most cases, I would agree. However, if you live in a house built earlier than the 1950s, it may still have pipes soldered with lead. In March 2001, Dr. Richard Mass, a scientist and internationally renowned specialist who studies lead in water, was interviewed on CBC's *Marketplace*; the program's researchers also did their own testing for lead in tap water across Canada. They found varying levels of lead in houses built before as well as after 1970.[114] Samples were taken from water that had been flushed (or run from the tap) for three minutes. Dr. Mass suggested that running the tap eliminates the standing lead level, and that it's the standing lead level that gives a more accurate measurement. Running the tap before filling up your glass may work first thing in the morning, but this needs to happen each time you turn on the tap, as 30 percent of the lead deposited in your water overnight makes its way into your tap water if the tap hasn't been allowed to run for ten minutes.

There's no safe level of lead exposure for anyone, at any age. However, infants and children are most at risk because the first years are such a crucial time of development. Dr. Mass noted on *Marketplace*, "We recognize now that there is no threshold dose below which lead does not cause neurologic damage."[115] Lead toxicity has a cumulative effect, causing neurological disorders, learning difficulties, emotional instability, aggression, decreased calcium deposition into bone, low sperm count, and sterility; as well, it has an antagonistic effect on important minerals such as zinc and iron, possibly leading to anemia. Wait times to have your water tested for lead can be lengthy, but it's important nonetheless. Contact your local water provider for further details.

Chlorine is used to clean our tap water, ridding it of disease-causing bacteria and making it safe to drink. Or does it? Chlorine has solved one problem but created another. Chlorine in tap water has been associated with asthma, eczema, and higher rates of miscarriage and birth defects. Chlorine also kills the beneficial bacteria in the gut, leading to the potential for digestive and immune problems. Bottled water and filters of all kinds have become more popular in recent years. It's worth investigating what's in your tap water and the different types of filter systems available. I recommend using at least a carbon filter to remove some chlorine and other contaminants.

For your baby, avoid distilled water, which has no trace minerals and thus might contribute to deficiencies of certain minerals. Reverse osmosis, with calcium and magnesium added after filtering, is my preferred method of cleaning water. It's safe and easy and doesn't require boiling or filtering. See the Resources page on SproutRight.com for recommendations.

WATER VERSUS JUICE

Your baby needs only two types of fluids at this stage—breast milk or formula and water—which provide most of her nourishment and hydration. I strongly encourage you to avoid giving juice to your baby until absolutely necessary. That may be closer to two years of age, if at all. If you feel that your baby is dehydrated and needs extra fluids during sickness, very hot weather, or a bout of constipation, add only a splash of juice to the sippy cup. Juice is a concentrated source of sweetness without fibre, and your baby just doesn't need it.

CHUNKY MEALS FEEDING CHART

Use the following table as a guideline to help you create a milk and solids schedule as you introduce some of the recipes that follow. It shows how to introduce and test new, textured purées for five days—in this case, lentil purée. All food eaten at other meals should already have been tested and be on the safe list. Offer water in a sippy cup throughout the day, and continue to give either breast milk or formula upon rising and at bedtime.

	BREAKFAST	SLEEP	LUNCH	SLEEP	DINNER
Day 1	Avocado and Pear Purée (page 144), Blueberry Purée (page 133), or Banana Purée (page 134)	Milk*	Milk + Lovely Lentils (page 165)	Milk	Milk + Zucchini Purée (page 138) mixed with amaranth or millet puffs
Day 2	Pea and Mint Purée (page 143)	Milk	Milk + Broccoli Purée (page 135) mixed with quinoa puffs	Milk	Milk + Lovely Lentils (page 165)
Day 3	Sweet Potato Purée (page 136) with cinnamon	Milk	Lovely Lentils (page 165)	Milk	Broccoli Purée (page 135) or Green Bean Purée (page 141) and Dried Apricot Purée (page 136)
Day 4	Lovely Lentils (page 165)	Milk	Milk + Green Bean Purée (page 141)	Milk	Avocado and Pear Purée (page 133)
Day 5	Oat Cereal (page 142) mixed with Spiced-Up Apples (page 177)	Milk	Lovely Lentils (page 165)	Milk	Carrot and Parsnip Purée (page 147)

Milk is either breast milk or formula.

RECEIPES

CHUNKY PURÉES AND MASHES

SUPER-CHUNKY MEALS AND MASHES

LOVELY LENTILS MAKES ABOUT 3 CUPS (750 ML)

DAIRY-FREE • EGG-FREE • GLUTEN-FREE • NUT-FREE • VEGAN • VEGETARIAN • WHEAT-FREE

Red lentils are super easy to cook with and will keep your baby going. For toddlers, you can serve this purée as a sauce for noodles. It's wonderful on its own, mixed with rice, or served as a soup for mom and dad with extra lentils and broth.

2 cups (500 mL) peeled and chopped
   butternut squash

2 cups (500 mL) filtered water

½ cup (125 mL) red lentils, rinsed well

3 medium carrots, peeled and chopped

2 stalks celery, chopped

1 small yellow onion, chopped

1 tablespoon (15 mL) extra virgin olive oil

1 to 2 tablespoon (15 to 30 mL) chopped fresh
   flat-leaf or curly parsley

Handful of baby spinach, roughly chopped
   (optional)

1. Combine the squash, water, lentils, carrot, celery, onion, and olive oil in a medium saucepan.

2. Bring to a boil, cover, and reduce heat to low. Simmer with the lid on until vegetables are fork-tender, about 20 minutes.

3. Mash or purée with parsley and spinach (if using) to desired consistency.

4. Store the purée in an airtight container in the fridge for up to 3 days or in the freezer in ice cube trays or baby-safe food containers for up to 3 months.

TIP: Substitute Meat Broth (page 129) or Vegetable Broth (page 130) for the water for more nutrients and taste.

NUTRITIONAL INFORMATION These lentils are a good source of protein, beta carotene, fibre, potassium, and vitamins C and E.

CHEEKY CHICKPEAS MAKES ABOUT 3 CUPS (750 ML)

DAIRY-FREE • EGG-FREE • GLUTEN-FREE • NUT-FREE • VEGAN • VEGETARIAN • WHEAT-FREE

This is an absolute favourite of both babies and parents. The variety of flavours, including onion, cilantro, and lemon, will have your baby's taste buds awake and dancing! It's a firm favourite and a staple for many families.

1½ cups (375 mL) filtered water

1 can (14 ounces/398 mL) chickpeas, drained and rinsed

2 medium sweet potatoes, peeled and chopped into small cubes

1 small onion, finely chopped

2 stalks celery, chopped

1 medium carrot, peeled and chopped into small cubes

1 tablespoon (15 mL) extra virgin olive oil

2 tablespoons (30 mL) chopped fresh cilantro (or 1 teaspoon/5 mL dried)

1 teaspoon (5 mL) fresh lemon juice

1. Combine the water, chickpeas, sweet potatoes, onion, celery, carrot, and olive oil in a medium saucepan.

2. Bring to a boil, cover, and reduce heat to low. Simmer with the lid on until vegetables are fork-tender, about 20 minutes.

3. Remove from the heat and add the cilantro and lemon juice. Mash or purée to desired consistency, adding water if necessary.

4. Store the purée in an airtight container in the fridge for up to 3 days or in the freezer in ice cube trays or baby-safe food containers for up to 3 months.

TIP: Substitute Meat Broth (page 129) or Vegetable Broth (page 130) for the water for more nutrients and taste.

NUTRITIONAL INFORMATION Chickpeas, or garbanzo beans, are a good source of folate, manganese, fibre, protein, and copper.

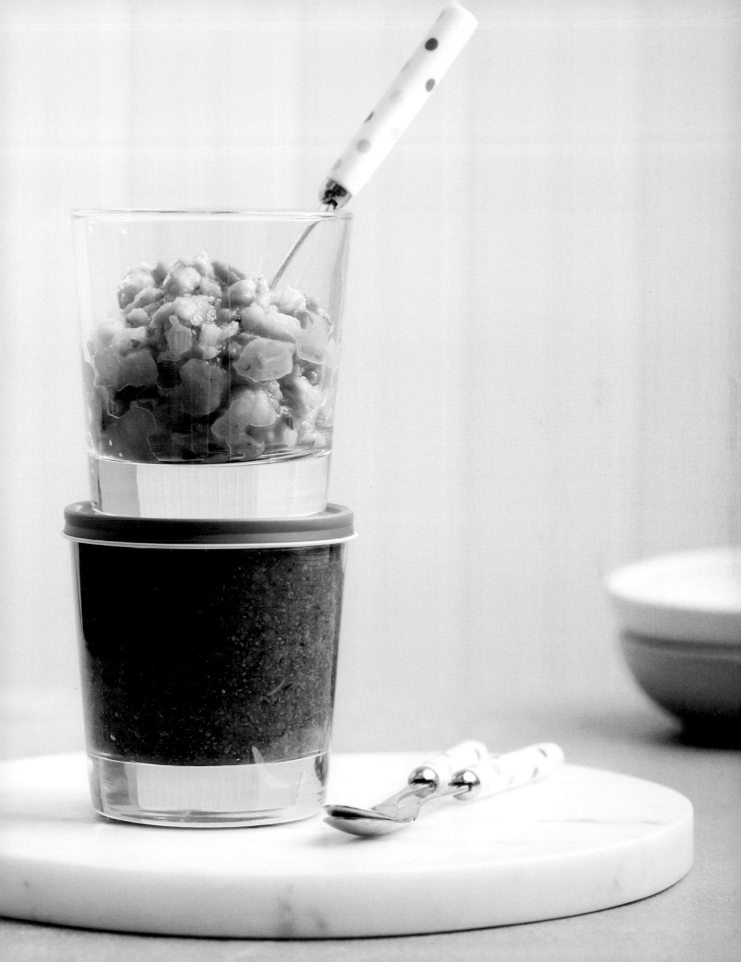

AMAZING SWEET AMARANTH MAKES ABOUT 3 CUPS (750 ML)

DAIRY-FREE • EGG-FREE • GLUTEN-FREE • NUT-FREE • VEGAN • VEGETARIAN • WHEAT-FREE

This is what adults would consider a hot breakfast cereal. It's not just for babies; I still make this purée for myself by simply keeping the skin on the fruit and not puréeing.
The sweetness of the fruit combined with cinnamon and ginger is warming and delicious!

2 cups (500 mL) filtered water

1 cup (250 mL) amaranth, rinsed in a fine-mesh sieve

2 pears, peeled, cored, and chopped

2 apples (Fuji, Gala, or Pink Lady), peeled, cored, and chopped

¼ cup (60 mL) frozen blueberries

1 teaspoon (5 mL) ground cinnamon

1½-inch (4 cm) piece fresh ginger, finely chopped or grated

1. Add the water, amaranth, pear, apple, blueberries, cinnamon, and ginger to a medium saucepan.
2. Bring to a boil, cover, and reduce the heat to low. Simmer, stirring often, until the amaranth is tender, about 20 minutes.
3. Purée to desired consistency or leave chunky.
4. Store the purée in an airtight container in the fridge for up to 3 days or in the freezer in ice cube trays or baby-safe food containers for up to 3 months.

TIP: **1.** Amaranth has a sticky texture, and care should be taken not to overcook it, as it can become gummy. After this dish is frozen or refrigerated, you'll need to add more water to thin it out when reheating. **2.** Substitute Meat Broth (page 129) or Vegetable Broth (page 130) for the water for more nutrients and taste.

NUTRITIONAL INFORMATION Botanically, amaranth isn't really a grain, but it has the nutritional profile of one. It surpasses whole wheat in calories, protein, iron, zinc, copper, and nearly all nutrients and is the grain highest in folic acid, calcium, and vitamin E. Also, like wheat, amaranth is rich in the amino acid lysine. It even contains a bit of vitamin C. It also has three times as much calcium as a glass of milk!

IMMUNE-BOOSTING PURÉE MAKES ABOUT 2½ CUPS (625 ML)

DAIRY-FREE • EGG-FREE • GLUTEN-FREE • NUT-FREE • VEGAN • VEGETARIAN • WHEAT-FREE

This dish is incredibly popular with the whole family. Serve some to baby and have the rest as a side with your dinner. The vitamin C in the apples and turnip or rutabaga helps the absorption of iron from the raisins, and garlic is an incredible immune booster. A parent told me that she served this with Thanksgiving dinner and everyone loved it!

1½ cups (375 mL) filtered water

2 apples (Fuji, Gala, or Pink Lady), peeled and chopped into small cubes

1 large turnip or medium rutabaga, peeled and chopped into small cubes

1 medium parsnip, peeled and chopped into small cubes

1 medium carrot, peeled and chopped into small cubes

1 clove garlic, chopped

2 tablespoons (30 mL) Thompson raisins

1. Add the water, apple, turnip or rutabaga, parsnip, carrot, garlic, and raisins to a medium saucepan.

2. Simmer for 30 to 40 minutes or until tender, adding extra water if necessary. Mash or purée to desired consistency.

3. Store the purée in an airtight container in the fridge for up to 3 days or in the freezer in ice cube trays or baby-safe food containers for up to 3 months.

TIP: Substitute Meat Broth (page 129) or Vegetable Broth (page 130) for the water for more nutrients and taste.

NUTRITIONAL INFORMATION This purée is a good source of vitamin C, fibre, calcium, potassium, and iron.

COLOURFUL QUINOA MAKES ABOUT 4 CUPS (1 L)

DAIRY-FREE • EGG-FREE • GLUTEN-FREE • NUT-FREE • VEGAN • VEGETARIAN • WHEAT-FREE

Quinoa makes a savoury but sweet purée with quite a bit of texture. Set some aside before puréeing for the rest of the family to enjoy as a meal or a side dish.

2 cups (500 mL) filtered water

1 cup (250 mL) quinoa, rinsed well

1 medium butternut squash, peeled
  and chopped

4 asparagus spears, ends broken
  off and chopped

6 pitted prunes, chopped

2 tablespoons (30 mL) chopped fresh parsley
  (or 1 teaspoon/5 mL dried)

1 garlic clove, chopped

1. Combine all ingredients in a medium saucepan, bring to a boil, cover, and reduce the heat to low. Simmer for 30 to 40 minutes or until soft.

2. Remove from heat and let cool. For a mushier consistency, add a bit of extra water at the end, stir, and let it be absorbed as the quinoa cools. Mash or purée to desired consistency.

3. Store the purée in an airtight container in the fridge for up to 3 days or in the freezer in ice cube trays or baby-safe food containers for up to 3 months.

TIP: **1.** Substitute Meat Broth (page 129) or Vegetable Broth (page 130) for the water for more nutrients and taste. **2.** Substitute 1 cup (250 mL) chopped green beans for the asparagus.

NUTRITIONAL INFORMATION This purée is a good source of protein, calcium, phosphorus, iron, and vitamins B and E.

SWEET POTATO WITH CORN AND RED PEPPER

MAKES ABOUT 3 CUPS (750 ML)

DAIRY-FREE • EGG-FREE • GLUTEN-FREE •
NUT-FREE • VEGAN • VEGETARIAN • WHEAT-FREE

This intriguing purée has a richness from the blackstrap molasses and a sweetness from the corn and red pepper. It's a powerhouse of nutrients, antioxidants, and immune-boosting properties.

2 medium sweet potatoes, peeled and
  chopped into cubes
1 cup (250 mL) fresh or frozen corn kernels
½ sweet red pepper, seeded and chopped
1 tablespoon (15 mL) blackstrap molasses

1. Steam the sweet potato for about 15 minutes.
2. Add the corn and red pepper. Continue to steam until the vegetables are fork-tender, about 5 minutes.
3. Transfer the vegetables to a bowl. Mix in the molasses and mash or purée to desired consistency, adding water if necessary.
4. Store the purée in an airtight container in the fridge for up to 3 days or in the freezer in ice cube trays or baby-safe food containers for up to 3 months.

NUTRITIONAL INFORMATION This purée is a good source of vitamin B1, vitamin B5, folate, fibre, vitamin C, phosphorus, manganese, iron, calcium, copper, magnesium, and potassium.

STEAMED VEGETABLE FINGER FOODS

DAIRY-FREE • EGG-FREE • GLUTEN-FREE •
NUT-FREE • VEGAN • VEGETARIAN • WHEAT-FREE

Steamed vegetables make healthy and tasty finger foods for your baby. Remember, enjoying pieces of food at mealtime is a learning experience and a way for babies to practise their pincer grip, as opposed to the full-hand grab, so expect a lot to land everywhere but in their mouth!

Your choice of:
Broccoli, stem peeled to remove outer
  fibrous layer (use the stem and florets)
Carrots
Cauliflower, stem removed
Beets
Green beans
Asparagus, ends trimmed

1. Peel or scrub the vegetables of your choice and chop them into pieces that are easy to pick up with little fingers.
2. Steam until tender.
3. Leftover vegetables can be frozen in ice cube trays or on a baking sheet, then transferred to a freezer storage bag. To use frozen vegetables, defrost them in the fridge overnight or drop a handful into boiled water and cook until thawed. Drain and serve.

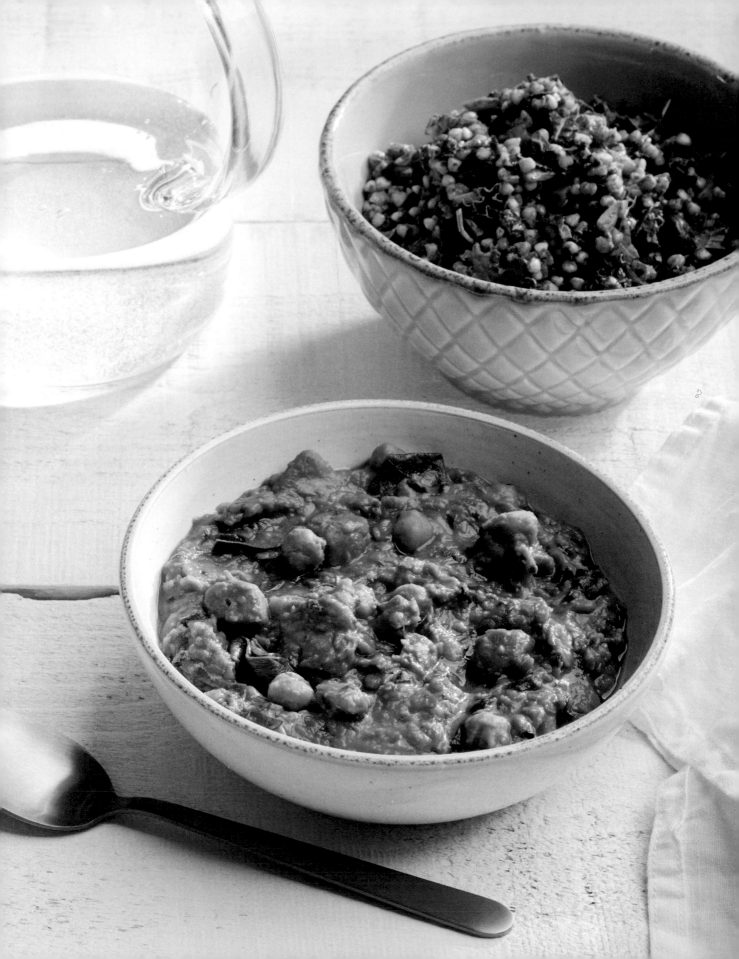

DELICIOUS LENTIL DHAL MAKES 4 CUPS (1 L)

DAIRY-FREE • EGG-FREE • GLUTEN-FREE • NUT-FREE • VEGAN • VEGETARIAN • WHEAT-FREE

Many people are surprised that their babies can eat spices like turmeric and cumin, but these add wonderful flavours—and turmeric is an anti-inflammatory, too. Parents can eat this served over brown rice with a dollop of yogurt.

3 cups (750 mL) filtered water

1 cup (250 mL) red lentils, rinsed well

1 medium sweet potato, chopped into small cubes

1 small yellow onion, finely chopped

1 tablespoon (30 mL) extra virgin olive oil

1 teaspoon (5 mL) ground turmeric

1 teaspoon (5 mL) ground cumin

1 clove garlic, minced

Handful of fresh cilantro leaves

1 cup (250 mL) packed baby spinach, finely chopped

2 Swiss chard leaves, finely chopped

1 can (14 ounces/398 mL) chickpeas, drained and rinsed

1. Combine the water, lentils, sweet potato, onion, olive oil, turmeric, cumin, garlic, and cilantro in a medium saucepan. Bring to a boil, cover, and reduce heat to low. Simmer for about 20 minutes.

2. Add the spinach and Swiss chard and simmer for 2 minutes longer. Stir in the chickpeas and simmer for an additional 3 minutes. Leave chunky or purée slightly to desired consistency.

3. Store the purée in an airtight container in the fridge for up to 3 days or in the freezer in ice cube trays or in baby-safe food containers for up to 3 months.

TIP: Substitute Meat Broth (page 129) or Vegetable Broth (page 130) for the water for more nutrients and taste.

NUTRITIONAL INFORMATION This dhal is a good source of vitamin C, vitamin A, magnesium, calcium, potassium, protein, and fibre.

FRUITY CURRY BUCKWHEAT MAKES ABOUT 3 CUPS (750 ML)

DAIRY-FREE • EGG-FREE • GLUTEN-FREE • NUT-FREE • VEGAN • VEGETARIAN • WHEAT-FREE

Don't let the curry powder keep you from making this dish for your baby—it's deliciously sweet, and babies love it! Containing buckwheat, this gluten-free purée is easy to digest and a very good source of protein, B vitamins, iron, and calcium. Use buckwheat groats, not toasted buckwheat or kashi.

2 to 2½ cups (500 to 625 mL) filtered water

3 nectarines or 1 large mango, finely chopped

⅓ cup (75 mL) Thompson raisins or sultanas

½ medium yellow onion, finely chopped

1 clove garlic, finely chopped

1 to 2 teaspoons (5 to 10 mL) curry powder

1 to 2 teaspoons (5 to 10 mL) ground cinnamon

1 cup (250 mL) buckwheat groats, rinsed

2 curly kale leaves, stems removed and finely chopped

1. In a medium saucepan, combine the water, nectarine, raisins, onion, garlic, curry powder, and cinnamon. Bring to a boil, then stir in the buckwheat and kale.

2. Simmer, stirring frequently, for about 10 minutes or until the buckwheat is soft. The mixture can be left chunky or puréed for a smoother texture.

3. Store in an airtight container in the fridge for up to 3 days or in the freezer in ice cube trays or baby-safe food containers for up to 1 month.

TIP: Substitute Meat Broth (page 129) or Vegetable Broth (page 130) for the water for more nutrients and taste.

NUTRITIONAL INFORMATION Buckwheat is a gluten-free grain from the rhubarb family. It contains protein and B vitamins and is rich in phosphorus, potassium, iron, and calcium.

BEAN AND RICE SURPRISE STEW MAKES ABOUT 3 CUPS (750 ML)

DAIRY-FREE • EGG-FREE • GLUTEN-FREE • NUT-FREE • VEGAN • VEGETARIAN • WHEAT-FREE

This recipe creates a more challenging texture, which is perfect for self-feeding and great for the whole family. The combination of beans and rice makes this dish a complete protein.

2 cups (500 mL) filtered water

½ cup (125 mL) brown rice, rinsed

½ cup (125 mL) chickpeas or adzuki beans, rinsed

1 medium carrot, peeled and chopped

1 stalk celery, chopped

1 to 2 kale leaves, stems removed and finely chopped

1 small yellow onion, finely chopped

1 clove garlic, minced

1 medium sweet potato, peeled and chopped

1 tablespoon (15 mL) fresh flat-leaf or curly parsley, or cilantro

1. Combine all ingredients in a medium saucepan and bring to a boil. Cover and simmer until the rice is cooked and the vegetables are fork-tender, about 25 to 30 minutes. Leave chunky, mash, or purée slightly to desired consistency.
2. Store this dish in an airtight container in the fridge for up to 3 days or in the freezer in ice cube trays or baby-safe food containers for up to 3 months.

TIP: Substitute Meat Broth (page 129) or Vegetable Broth (page 130) for the water for more nutrients and taste.

NUTRITIONAL INFORMATION This stew is high in fibre, protein, manganese, potassium, iron, B vitamins, vitamin A, and vitamin C.

BROWN RICE PUDDING   MAKES ABOUT 3 CUPS (750 ML)

DAIRY-FREE • EGG-FREE • GLUTEN-FREE • NUT-FREE • VEGAN • VEGETARIAN • WHEAT-FREE

This is a rich, warming, and delicious dish. It's sweet but has a contrasting nuttiness from the short-grain brown rice. Making it with coconut milk keeps it dairy-free for those with sensitivities and those who want to limit their dairy intake. It can be served as a meal or as a dessert.

1½ cups (375 mL) filtered water

¾ cup (175 mL) short-grain brown rice, rinsed

1 can (14 ounces/398 mL) coconut milk

¾ cup (175 mL) vanilla rice milk

6 unsulphured dried apricots, chopped

2 tablespoons (30 mL) chopped Thompson raisins or sultanas

1 teaspoon (5 mL) ground cinnamon

One ¾-inch (2 cm) piece fresh ginger, peeled

1. In a medium saucepan, bring the water and rice to a boil. Cover and simmer until all the water is absorbed and the rice is nearly cooked. **2.** Add the coconut milk, rice milk, apricots, raisins, cinnamon, and ginger to the saucepan and bring to a boil. Reduce the heat and simmer, stirring often, until the mixture thickens and the rice is tender, about 10 to 15 minutes. **3.** Remove the ginger and serve or freeze in a container for up to 1 month.

TIP: **1.** Substitute Meat Broth (page 129) or Vegetable Broth (page 130) for the water for more nutrients and taste. **2.** Use California rice, as it's lower in arsenic (see page 119).

NUTRITIONAL INFORMATION Brown rice is a whole grain that's a great source of fibre, manganese, selenium, magnesium, and B vitamins.

FABULOUS FRESH FRUIT PURÉE

MAKES 2 CUPS (500 ML)

DAIRY-FREE • EGG-FREE • GLUTEN-FREE •

NUT-FREE • VEGAN • VEGETARIAN • WHEAT-FREE

This fresh, raw purée is super yummy and sure to please. Mom can make a little extra for herself and add some milk and protein powder for a healthy breakfast or snack. This is also a great purée to sneak some raw garlic into, if baby is getting sick. Garlic is incredibly immune boosting, and hiding it in this dish is a great way to support baby's immunity.

1 ripe avocado

1 ripe pear, cored

1 large ripe banana

⅔ cup (150 mL) frozen wild blueberries

1. Cut the avocado in half, remove the pit, and spoon out the flesh. Cut the pear and banana into 1-inch (2.5 cm) pieces. Purée all ingredients in a food processor or with a hand blender until smooth.

2. Store the purée in an airtight container in the fridge for up to 2 days or in the freezer in ice cube trays or baby-safe food containers for up to 2 weeks.

TIP: To increase the texture, purée ½ cup (125 mL) of the blueberries and simply stir in the rest.

NUTRITIONAL INFORMATION This purée is a good source of fibre, vitamin C, potassium, folic acid, and vitamin E.

SPICED-UP APPLES

MAKES ABOUT 2 CUPS (500 ML)

DAIRY-FREE • EGG-FREE • GLUTEN-FREE •

NUT-FREE • VEGAN • VEGETARIAN • WHEAT-FREE

This is a great purée to add to plain, organic or grass-fed full-fat yogurt. For a subtle twist, try replacing half of the apples with pears.

8 medium apples (Gala, Fuji, or Pink Lady)

½ teaspoon (2 mL) ground cinnamon

¼ teaspoon (1 mL) grated lemon zest or juice

Pinch of ground ginger

Pinch of ground nutmeg (optional)

1. Peel, core, and chop the apples into small cubes.

2. Steam the apple until fork-tender.

3. Transfer the apple to a bowl and stir in the cinnamon, lemon zest, ginger, and nutmeg (if using). Purée to desired consistency.

4. Store the purée in an airtight container in the fridge for up to 3 days or in the freezer in ice cube trays or baby-safe food containers for up to 3 months.

NUTRITIONAL INFORMATION This purée is a good source of fibre, vitamin C, and flavonoids.

FINGER FOOD PANCAKES MAKES ABOUT 24 MINI PANCAKES

DAIRY-FREE • EGG-FREE • GLUTEN-FREE • NUT-FREE • VEGAN • VEGETARIAN • WHEAT-FREE

This is a great recipe that the whole family can enjoy either as finger food or dipped in Yummy Carrot Spread (page 180) or Delicious Lentil Dhal (page 173). Older kids will love this for breakfast, drizzled with maple syrup. These pancakes freeze well and can be stored in the freezer for up to 2 weeks. For a slightly different flavour, replace the rice milk with vanilla unsweetened almond milk.

1 cup (250 mL) brown rice flour

¼ cup (60 mL) potato starch

¼ cup (60 mL) tapioca starch

2 teaspoons (10 mL) baking powder

1 tablespoon (15 mL) ground chia seeds
  or powder

1 egg

1 cup (250 mL) vanilla unsweetened rice milk

2½ tablespoons (37 mL) pure maple syrup

3 tablespoons (45 mL) sunflower oil, plus
  more for cooking

1. In a medium bowl, stir together the brown rice flour, potato starch, tapioca starch, baking powder, and ground chia seeds.
2. In a small bowl, whisk together the egg, rice milk, and maple syrup. Slowly whisk in the sunflower oil. Add the wet ingredients to the dry ingredients and mix thoroughly.
3. Heat a medium skillet or griddle over medium-high heat and lightly coat with sunflower oil. Pour 1 tablespoon (15 mL) batter per pancake into the frying pan. Cook each side of the pancakes until golden brown.
4. The pancakes can be stored in an airtight container in the fridge for 3 days or in the freezer for up to 2 weeks.

TIP: **1.** For an egg-free option, replace the egg with 3 tablespoons (45 mL) water mixed with 1 tablespoon (15 mL) ground flaxseed. Let sit for a few minutes and add to the wet ingredients. This vegan option produces a gummier texture, but the pancakes are still delicious. This can also be made with only egg yolk if your baby is sensitive to egg white. **2.** Sprinkle cinnamon into the batter and serve the pancakes with fruit purée. Or try adding grated carrot to the batter for some extra vegetable power.

NUTRITIONAL INFORMATION Chia seeds are one of nature's superfoods. They are a complex protein offering all eight amino acids, and they are also high in fibre, omega-3 and omega-6 fatty acids, calcium, iron, folate, potassium, magnesium, and antioxidants. Grinding them just before use, rather than purchasing ground chia seeds, helps to minimize oxidation of fats and nutrients.

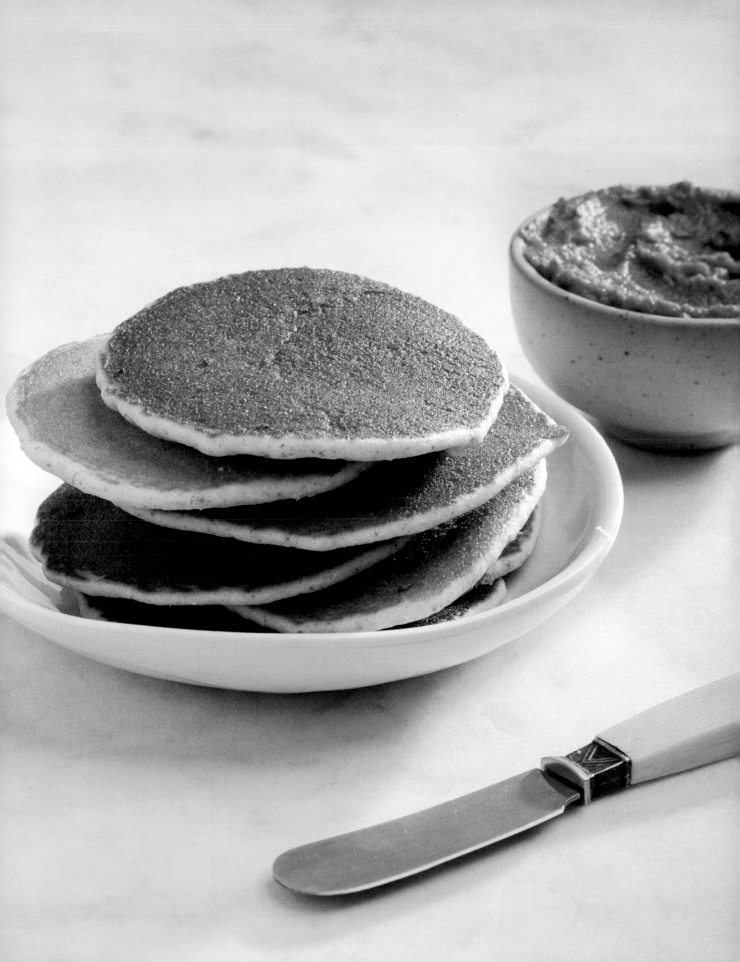

YUMMY CARROT SPREAD MAKES ABOUT 1½ CUPS (375 ML)

DAIRY-FREE • EGG-FREE • GLUTEN-FREE • NUT-FREE • VEGAN • VEGETARIAN • WHEAT-FREE

This is a very versatile spread that can be eaten straight up or spread over Finger Food Pancakes (page 178) or rice cakes. For toddlers, serve it as a dip with raw veggies and crackers. This also makes a great sandwich spread that the whole family will enjoy.

8 medium carrots, peeled and diced

1 clove garlic

1 tablespoon (15 mL) tahini or sunflower
  seed butter

1 tablespoon (15 mL) chopped fresh cilantro
  or basil

1 tablespoon (15 mL) extra virgin olive or
  flaxseed oil

1 teaspoon (5 mL) fresh lemon juice

1. Steam the carrots until fork-tender. Remove from the heat and let cool for a few minutes.

2. In a small bowl, combine the carrot with the garlic, tahini, cilantro, olive oil, and lemon juice. Purée until the consistency of a slightly chunky spread.

3. Best consumed within 3 days, this purée can also be frozen, although the texture may change slightly. Freeze in ice cube trays or baby-safe food containers for up to 1 month.

NUTRITIONAL INFORMATION Carrots are an excellent source of antioxidant compounds and the richest vegetable source of the pro–vitamin A carotenes.

BEANY GREEN DIP MAKES ABOUT 1½ CUPS (375 ML)

DAIRY-FREE • EGG-FREE • GLUTEN-FREE • NUT-FREE • VEGAN • VEGETARIAN • WHEAT-FREE

This dip is bursting with fresh flavour and green goodness! It can sometimes be difficult to get greens into your child's diet, as they can be a choking hazard or they're not liked. This dip has such a fresh taste, and it's well loved. Dip a large carrot into it and let your baby suck the dip off or just serve it from a spoon.

1 can (14 ounces/398 mL) cannellini beans, drained and rinsed
1 clove garlic, roughly chopped
⅓ cup (75 mL) fresh basil or cilantro, roughly chopped
¼ cup (60 mL) extra virgin olive oil, hemp oil, or flaxseed oil
4 teaspoons (20 mL) fresh lemon juice
¼ teaspoon (1 mL) sweet paprika
¼ teaspoon (1 mL) ground cumin
Handful of dinosaur kale or other leafy green, chopped

1. Purée all ingredients in a food processor or with a hand blender—then it's ready to eat!
2. This dish is best eaten fresh. Refrigerate in an airtight container for up to 4 days or freeze in baby-safe food containers for up to 1 month.

NUTRITIONAL INFORMATION This dip is a good source of fibre, protein, iron, magnesium, folate, vitamin A, and calcium.

HUMMUS MAKES ABOUT 2 CUPS (500 ML)

DAIRY-FREE • EGG-FREE • GLUTEN-FREE • NUT-FREE • VEGAN • VEGETARIAN • WHEAT-FREE

Hummus is fantastic served on its own or spread on a rice cake. Instead of raw garlic, you can use roasted garlic for a sweeter, milder flavour. Remember that you're not adding salt, so don't expect this to taste like store-bought hummus.

1 can (14 ounces/398 mL) chickpeas, drained
4 tablespoons (60 mL) extra virgin olive oil
2 tablespoons (30 mL) filtered water
2 tablespoons (30 mL) tahini
2 tablespoons (30 mL) fresh lemon juice
1 clove garlic

1. Place the chickpeas, olive oil, water, tahini, lemon juice, and garlic in a food processor or high-speed blender and blend to desired consistency, adding extra water to thin it out or extra olive oil for more flavour. Serve immediately.
2. Store the hummus in an airtight container in the fridge for up to 4 days or freeze in ice cube trays or baby-safe food containers for up to 1 month.

TIP: **1.** To roast garlic, slice the top off a whole garlic bulb and place the bulb in aluminum foil. Drizzle with extra virgin olive oil, wrap the foil together, and bake in a 350°F (180°C) oven for about 20 minutes or until the cloves are tender. Let cool, then "squish" the garlic cloves out of the bulb. **2.** This recipe can also be made with cannellini beans or navy beans instead of chickpeas.

NUTRITIONAL INFORMATION This hummus is a good source of fibre, calcium, magnesium, iron, folate, manganese, copper, and protein.

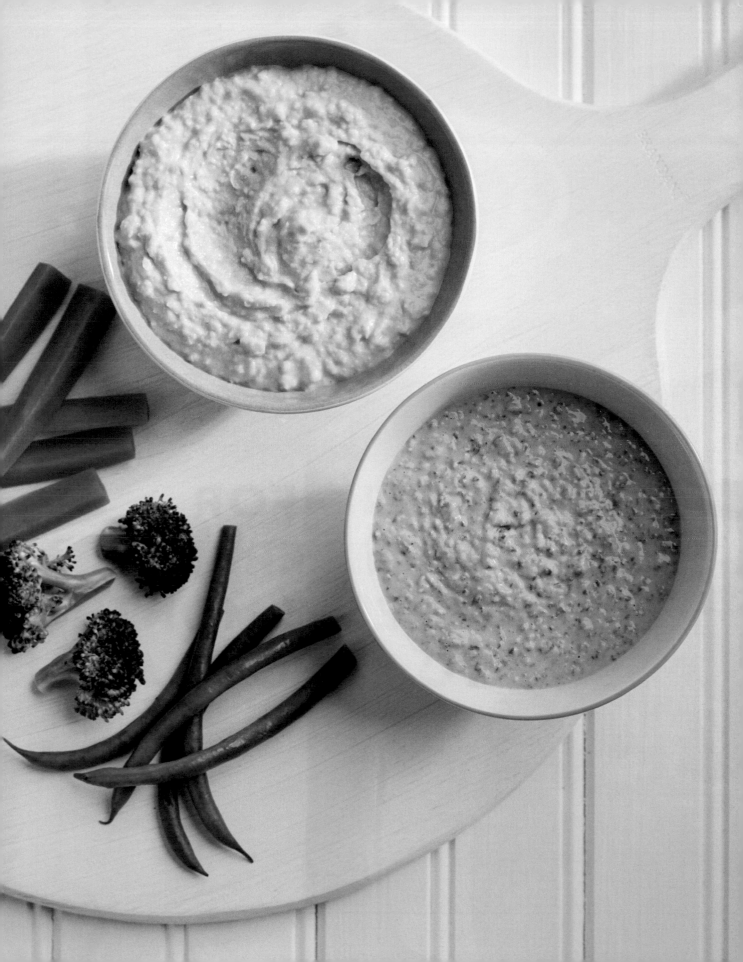

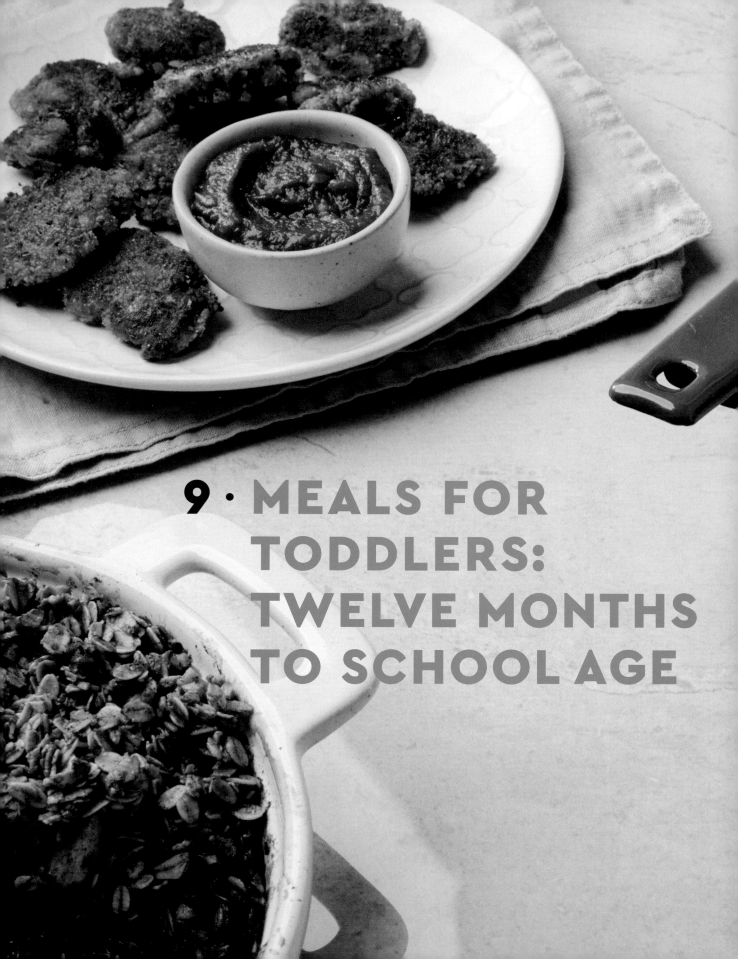

9 · MEALS FOR TODDLERS: TWELVE MONTHS TO SCHOOL AGE

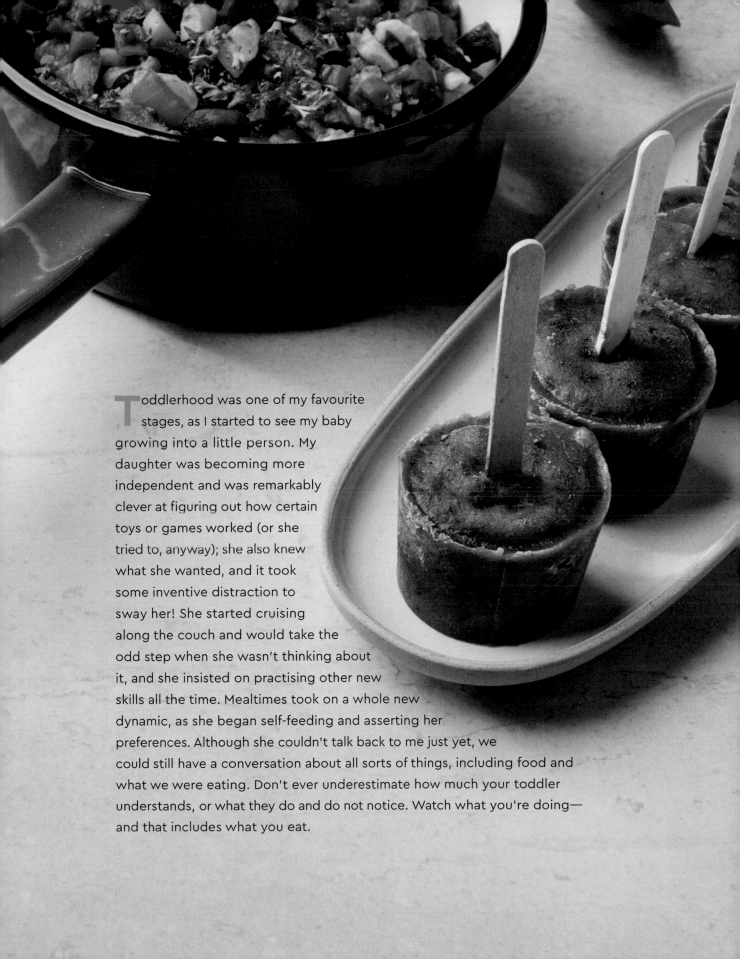

Toddlerhood was one of my favourite stages, as I started to see my baby growing into a little person. My daughter was becoming more independent and was remarkably clever at figuring out how certain toys or games worked (or she tried to, anyway); she also knew what she wanted, and it took some inventive distraction to sway her! She started cruising along the couch and would take the odd step when she wasn't thinking about it, and she insisted on practising other new skills all the time. Mealtimes took on a whole new dynamic, as she began self-feeding and asserting her preferences. Although she couldn't talk back to me just yet, we could still have a conversation about all sorts of things, including food and what we were eating. Don't ever underestimate how much your toddler understands, or what they do and do not notice. Watch what you're doing—and that includes what you eat.

WHAT'S YOUR TODDLER EATING NOW?

Your baby has hopefully had a great appetite until now (other than when sick or teething), but you might see that change. His weight will likely plateau as he becomes a busybody and gets into everything except what might be on his plate. Grazing or snacking becomes more important now as his milk intake declines, making way for more nutrients and calories from food. Ideally, mealtimes continue to be a lot of fun, with a wide variety of tastes and textures on the menu. But perhaps your toddler has limited tastes for certain foods. I encourage you to keep trying with foods that he isn't sure about or dislikes. What he will eat in terms of flavours and textures can change daily, and if it's not on the menu, you won't know if it could be his next favourite food.

By around one year of age, your toddler may be eating a long list of foods, including many colourful fruits and vegetables, some grains and breads, beans, pulses (lentils) and legumes, dairy, eggs, meat, and fish. If any of these haven't been offered yet, you can start to introduce them any time now. Honey is on the safe list now, though it's good to limit sweetness. Texture is often a hurdle that your toddler will need some time to get over. Keep experimenting with an array of colourful vegetables mixed with beans and rice or with something new like buckwheat (see Fruity Curry Buckwheat on page 174), which may have had too much texture when you tried it last; try it again and see what happens! Your toddler may now gobble up cooked quinoa with vegetables before it's puréed (see Colourful Quinoa on page 170), or it could still have too much texture. You can only move at your child's pace. Although your friend's toddler may be eating anything and everything, don't think that your baby should be doing the same. We all have different preferences for textures and flavours, and this also applies to your toddler.

RAISING A VEGETARIAN OR VEGAN TODDLER

I have counselled many parents who prefer that their children be raised with the same dietary philosophy as the rest of the family. Eating a vegetarian diet can be healthy, as long as you know how to create a meal with complex protein and ensure that the common nutrient deficiencies (iron; zinc; vitamin B12; omega-3 essential fats, including docosahexaenoic acid [DHA]) are covered. My recommendation to start your child on meat broth may not fit in with a vegetarian or vegan family's philosophy. If it does, even if only in the early days, then that will provide many healing and nourishing nutrients and fat for your baby. Egg yolk is an iron-rich food suitable for vegetarians but not vegans. All of the parents I've seen in my office, even vegan ones, have given their babies and children eggs up to a point. If you're raising your child on a vegan diet, supplement with DHA from a vegan (possibly algae) source as well as with vitamin B12 and learn which foods supply iron and zinc. It's easy for your little one to become deficient in these nutrients, and with such a huge growth rate between eighteen months and three years, she needs nutritional support to reach her full potential.

Vegetarians often lack protein in their diet, but offering protein-rich eggs and fish, if you're able to, can cover this concern. Protein provides the building blocks (amino acid) for cell growth and repair, supports a strong and healthy immune system, and stabilizes blood sugar. Animal protein offers minerals such as iron, zinc, and vitamin B12 in more absorbable forms than vegetarian protein, but you can make up for this difference by eating smart. Serving foods high in vitamin C like colourful peppers and sweet potato alongside iron-rich beans, lentils, quinoa, amaranth, soy, blackstrap molasses, and sunflower, pumpkin, and sesame seeds increases iron absorption. Moving to a full vegetarian diet at school age or adolescence may be a better nutritional choice; however, your toddler may have decided that meat isn't on his menu just yet. To ensure adequate calorie intake from a vegetarian diet, some higher-fat foods need to be eaten. Nuts and seeds, coconut milk or oil, eggs, and dairy products are all great choices. Your busy toddler needs a constant supply of calories. Fats provide higher calories (9 calories per gram) than protein or carbohydrate (4 calories per gram). Although carbohydrates are also important, these are easy foods to get into the diet (fruits, vegetables, cereals, and grains). I'm not sure I've ever come across a child (or an adult) who was lacking carbohydrates in their diet. Make sure that protein, fat, and carbohydrates are offered to your toddler every day. See more in the plant-based diet section in Chapter 10 (page 236).

WHAT YOU NEED TO KNOW ABOUT SOY

Soy products are not always the best protein option for vegetarian diets. Items such as tofu, tempeh, soy milk, edamame, miso, soy oil, and soy sauce have the potential to be allergenic, and they also contain a compound called phytate. Phytate binds with minerals such as iron, zinc, and calcium and interferes with their absorption by the body, which isn't ideal for supporting strong bone growth, especially for vegetarians trying to eat iron- and zinc-rich foods. Furthermore, almost all nonorganic soy is genetically modified, which, as discussed in Chapter 5, may bring negative health issues in the future.

IT'S OKAY TO PURÉE

As your baby reaches age one, you may expect that her eating will change dramatically and that she'll start eating family meals or food from your plate. But please don't worry if she still wants her purée or prefers her own food. Purée can be made with so many great foods, nutrients, herbs, and spices that you otherwise wouldn't be able to get your toddler to eat, so I'd encourage serving it for as long as you can. Leafy greens, which are packed with nutrients, are difficult to give without puréeing because they're a choking hazard. Try adding spinach, chard, kale, parsley, cilantro, or maybe a vegetable that's not a favourite, such as broccoli or cauliflower, to a purée. The purées will eventually get chunkier and lumpier, and before you know it, your toddler will have transitioned to table food and you'll be cooking one meal for the whole family. Then all you'll need to do is make healthy family meals! There's a whole chapter coming up to help you with just that.

TIME FOR THE SWITCH TO MILK

Health Canada recommends that parents start giving milk to their children at nine months of age. I'm not totally on board with that recommendation. I believe that such a recommendation needs to consider baby's overall diet first. At about one year, formula-fed babies will transition from formula to milk, which will provide needed calories and nutrients throughout the day. Formula is needed until one year because it makes up baby's main source of nutrition. If your one-year-old is still on a limited diet or not a great eater, you can choose to keep him on formula until thirteen or fourteen months or until his diet expands and he eats more. If breastfeeding, you can continue nursing morning and night or more often if you're at home with your toddler. Or, you may choose to wean him completely from the breast at this point, whether or not you're heading back to work. I encourage you to keep breastfeeding for as long as possible.

Either way, you can introduce a drink of milk at age one. A bottle or nursing first thing in the morning and before bed is recommended until close to two years of age. Between twelve and eighteen months, your baby's milk intake should start to decrease as her food intake increases. Ideally, your toddler will be eating three meals a day plus snacks and working toward decreasing her milk to about 16 ounces (475 mL) per day, or maybe less.

If your toddler is drinking three or four bottles of formula or milk a day, start to decrease the amount you offer. With a full belly of milk, he isn't going to be as hungry for a plate of fruits, vegetables, carbohydrates, and protein-rich foods, and you might think he's being a picky eater and doesn't want to eat when in fact he's satiated with milk. Drinking too much milk also lowers the amount of nutrients that can be gained from other foods and can decrease iron status; milk offers a certain nutrient profile, but your toddler needs more than just calcium, vitamin D, and fat from milk in his diet.

MILK OPTIONS

I know what you're thinking: *Options . . . what options?* Well, not everyone does well with dairy or cow's milk, so you might need to choose another kind. I've mentioned before that milk is the number-one allergic food in the world, so if your child doesn't do well with it, it's not just her. Whether you can't offer it because of a reaction to dairy in the past or you don't want to offer your toddler as much as she might choose to drink, calories from milk can still make up for the daily intake of both energy and fluid. Higher fat milks are recommended for all toddlers until age two.

Your options are:

- Homogenized (3.38%) cow's milk, preferably organic
- Goat's milk (3.25%), preferably organic
- Sheep's milk (6%)
- Almond milk, coconut milk, coconut and almond milk, cashew milk, or hemp milk, all preferably organic and some homemade

COW'S MILK If tolerated, cow's milk is a good source of calcium, vitamin D, and protein. Watch for possible signs of sensitivity such as diarrhea, rash (including eczema), runny nose, ear infection, or a constant cold. These symptoms may occur with increasing amounts of milk. An allergy to milk will show more severe reactions, including hives, vomiting, blood in the stool, and local swelling. Children who are intolerant to cow's milk are often able to consume goat's milk without any symptoms.

GOAT'S MILK Goat's milk is naturally homogenized, which may make the fat easier to digest.[116] Also, goat's milk proteins have a slightly different amino acid structure than cow's milk, so an allergy is less likely. Goat's milk is a very good source of calcium, protein, phosphorus, potassium, vitamin B2, and the amino acid tryptophan. A common concern with drinking goat's milk is that it's low in folic acid. Check the packaging to ensure that it has been fortified with folic acid (most brands are).

SHEEP'S MILK Sheep's milk is more nutritious and better tolerated than cow's or goat's milk. Many common symptoms of diarrhea, nausea, vomiting, rash, migraine, and congestion disappear when drinking sheep's milk. It's high in protein and rich in calcium, magnesium, phosphorus, potassium, zinc, folate, and vitamins A, C, D, and B12. Although it has a high fat content, 25 percent is medium chain triglycerides—healthy fats that are easily digested, are not stored in the body as fat, and also help to reduce cholesterol. Sheep's milk may not be as easy to find as goat's milk, but if your local health food store sells sheep's milk products, such as cheese or yogurt, they may be able to order it for you.

The following table compares the nutrients in cow's, goat's, and sheep's milk.

NUTRIENTS	COW'S MILK (3.38%)	GOAT'S MILK (3.25%)	SHEEP'S MILK (6%)
Serving	1 cup (250 mL)	1 cup (250 mL)	1 cup (250 mL)
Energy	155 calories	167 calories	256 calories
Protein	8 g	9 g	15 g
Carbohydrates	12 g	11 g	13 g
Fat	8 g	10 g	17 g
Saturated fat	5.4 g	6.5 g	11 g
Calcium	291 mg	326 mg	483 mg
Iron	0.1 mg	0.12 mg	0.15 mg
Sodium	103 mg	122 mg	108 mg

NUTRIENTS	COW'S MILK (3.38%)	GOAT'S MILK (3.25%)	SHEEP'S MILK (6%)
Potassium	369 mg	499 mg	365 mg
Magnesium	26 mg	34 mg	75 mg
Phosphorus	235 mg	270 mg	332 mg
Vitamin A	72 RAE	136.64 RAE	360 IU
Vitamin D	2.7 mcg	0.73 mcg	2.2 mcg
Folate	13 DFE	2.4 mcg	1.35 mcg
Vitamin B12	1.13 mcg	0.16 mcg	0.711 mg
Riboflavin (vitamin B2)	0.47 mg	0.34 mg	1 mg

DFE: Dietary folate equivalents. Used because of the different bioavailability of folates and folic acid. 1 mcg DFE = 1 mcg food folate = 0.5 mcg folic acid taken on an empty stomach = 0.6 mcg folic acid from fortified food or as a supplement taken with meals.

IU: International unit.

MCG: Microgram (sometimes seen as µg).

RAE: Vitamin A and carotenoids are measured differently. Animal foods contain vitamin A, and vegetables and legumes contain beta carotene (carotenoids). Using the measurement RAE helps to account for these differences. Here is the formula: 1 mcg vitamin A = 12 mcg carotenoids = 1 RAE.

ALMOND MILK Almonds are a powerhouse of nutrients, including heart-healthy monounsaturated fats, which are associated with a reduced risk of heart disease. Almonds are a very good source of vitamin E, omega-6 fatty acids, calcium, phosphorus, manganese, magnesium, copper, and vitamin B2. I recommend making your own almond milk or looking for unsweetened options, as commercial milks can be high in sugar and additives, as well as not provide nearly the same benefits as whole almonds. If you look at the label of most ready-to-drink almond milks, they're made with blanched almonds (without the nutritious skins) and contain high levels of sugar. There's also an ingredient to avoid, carrageenan, which has been has been associated with malignancies and other stomach problems, diabetes, and more.[117] If you're feeding your toddler almond milk, you'll need to add 4 tablespoons (60 mL) of full-fat coconut milk to 4 cups (1 L) of almond milk to increase the amount of saturated fat and calories so that the nutritional profile is more like that of cow's or goat's milk.

RICE MILK Rice milk alone is not suitable for a toddler as a replacement for cow's milk. It could be added to smoothies and combined with other nut milks like cashew milk or even oat milk if the taste isn't loved. Rice milk is fortified with calcium but lacks the fat needed for extra calories. Rice milk could be mixed with almond milk or cow's milk from about eighteen months of age as long as the overall diet contains extra fat to make up for getting less from the milk.

MILK REFUSAL

I've seen many toddlers who choose not to drink milk at all. It doesn't matter what vessel it comes in—bottle, sippy cup, or glass with a straw—they just don't take to it. If this is the case with your toddler, please don't be concerned. Look at the rest of his dairy intake from, say, yogurt, cheese, or cottage cheese—if any of those foods are a part of his diet, he's covered. Although milk is seen as an important drink for the calories it provides, these can easily be made up with foods instead.

HEALTHY TODDLER SNACKS

Snacking is incredibly important for your toddler. Breast milk or formula may have been her main snack (and may still be), but now it's time to offer food as snacks and reduce the amount of milk (if she's still drinking more than 16 to 24 ounces/475 to 710 mL per day). Her busy body needs a constant source of nourishment and calories. Her little stomach can't hold enough food to keep her going from breakfast until lunch or lunch until dinner, especially when her intake at mealtime might sometimes be hit and miss.

Be careful about stocking up on packaged snacks and taking Goldfish crackers everywhere you go. Most toddlers and kids can go a bit longer than half an hour without food (if books had emojis, I'd put a winky face here). I took snacks with me when my kids were young. I didn't buy packaged, though, and stuck to a lot of what's listed below: fruits and vegetables. Often brown rice toast with almond butter and apple butter did the trick. I'd cut it up and then my daughter could take small squares from the container with her amazing pincer grip.

Getting the quantity of snacks right so that mealtime isn't affected is sometimes a challenge, but keeping to a routine of snacks and mealtimes helps toddlers' bodies tremendously in maintaining a good blood sugar balance.

Snack trays with flip lids are a great invention. In our house it was as much fun to flip the lids open and shut as it was to find out what was in each compartment. And then there was the fun of discovering what the picture stamped on the container under the eaten food was. It all helps to create healthy associations with food.

Snacks of fruits and vegetables cut into pieces that aren't easily choked on are preferable to cookies, chips, or sweet treats. Hummus (page 182), baba ganoush, or my Beany Green Dip (page 181) are often good fun and can be packed with nutrients. Whether your toddler eats it straight up or as a dip with the cracker or carrot stick acting as a spoon, if it goes down the hatch, it's all good!

Some healthy snack suggestions include:

- Fresh or frozen wild blueberries
- Cut-up grapes
- Banana slices (cut in half or quartered), plain or with a dollop of almond butter or tahini on top
- Plain full-fat yogurt (Greek is higher in protein) mixed with fruit purée or frozen blueberries and chia seeds
- Rice cakes or Oatcakes (page 318) with Hummus (page 182), baba ganoush, Beany Green Dip (page 181), Pure Green Hummus (page 309), tzatziki, Yummy

Carrot Spread (page 180), or almond butter topped with apple butter or fruit spread (jam sweetened with juice)

- Dried fruit such as raisins, apples, or apricots with cow's, goat's, or sheep's milk cheese
- Super Toddler Smoothie (page 205)
- Smoothie bowl made as above with much less milk
- Rice, millet, or quinoa puff cereal
- Organic Rice Crisp Surprise Squares (page 229)
- Go Faster Granola Bars (page 231)
- Sneaky Little Muffins (page 225), Zucchini Spice Muffins (page 317), Pumpkin Muffins (page 316), or Mini Blueberry Muffins (page 315)
- No-Mess Fruity Ice Pops (page 232)
- Fruity Frozen Yogurt (page 232)
- Steamed veggie sticks: carrot, parsnip, beets, or even broccoli
- ⅓ to ½ banana sliced down the middle, peanut butter, chopped nuts or fruit, and drizzle of maple syrup
- Apple slices with warm nut butter dip (gently warm 1 to 2 tablespoons/15 to 30 mL of preferably organic nut butter and add a small amount of maple syrup or honey)
- Frozen yogurt blueberries: toss blueberries in yogurt, spread out on a flat pan, and freeze
- Baked or lightly steamed broccoli florets
- Quesadilla (like the Bean and Veggie Kamut Quesadillas on page 220)
- ½ banana spread with peanut butter and rolled in Crunchy Granola (page 263)
- Mini Frittata (page 257)
- Seeds of Success Smoothie (page 253)
- Sweet Blue Smoothie (page 253)
- Apple Cinnamon Baked Pancakes (page 254)
- Blender Pancakes (page 255)
- Crunchy Granola (page 263)
- Chia Pudding (page 259)
- Bite-Size Fruit Balls (page 319)
- Chocolate Chip Cookies (page 311)
- Avocado fries: avocado cut into french fry shapes

SNACKS AND BABY'S TEETH

I interviewed three dentists for their views on childhood cavities and how they seem to be increasing, and they all agreed that snacking or grazing all day is not good for oral health. They commented that dried fruits are healthy but sticky and can hang around on the bite surface of premolars or molars or get stuck between teeth. All three preferred that snacks be eaten at one sitting and finished before moving on. Eating changes the pH of the mouth to acid, whereas an alkaline environment protects teeth from bacteria and therefore cavities. Eating a piece of cheese or a carrot stick at the end of a snack helps to alkalize the mouth after eating raisins, for instance. Dr. Dana Colson explains, "The mouth doesn't recognize the difference between all the different sugars. Honey, refined sugar, sugary drinks, candy, and raisins—they can all have the same end result. Plaque takes the sugar and turns it to acid and then causes destruction of enamel."[118] Brushing or even wiping the teeth after sticky snacks is essential to fight off cavities.

UPSIDE-DOWN BOWL NIGHT

In our home, we've always encouraged food that's "good for your body" and helps you grow big and strong, run faster, and play longer. It gives food a use, as opposed to the emotional persuasion of "please eat what mom and dad made for you that took us hours to prepare!" Use simple language to plant seeds in their minds that will grow into an awareness of what's healthy to eat and what needs to be eaten in moderation. So far, my daughters are super-healthy kids who have a great approach to nutritious eating. It's not just organic kale and broccoli around our house, though, and sometimes it can take a bit of coaxing to get the girls to eat what I'd like them to. When they were little, their dad loved to get involved and chop apples into moon and star shapes and cucumbers into butterflies. It was a creative way to get them interested in eating healthier foods. He also invented what is now a funny tradition: Upside-Down Bowl Night. As soon as it's mentioned, all the food on the girls' dinner plates is gobbled up! Here's how you can go about it for your toddlers. Start with a plate with something really good on it, such as pure fruit sorbet, fresh local strawberries, frozen yogurt, or Sprout Right Divine Cookies (page 224). Next, turn a cereal bowl upside down over the yummy stuff. Put something that you want your toddler to eat—fruit or a food you're seeing resistance to (I've used broccoli)—on the top of the upside-down bowl. Your children have to eat what's on top of the bowl before whatever is underneath it can be revealed. Then everyone at the table has to turn their bowl right side up at the same time for the big reveal. The anticipation gets everyone eating what's on top, so don't shy away from something super healthy! It's really a fun, creative, and smart way to eat. Try it out as your toddler gets older and can understand what's happening. We save this as a treat for weekends or when friends come over now, as our girls wanted it every night.

ANY FOODS STILL TO AVOID?

There aren't any foods that could harm your toddler, unless the food a choking hazard or your toddler has a food allergy. Remember that food intolerance or sensitivity can happen at any time, as it's more common when intake of a specific food increases or is eaten daily or multiple times a day. Wheat and dairy are both common food sensitivities (and allergies), along with egg, corn, soy, sugar, chocolate, and sometimes the gluten-containing grains (rye, barley, kamut, spelt, and, some say, oats). As dairy increases in the diet from yogurt, cheese, and milk, your child might show symptoms of a constant runny nose because dairy products are mucus-forming. Although it typically leads to gassiness and constipation, wheat also may cause a constant runny nose. Every now and then, write down a few days of what your child has eaten in a food diary and see which symptoms might correlate with foods that are eaten every day or at more than one meal a day. Wheat, dairy, and corn are often hiding in packaged foods, from cookies to ice cream to "healthy" snack bars. (See Chapter 5 for more on allergy and intolerance.)

Avoid sugar as much as possible. Your toddler doesn't need it in the amount that's found in so many foods. Read labels and look out for cane juice or syrup or any other description of cane sugar. It's still sugar, though it's not always presented as such. Look at the ingredients list, not just at the nutritional composition.

Carbohydrate foods, such as rice cakes, will show as "sugar" in the nutritional composition chart, although they may not contain refined sugar. Carbohydrates break down to sugar, so that will show up on the label. Otherwise, sugar is added to two-thirds of packaged foods and drinks in Canada[119] and can certainly encourage a sweet tooth in your toddler, leading him to refuse more nutritious foods for a healthy body. There's cane syrup in gummy vitamins for children—that's a combination most dentists would love to ban. Along with causing cavities, sugar slows down the immune system's response to foreign invaders and bacterial infections; can trigger behavioural problems; and may create blood sugar imbalances, feed yeast and fungus situations, and keep your toddler going for only short periods when what he needs is a continuous energy supply.

IMPORTANT NUTRIENTS FOR SUPER-HEALTHY TODDLERS

Essential nutrients in the toddler years are B vitamins, essential fatty acids (omega-3 and omega-6), vitamin C, and zinc. B vitamins provide energy, vitamin C contributes to a strong immune system (as does zinc), and zinc is important for growth.

Essential fatty acids (EFAs) (especially DHA) support development of nerve cells in the spine and brain. As your toddler becomes more active and dexterous with her limbs, her nutrient intake needs to increase to support the nervous system's development, allowing for speed and agility of movement as well as sharp mental focus. Eighteen months to three years of age is one of the most rapid growth periods for the spinal column (other than in utero) as the muscular system around it develops to support the full range of flexibility. Studies show that higher levels of EFAs in the diet can increase IQ, mental focus, and concentration and help to reduce symptoms of hyperactivity.

PICKY EATERS

You may have experienced challenges with feeding your toddler, or you may be lucky and have a great eater. It's common for your toddler to show his likes, preferences, and dislikes and to change them weekly! Your job is to be creative, come up with new foods in different forms, and continue to reinvent.

When should you worry? If your toddler is eating only a few foods, is suffering from recurrent colds and infections, has behavioural problems (possibly due to low blood sugar), or is losing weight, it's time to seek help. Tissue salts, mineral salts that are very low dose but have high absorbability, can be used to increase nutrient status as well as mineral absorption from foods. Picky eating can often be a vicious cycle of not eating and then failing to get the essential nutrients that stimulate appetite. Be sure to rule out iron deficiency, which can lead to lack of appetite. That may need a blood test from your doctor. It's not a nice thought, but it's better to know about it before it becomes a chronic deficiency.

I asked Liza Finlay, a registered psychotherapist, associate faculty member at Adler Graduate School, and author, about picky eaters, and she had this to say:

> *Chasing your kids around saying, One more bite! is a great way to ensure that they are not going to eat. It sets up a power struggle; it makes the parent the boss of the food, and the only leverage the child has is to keep his or her lips tightly shut or run from the table! Also, it sets up a rather dangerous precedent in which others dictate what your body needs. We want kids to tune in to the signals their bodies are sending them about hunger and satiety.*
>
> *So, the less you say about it the better. Your child's intrinsic desire to belong will ensure that she or he observes what others in the family and peer group are eating and follow suit. That means you should:*
> - *Model healthy, adventurous eating*
> - *Serve foods family-style, making it easier for your child to try, say, butter chicken alongside plain rice*
> - *Make the table an enjoyable place to be—less hounding, more engaging conversation and laughter*[120]

IDEAS FOR DEALING WITH PICKY EATERS

Try to identify why your child refuses to eat. Refusing food may be an emotional plea for attention or a way of rebelling against change, such as mom going back to work. If a toddler doesn't want mom to leave, she might refuse breakfast, knowing that mom will stay longer to feed her. It's her way of controlling the situation, especially when she sees a reaction. These issues may need to be addressed on a different level than just eating.

Make mealtimes relaxing and fun. Involve your toddler in meal preparation and cooking. Give foods names (such as "trees" for broccoli) or associate them with a favourite character. Maximize on textures he likes—the dry texture of bread, chewy noodles, or wet oatmeal. Sit with your toddler at each meal, eat with him, and encourage him when he eats something. If he's old enough, ask for a certain amount of bites before he leaves the table and have the fanfare ready when he achieves it. Don't make eating a struggle. That will kill his appetite, and the battle won't necessarily go the way you want it to.

"My toddler will only eat . . ." I've heard it hundreds of times from parents. "My toddler will only eat cheese, bread, chicken pieces, or french fries." If it's not in the house or offered when you're out, then it can't be eaten. It's that simple. Your toddler may have a strong personality and insist on what he wants, but you're still in charge, so don't offer what you don't want him to eat. If you're out and about and are stuck for something to eat, don't venture into a fast-food restaurant with limited healthy choices—go down the road for falafel or sushi (vegetarian, as he might not be ready for raw fish) or simply pick up some fruit or raisins to keep him going until you can find some healthy food. The only way a toddler will start to eat unhealthy food is if you allow it.

To be sure that your toddler isn't living on air (as it sometimes seems), look at what she has eaten in a whole day or over a few days, rather than at just one meal. If she's at daycare or isn't with you during the day, when was her last snack of the day? Quite often, by the time she is back with you at the end of the day, she's had enough food and dinner really isn't needed. Be sure to ask the daycare provider how much she ate that day, and be aware of what she ate yesterday. If yesterday was a food-filled day, she may hardly touch her plate today. Again, a food diary with times of snacks or meals can really help to alleviate your stress and lessen mealtime pressure. Start talking about why she is eating and how the foods will help to make her strong and keep her healthy. Relate that information to something that makes sense to her: "Wow, you were running so fast at the park today. I wonder if it was because of your healthy broccoli and eggs at lunch?" or "I know you want to play at the park, but that takes energy, so let's finish your food because that's energy right there!" It must be relevant for them to understand why on earth you want them to eat when they have, in their own minds, already moved on to the next thing.

Psychotherapist, parenting expert, author, and speaker Alyson Shafer, who is also a great friend, helped me via her three books when I was trying to figure out this parenting thing. I asked her for some strategies for kids who refuse to eat what's put in front of them. In addition to some of the ideas above, Shafer suggests the following:

> Serve very small amounts. Two carrots is fine. Arrange the food on the plate to look like a picture. Now those carrots are flower petals, and who doesn't think it's silly to eat flower petals? Serve the foods they like the least at the times of day when they are hungriest. If vegetables are not their thing, put out a plate of veggies after they come home from daycare and before dinner. If they don't like broccoli, try it raw, cooked, roasted, puréed, and inside a lasagna until you find ways your child might enjoy it more. See if they would take a "polite bite" instead of forcing them to eat. A respectful single bit to try a new flavour without being too forceful is a cooperative approach to take with your child's developing palate.[121]

I love the "polite bite" concept. This is certainly something that can be used as they get older, so they know they have to try just one bite.

Here are some other healthy-eating ideas:

• Encourage snacking every couple of hours. If mealtimes aren't going well, offer snacks of pieces of chicken and peas, for instance. Toddlers need about 40 calories per inch (2.5 cm) of height per day. They burn calories quickly, so need constant topping up.

- Have friends over to show them how it's done. Children are influenced by what others do even at a young age, so seeing their friends clean their plates might just inspire them to try, too.
- Be inventive with the way you cut up food. Make special shapes and give them names. Apples can be a moon, broccoli can be a tree with branches and green flowers, cucumber can be cut into stars, and so on.
- Sneak fruits or vegetables into everything! Chop or process them very small and add to Super Burgers (page 217), put under the cheese topping of Veggie Pesto Pizza (page 212), and blend into bean dips like Beany Green Dip (page 181), puréed soup like Sweet Potato and Coconut Soup (page 215), or pasta sauce. This way your child can't easily identify or pick out what she doesn't want to eat. While you're in a phase with your child where she won't eat a certain colour, this will work until she's through the phase.
- Serve their meals or snacks at their own table. A kid-size table may be more appealing than the big table or high chair. Let them know that big girls and boys can sit at their own table, but only if they eat what's on their plates.
- Don't worry about which meal happens when. We are accustomed to eating breakfast-type foods in the morning, but it's not necessary to follow that schedule. Still aim for a variety of foods, not just cereal for breakfast, lunch, and dinner. If they're not eating much, make what does get eaten count.
- If your toddler is inconsistent with foods that you have lovingly prepared, don't take it personally, and don't stop offering the same or new foods. Some days I don't feel like a certain food. That doesn't mean I won't ever eat it again. Offer it a couple of days later and keep it in the rotation of meals, just not as often.

OFF TO DAYCARE: AVOIDING SICKNESS AND DEALING WITH SOMEONE ELSE'S MENU

Daycare is one of the most dreaded situations among the parents I speak with. Being home for almost a year and watching your baby grow up into a little person is precious. And now it's time to drop him off at the door of a place you put your trust in and walk away, praying that it's all going to be okay. The transition can be heart-wrenching at first, but it quickly improves as your toddler realizes what fun daycare is.

When you're doing the rounds of daycares or making child care arrangements, ask to see a menu of the food served. If you aren't sure about some of the foods on the menu, ask if you can bring your own food. Most daycare centres don't permit nuts and other potential allergens, so know that you'll have to stick to a list if you're allowed to bring your own foods. The usual safe options are sunflower, pumpkin, and sesame seed butters instead of peanut or almond butter. If organic is important to you, ask how much of the food is organic and how much wheat and dairy is served. When I counsel daycares to improve their menus, I spend most of my time suggesting grain alternatives to wheat. It's in just about everything and is offered three to four times a day in the form of bread, buns, cookies, crackers, cereal, and muffins. What do they give the children to drink? How easy would it be to give them water instead of juice, and do you want them having milk? All of these questions need to be answered to help you decide which child care situation is best for your toddler. I've heard of parents turning down a daycare spot because hot dogs, chicken nuggets, and Jell-O were on the menu. I'm astounded that anyone would think that's an appropriate diet for a growing child, and kudos to those parents for saying no thank you.

BOOSTING THAT IMMUNE SYSTEM

Once you have the food situation figured out, it's time to boost the family's immune system. Parents of kids in their first year of daycare tell me that they can't believe how sick they are in that first year. Illness is constant throughout winter in particular. Be prepared for everyone to come down with some sort of sickness within the first couple of weeks of daycare. As I discussed in Chapter 5, your baby's or toddler's immune system needs to be put through its paces, so the sneezes and wheezes that accompany children in daycare do serve a purpose! Hold on to that knowledge as you crack open another box of tissues and drink another coffee to get through the day! It's crazy how long a cold can last or that you can be sick from September to March. I remember that when my youngest was just over a year old, she and I were both sick for a whole month (as well as off and on for most of the winter). Luckily, neither of us got a secondary infection (ear, chest, or throat infection) that required antibiotics. Our immune systems worked really hard to keep the illness under control with the support of loads of probiotics, vitamin C, garlic (added to the Fabulous Fresh Fruit Purée on page 177), echinacea, a good multinutrient, and rest.

My definition of a strong immune system is one that's able to fight off illness and diseases that come your way through viruses, bacteria, fungi, or parasites. Colds and sickness will happen (especially during teething episodes, when the immune system is busy thinking that the erupting tooth is a foreign invader), but if the immune system is able to prevent any secondary infection such as ear, chest, or sinus infections, the battle has been won. Going to the doctor and leaving without a prescription for antibiotics is a sign of a strong immune system and also that your child is suffering from a virus (it's far more common to be given antibiotics, though). That means the body is dealing with the sickness and isn't allowing it to become a bacterial issue. We still want to feed the immune army with the nutrients they need to carry out the battle. Everyone in the family should include the items discussed below in his or her diet and think about taking some extras in supplement form.

PROBIOTICS

With more than 80 percent of our immune system found in our digestive system, ensuring a healthy amount of friendly bacteria or probiotics in the digestive tract will boost the immune system (see Chapter 5). At the first sign of any sickness, take an increased amount of probiotics. Even better, take an increased level all winter long. I've listed some of the ones I find help my clients the most on the Resources page at SproutRight.com. If antibiotics are prescribed, keep taking probiotics but take them three hours away from the antibiotic dose. Then, once the course of antibiotics is finished, increase the amount of probiotics by doubling or tripling the usual dose for one month. If probiotics are taken, research shows that it can take between one and four years to repopulate the digestive system with a healthy colony, and this period is much longer if probiotics aren't taken. Specific strains of probiotics called *Lactobacillus sporogenes* and *Saccharomyces boulardii* both survive antibiotics, lessening the antibiotic-associated diarrhea symptoms. This means they are better options during a course of antibiotics. Then, you can do a higher dose afterwards. Eating a pot of yogurt or kefir daily when sick isn't advisable, as dairy is so mucus forming and can contribute to the existing buildup of mucus in the nose, chest, sinuses, or ear canal. Probiotic supplements are a better option here.

VITAMINS A AND C

Think reds, oranges, and yellows. Try to eat a variety of colourful fruits and vegetables—they have antioxidants that fight disease, help wounds heal, and support the immune system. Adults can take between 2000 and 4000 mg of vitamin C per day—more if you're getting sick—and toddlers can take between 200 and 400 mg per day in divided doses. This is in addition to what's consumed in the diet. The only side effect of taking too much vitamin C is gas or diarrhea (which is handy for constipation!). If you see these side effects, ease off the vitamin C for a day or so.

ZINC AND IRON

Zinc and iron are needed for healthy immune function and red blood cells. Good sources of iron and zinc include meat, especially organ meats, seafood, particularly oysters and herring; beans; sunflower and pumpkin seeds; whole grains like oats, amaranth, quinoa, and brown rice; lentils; dried fruit such as figs; blackstrap molasses; mushrooms; green leafy vegetables; kelp; beets; asparagus; avocados; cucumbers; parsley; and bananas. Iron should not be supplemented unless deficiency is diagnosed by blood test. A symptom of zinc deficiency (and deficiency of other minerals) is white marks on the fingernails. If you notice this, a supplement is necessary to correct the deficiency. UNDA Gammadyn zinc liquid provides a safe level for anyone.

GARLIC

Garlic (especially raw) is a superfood! It inhibits the common cold virus, promotes the growth of healthy intestinal flora, and eliminates "bad" bacteria and yeasts. For the common cold, sore throats, and sinus headaches, add raw garlic to anything. For a cure-all garlic remedy, boil a cup (250 mL) of water and add lemon juice to taste and a teaspoon (5 mL) of raw honey. Using a garlic press, squeeze in one clove garlic and drink the whole mug. For your toddler, share your mug with her or tip a bit into her own mug and encourage that she drink the garlic, too. Do this a few times a day and you'll be better in no time (and don't worry about smelling of garlic—you won't see anyone anyway, since you're at home with your toddler). A drop of garlic oil or St. Francis Herb Farm's Ear Oil in the ear canal once a day helps clear ear infections. To prepare garlic oil, crush several cloves of garlic and soak in ¼ cup (60 mL) olive oil for at least an hour and up to three days. Then strain the oil through cheesecloth or drain off a few drops of the oil with a dropper (no garlic, just oil), drop them into the ear canal, and seal with a bit of cotton wool. Repeat as needed.

PROTEIN

The amino acids in protein are the building blocks of the cells in your immune system, and they help create protective white blood cells and antibodies. Choose lean protein from the following sources: fish, chicken, turkey, eggs, beans, whole grains, legumes, quinoa, tempeh, nuts, and seeds. My family's favourite meal when the girls are sick is a boiled egg and soldiers (toast cut into finger strips) and Immune-Boosting Soup (see recipe on page 297). When I make it for dinner, they feel special and I know they're getting a meal that helps their bodies fight off illness. If you can't get food into your toddler, try a smoothie with hemp protein powder in a sippy cup with the valve removed.

ECHINACEA

Echinacea is known as an herbal antibiotic that helps boost the immune system. Echinacea works best at the beginning of a cold. If you're already sick, it's not as effective. Long-term use isn't advised, as it loses its effectiveness; use it for five days to one week, then take a break for the same amount of time. Liquid echinacea for children is readily available at supplement and health food stores. I recommend UNDA Echinasyr in my toddler and preschool immune-boosting programs on SproutRight.com.

BOIRON'S CORYZALIA

Coryzalia, by Boiron Laboratories, is a homeopathic remedy for babies from six to thirty-six months of age (I used it for my daughters from two months) that helps to relieve nasal congestion and runny nose. Homeopathy is completely safe during pregnancy and for breastfeeding mothers.

CASTOR OIL

Castor oil, rubbed on the chest, front, and back before bed, helps boost the immune system and "drain" the respiratory system. It's a simple and effective remedy that works especially well with coughing. The oil can also be rubbed over the neck for a sore throat and from the back of the neck to the back of the ear to help drain the ear canal. It's also good for helping to alleviate constipation when rubbed on the abdomen.

MEAL PLANNING

On the following page are two meal plans to give you an idea of what your toddler can be eating at this stage development. It also includes meals for the whole family that your toddler can enjoy too. When following the meal plans, continue to offer water throughout the day. You may offer milk upon rising and at bedtime, and some moms may continue to breastfeed at the beginning and end of each day. If giving milk, I recommend full-fat organic cow's, goat's, or sheep's milk or homemade almond milk (see recipe on page 203).

Toddler (Twelve Months–Plus) Meal Planner

	BREAKFAST	SNACK	LUNCH	SNACK	DINNER
Day 1	Amazing Sweet Amaranth (page 168) (not puréed)	Dried fruit with cheese	Lovely Lentils (page 165) over brown rice pasta; Milk before nap	Rice cake with apple butter and almond butter	Veggie-Packed Chili (page 211) with baked potato
Day 2	Finger Food Pancakes (page 178) and Super Toddler Smoothie (page 205)	Rice cake and hummus	Bean and Rice Surprise Stew (page 175) (not puréed); Milk before nap	Yogurt with Spiced-Up Apples or Pears (page 177)	Bean Burgers (page 206) and Sweet Potato Fries (page 208)
Day 3	Lovely Soaked Muesli (page 204)	Apple slices and almond butter	Leftover Bean Burger patties (page 206) with carrot sticks and Hummus (page 182); Milk before nap	Rice cake with Yummy Carrot Spread (page 180)	Smarty Pants Fish Cakes (page 209) with Apple Butter Dip (page 208) and steamed veggie sticks

Family Meals with Your Toddler in Mind

	BREAKFAST	SNACK	LUNCH	SNACK	DINNER
Day 1	Toast and eggs and Super Toddler Smoothie (page 205)	Apple slices with cheese	Veggie Pesto Pizza (page 212)	Rice cake with fruit spread and almond butter	Super Burgers (page 212) with Sweet Potato Fries (page 208) and steamed broccoli
Day 2	Overnight Oatmeal (page 259) with cinnamon and chopped fruit	Rice cake and Hummus (page 182)	Leftover Super Burger (page 217) made into a wrap with sprouts and apple butter	Yogurt with Spiced-Up Apples or Pears (page 177)	Sweet Potato and Coconut Soup (page 215) with whole-grain bread and Hummus (page 182)
Day 3	Your Own Boxed Cereal (page 205) and scrambled eggs	Apple slices and almond butter	Leftover soup with veggie sticks and Hummus (page 182)	Veggie sticks with Beany Green Dip (page 181)	The Ultimate Lasagna (page 219) with slices of fresh peppers

RECICPES

TODDLER MEALS

ALMOND MILK MAKES ABOUT 4 CUPS (1 L)

DAIRY-FREE • EGG-FREE • GLUTEN-FREE • VEGAN • VEGETARIAN • WHEAT-FREE

This may seem like an unnecessary recipe since almond milk is so widely available, but as with all foods, homemade will yield more nutrients without questionable added ingredients. Commercial milks can be high in sugar and additives and don't provide nearly the same benefits as whole almonds. If you're feeding your child almond milk as a dairy alternative, you'll need to add a couple of tablespoons of full-fat coconut milk to increase the amount of saturated fat and calories, so that its nutritional profile will be more like that of cow's or goat's milk.

---

1 cup (250 mL) raw almonds (organic, if possible)

4 cups (1 L) filtered water

¼ cup (60 mL) sesame seeds (optional)

¼ cup (60 mL) full-fat coconut milk

2 teaspoons (10 mL) pure maple syrup

1. Soak the almonds in water overnight, or for at least 4 hours. Drain and rinse several times (you can skip soaking if you're in a rush, but it's an important step to get more nutrients).

2. In a high-speed blender, combine the almonds, water, sesame seeds (if using), coconut milk, and maple syrup. Blend for 4 to 5 minutes. Strain using a fine-mesh strainer lined with cheesecloth, a bag for making jelly, or a cloth milk bag (used for nut milks).

3. Store the milk in an airtight glass container in the fridge for up to 3 days. It can also be frozen for up to 2 weeks.

TIP: Before opening, shake the can of coconut milk thoroughly after warming it in a bowl of hot water. Freeze leftover coconut milk in ice cube trays for up to 1 month.

NUTRITIONAL INFORMATION Almonds are a very good source of vitamin E, omega-6 fatty acids, calcium, manganese, magnesium, copper, riboflavin (vitamin B2), and phosphorus. Sesame seeds are a powerhouse of calcium—they contain a much higher level than is found in milk.

LOVELY SOAKED MUESLI MAKES ABOUT 3 CUPS (750 ML) DRY MUESLI MIX

DAIRY-FREE • EGG-FREE • GLUTEN-FREE • VEGAN • VEGETARIAN • WHEAT-FREE

Soaking the grains and seeds releases enzymes that make them easier to digest. This is a quick, delicious, and nutritious breakfast!

1 cup (250 mL) gluten-free old-fashioned rolled oats

1 cup (250 mL) quinoa flakes

½ cup (125 mL) mixed seeds (flax, sunflower, and pumpkin), plus more for serving

¼ cup (60 mL) chopped unsulphured dried apricots, plus more for serving

¼ cup (60 mL) chopped Thompson raisins or sultanas, plus more for serving

1 apple (Fuji, Gala, or Pink Lady)

Almond, rice, coconut, or dairy milk (amount will depend on your serving size)

1. Combine the oats, quinoa flakes, mixed seeds, apricots, and raisins. Store in an airtight container in the fridge for up to 2 weeks or in the freezer for up to 1 month.

2. To prepare the soaked muesli, add a handful of the dry mixture to a cereal bowl. Grate half of the apple overtop and cover the mixture completely with your milk of choice. Cover the bowl and refrigerate overnight.

3. In the morning, add extra fresh fruit and milk, as desired, and serve.

NUTRITIONAL INFORMATION This muesli is a good source of manganese, selenium, iron, vitamin B1, fibre, magnesium, protein, phosphorus, vitamin C, and zinc.

YOUR OWN BOXED CEREAL

MAKES ABOUT 3½ CUPS (875 ML)

DAIRY-FREE • EGG-FREE • GLUTEN-FREE • VEGAN •
VEGETARIAN • WHEAT-FREE

There is nothing but good stuff in this cereal!
It also doubles as a great finger food snack—
simply leave out the millet puffs and ground
nuts and seeds, as they're too difficult for little
fingers to pick up.

1 cup (250 mL) Nature's Path Millet Rice Flakes or
   other low- or no-sugar flakes
¾ cup (175 mL) Breakfast O's cereal
¾ cup (175 mL) Nature's Path Rice Puffs
½ cup (125 mL) Nature's Path Millet Puffs
½ cup (125 mL) Thompson raisins or sultanas
½ cup (125 mL) ground nuts and seeds or
   chopped dried fruit
Almond, rice, coconut, or dairy milk (amount will
   depend on your serving size)

1. Mix all the dry ingredients together and store
in an airtight container for up to 2 weeks.
2. To serve, add milk or eat dry as a snack.

NUTRITIONAL INFORMATION In addition to being
organic, this cereal is gluten-free, making it easy
to digest; it's also low in salt and made with
natural fruit sugars.

SUPER TODDLER SMOOTHIE

MAKES ABOUT ¾ CUP (175 ML)

DAIRY-FREE • EGG-FREE • GLUTEN-FREE •
NUT-FREE • VEGAN • VEGETARIAN • WHEAT-FREE

Smoothies are a great way to get a lot of
nutrients into your toddler. Stir in fish oil to add
beneficial DHA.

½ cup (125 mL) almond, rice, coconut,
   or dairy milk
¼ cup (60 mL) frozen wild blueberries
½ ripe banana
¼ ripe pear, cored
1 tablespoon (15 mL) hemp protein, pea protein,
   bone broth protein, or whey powder
2 teaspoons (10 mL) flaxseed or hemp oil
2 teaspoons (10 mL) blackstrap molasses
   (optional)
Small handful of sunflower sprouts or baby
   spinach leaves

1. Add all ingredients to a blender and blend
until smooth. Serve immediately.

NUTRITIONAL INFORMATION This smoothie
is a good source of fibre, antioxidants, and
omega-3 fats, as well as protein that will keep
your baby going longer.

BEAN BURGERS MAKES ABOUT 24 MINI BURGERS

DAIRY-FREE • GLUTEN-FREE • NUT-FREE • VEGETARIAN • WHEAT-FREE

Easy for little hands to pick up, these burgers are also great dipped in Apple Butter Dip (page 208), Hummus (page 182), or tzatziki. Serve with Sweet Potato Fries (page 208)—yummy!

2 medium carrots

1 small yellow onion

1 clove garlic

Handful of fresh cilantro or flat-leaf or curly parsley, chopped

3 cups (750 mL) canned mixed beans

1 tablespoon (15 mL) extra virgin olive oil, plus more for cooking

1½ cups (375 mL) whole-grain or gluten-free breadcrumbs

2 to 3 eggs

1. In a food processor, pulse the carrots, onion, garlic, and cilantro until finely chopped. Add the beans and olive oil and pulse until combined.
2. Add the breadcrumbs and 2 of the eggs and pulse until the texture is uniform. If the mixture is too crumbly and dry, add the remaining egg and blend. Let sit for a few minutes. The mixture should hold together easily to form into patties.
3. Form into 24 small patties (about 2 inches/5 cm in diameter) or sausage shapes. Brush a nonstick grill or frying pan with olive oil and place over medium heat. Cook the patties about 5 minutes per side until golden brown. Alternatively, bake in the oven at 350ºF (180ºC) for 15 minutes, turning once halfway through.
4. Store patties in an airtight container in the fridge for up to 4 days or in the freezer in a container or large freezer bag with parchment paper in between layers of patties for up to 2 months.

TIP: **1.** Use 1 cup (250 mL) each canned chickpeas, kidney beans, and adzuki beans or your favourite beans instead of canned mixed beans. **2.** Substitute ½ cup (125 mL) ground seeds (sunflower seeds or pumpkin seeds) for ½ cup (125 mL) of the breadcrumbs for more nutrients and taste.

NUTRITIONAL INFORMATION These patties are a good source of fibre, protein, magnesium, potassium, iron, zinc, copper, manganese, and vitamin B3.

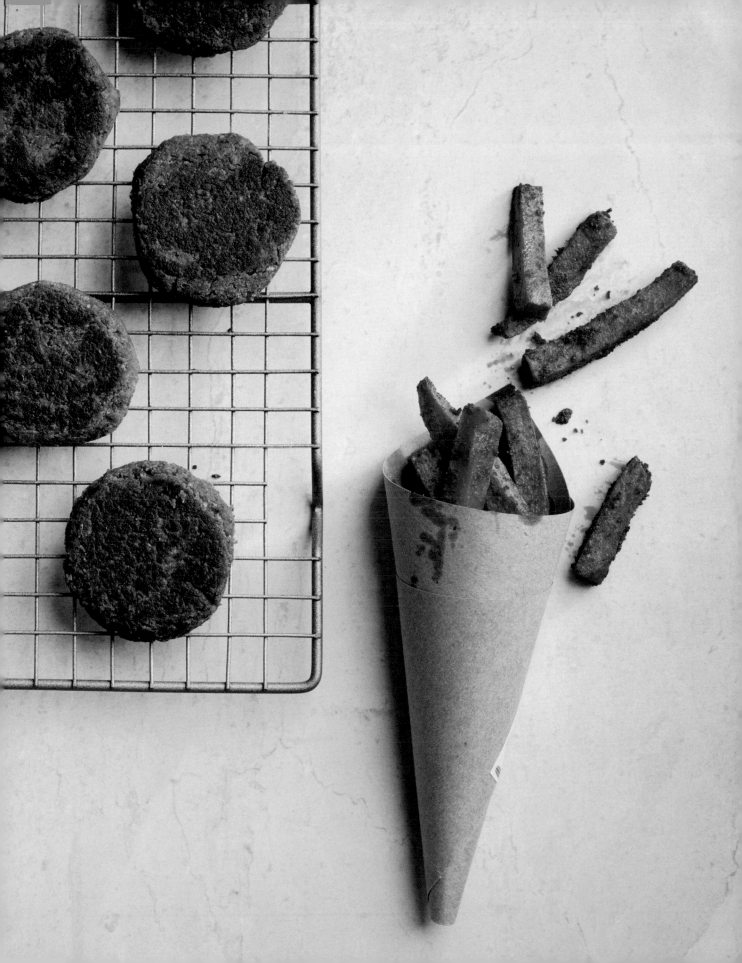

SWEET POTATO FRIES

SERVES 2 TO 4

DAIRY-FREE • EGG-FREE • GLUTEN-FREE •
NUT-FREE • VEGAN • VEGETARIAN • WHEAT-FREE

The trick with these fries is to put loads of garlic and paprika on them. They are a staple in so many homes! Although they're not crispy, the taste of the spice combination along with the sweetness of the potato make them an instant hit, and you'll love that they're baked, not fried, and contain no salt.

---

2 medium sweet potatoes or yams, peeled
2 tablespoons (30 mL) extra virgin olive oil
1 tablespoon (15 mL) garlic powder
1 tablespoon (15 mL) sweet paprika

1. Preheat the oven to 350°F (180°C). Line a baking sheet with parchment paper.
2. Cut the sweet potatoes into ½- × ½- × 2½-inch (1 × 1 × 6 cm) sticks either by hand or using a mandolin. Place the sweet potato sticks, olive oil, garlic, and paprika in a resealable plastic bag. Seal the bag and shake until the sweet potato sticks are coated completely.
3. Spread the sweet potato sticks out on the prepared baking sheet and bake for 20 minutes or until tender (they won't be as crispy as potato fries).

TIP: **1.** You can keep the skin on the sweet potatoes for extra nutrients and fibre. **2.** Parsnips, carrots, and potatoes are good substitutes for a change of pace, but sweet potato works best.

NUTRITIONAL INFORMATION Sweet potatoes are high in beta carotene, fibre, potassium, and vitamins C and E.

APPLE BUTTER DIP

MAKES ABOUT 1 CUP (250 ML)

DAIRY-FREE • EGG-FREE • GLUTEN-FREE •
NUT-FREE • VEGAN • VEGETARIAN • WHEAT-FREE

This dip is fabulous with the Smarty Pants Fish Cakes (page 209) and the Bean Burgers (page 206). It's a versatile sauce that can be used in both sweet and savoury dishes. I like to turn this into a stir-fry sauce by adding grated ginger and extra lemon and garlic. It's also delicious as a topping for roasted salmon.

---

1 cup (250 mL) apple butter (I like Filsinger's)
2 cloves garlic, finely chopped
2 tablespoons (30 mL) fresh lemon juice
2 teaspoons (10 mL) extra virgin olive oil

1. In a small bowl, stir together all the ingredients. Serve.
2. Store the apple butter in an airtight container in the fridge for up to 3 weeks.

NUTRITIONAL INFORMATION This healthy fruit sauce contains no sugar. Garlic is antibacterial and antiviral and therefore boosts the immune system. Apple butter contains fibre and flavonoids.

SMARTY PANTS FISH CAKES MAKES 12 TO 16 FISH CAKES

DAIRY-FREE • EGG-FREE • GLUTEN-FREE • NUT-FREE • WHEAT-FREE

This is a great way to introduce fish to your child, if you haven't already. Most toddlers like potatoes, so these fish cakes have a texture that's easy to like. Serve them with Apple Butter Dip (page 208).

1 pound (450 g) yellow potatoes, peeled

1 clove garlic, peeled and chopped in half

¼ cup (60 mL) fresh or frozen corn

¼ cup (60 mL) fresh or frozen peas

¼ pound (115 g) white fish fillet of your choice (see Tip)

2 heaping tablespoons (35 mL) chopped fresh dill or cilantro

1 cup (250 mL) gluten-free breadcrumbs or whole sesame seeds

TIP: White fish such as cod is mild tasting and best for new fish eaters, but wild salmon (non-GMO) is also an excellent choice and surprisingly loved. You can substitute 5 ounces (150 g) of drained canned fish for fresh fish. For more essential fatty acids, use canned wild salmon like the Safe Catch brand.

NUTRITIONAL INFORMATION These fish cakes are a very good source of protein, omega-3 fats (if using salmon), vitamin C, vitamin B6, copper, potassium, manganese, and fibre.

1. Preheat the oven to 400°F (200°C). Line a baking sheet with parchment paper.
2. Bring a medium pot of water to boil over high heat. Meanwhile, chop the potato into small cubes. Once the water is boiling, add the potato and garlic and cook until fork-tender, about 7 to 10 minutes.
3. Drain the potato and garlic, then mash them in a large bowl. Stir in the corn and peas (hot potato will defrost them, if using frozen). Let cool for 5 minutes.
4. Bake the fish on the prepared baking sheet for 10 to 12 minutes or until flaky.
5. Place the fish on top of the mashed potato mixture. Add the dill and gently mix together. Don't overmix, as potatoes can become gluey. Form the mixture into small burgers (each about 1½ inches/4 cm in diameter) and coat with breadcrumbs, shaking off excess. Fish cakes are cooked and ready to eat—serve immediately or reheat later in a frying pan or oven.
6. Store the fish cakes in an airtight container in the fridge for up to 3 days or in the freezer in a container or large freezer bag with parchment paper in between layers of fish cakes for up to 2 weeks.

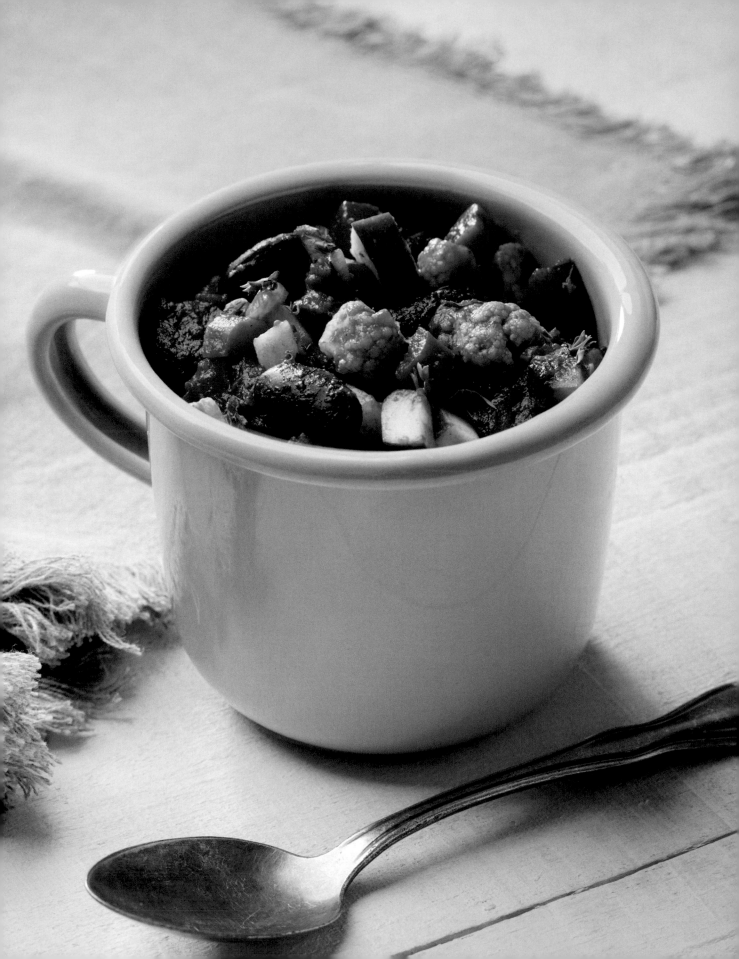

VEGGIE-PACKED CHILI MAKES ABOUT 6 CUPS (1.5 L)

DAIRY-FREE • EGG-FREE • GLUTEN-FREE • NUT-FREE • VEGAN • VEGETARIAN • WHEAT-FREE

Veggie chili is a staple for the whole family. Feel free to add other favourite veggies, such as peas or green beans, to those listed here. Serve with brown rice, baked potato, or noodles.

1 tablespoon (15 mL) extra virgin olive oil

1 medium onion, chopped

1 clove garlic, chopped

1 small eggplant or zucchini, chopped

1 head cauliflower, chopped

2 medium carrots, chopped

½ sweet red pepper, chopped

Handful of shiitake or button mushrooms

1 teaspoon (5 mL) chili powder

1 can (28 ounces/796 mL) diced tomatoes
   (see Tip)

5 black mission figs, finely chopped (optional)

1 can (14 ounces/398 mL) kidney beans, drained
   and rinsed

3 tablespoons (45 mL) chopped fresh flat-leaf
   or curly parsley

1. Heat the olive oil in a large saucepan over medium heat. Add the onion and garlic and sauté until soft. Add the eggplant or zucchini, cauliflower, carrot, red pepper, mushrooms, and chili powder and sauté for 5 minutes until vegetables just start to soften.
2. Add the tomatoes and figs (if using) and bring to a boil. Reduce the heat to low and simmer for 20 minutes. Stir in the kidney beans and parsley and cook for 10 minutes longer.
3. Serve over baked potato, rice, or noodles and top with shredded cheddar or mozzarella cheese (goat or cow dairy).
4. Store the chili in an airtight container in the fridge for up to 3 days or in the freezer for up to 1 month.

TIP: To avoid potential bisphenol A (BPA) in canned tomatoes, use a 24-ounce (710 mL) jar of tomato sauce and ¼ cup (60 mL) of water instead.

NUTRITIONAL INFORMATION This chili is a good source of molybdenum, folate, fibre, manganese, protein, thiamine (vitamin B1), phosphorus, iron, copper, magnesium, potassium, and vitamin K.

VEGGIE PESTO PIZZA MAKES 2 SMALL OR 1 LARGE PIZZA

EGG-FREE • GLUTEN-FREE • NUT-FREE • VEGETARIAN • WHEAT-FREE

Pizza is a great way to sneak in a ton of vegetables. Stack it thick, and whatever vegetables fall on the plate will be picked up by little fingers. The assembled unbaked pizza can be frozen, or leftovers can be enjoyed the next day for lunch.

2 cups (500 mL) packed fresh basil

½ cup (125 mL) packed fresh cilantro leaves

2 tablespoons (30 mL) sunflower seeds

2 teaspoons (10 mL) capers

4 Kalamata olives, pitted

4 sundried tomatoes

2 cloves garlic, peeled

⅓ cup (75 mL) extra virgin olive oil

Pinch of sea salt

2 small or 1 large pizza base (preferably gluten-free or spelt)

1 cup (250 mL) shredded goat's or cow's milk mozzarella cheese

Topping options (finely chopped)

Green beans

Corn

Asparagus

Shiitake or button mushrooms

Onion

Broccoli

Sweet red or yellow pepper

Baby spinach

Thompson raisins or sultanas

1. Preheat the oven to 400°F (200°C).

2. To make the pesto, add the basil, cilantro, sunflower seeds, capers, olives, sundried tomatoes, and garlic to a food processor and pulse a few times. Slowly add the olive oil in a constant stream while the food processor is running and blend until smooth. Stop a couple of times to scrape down the sides of the bowl with a rubber spatula. Add a pinch of salt to taste.

3. Top the pizza base or bases with a layer of pesto. Sprinkle with 2 tablespoons (30 mL) of the cheese and scatter with the desired toppings, covering all edges. Make it colourful and press the vegetables firmly onto the crust. Top with the remaining cheese.

4. Bake for 15 to 20 minutes or until the cheese is melted and the crust is crisp. Cut into slices and serve.

5. Store leftover pizza in an airtight container in the fridge for up to 3 days or in the freezer for up to 2 weeks.

NUTRITIONAL INFORMATION This pizza is a good source of fibre, protein, vitamin K, iron, calcium, and vitamin A.

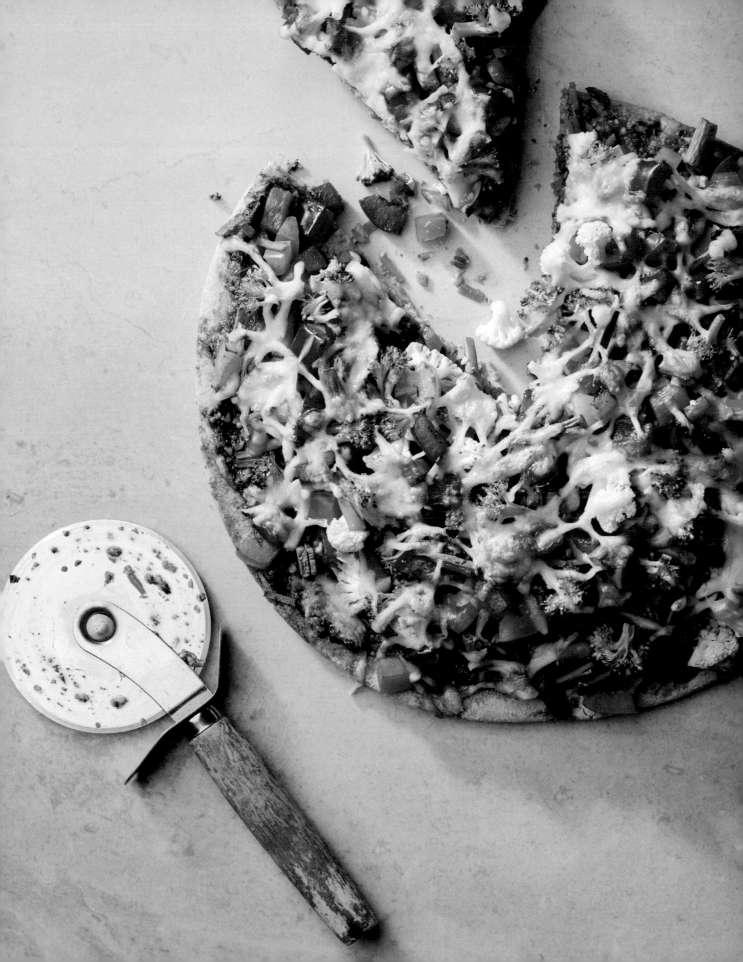

LENTIL SHEPHERD'S PIE SERVES 6 TO 8

EGG-FREE • GLUTEN-FREE • NUT-FREE • VEGETARIAN • WHEAT-FREE

This recipe is well loved by my family. It's a hearty and delicious meal that even meat eaters will enjoy. If you want to make individual servings, cook in a muffin tin (silicone works well), cool, freeze overnight, and then pop out the individual servings and store them in a freezer bag.

½ cup (125 mL) dried green or French lentils

1 slice kombu seaweed

1½ pounds (675 g) potatoes

1 tablespoon (15 mL) salted butter

1 tablespoon (15 mL) plain almond milk or 2% dairy milk

1 tablespoon (15 mL) extra virgin olive oil

1 large yellow onion, chopped

1 clove garlic, minced

2 carrots, peeled and diced

¾ cup (175 mL) chopped button or shiitake mushrooms

½ cup (125 mL) fresh or frozen peas

1¾ cups (425 mL) tomato sauce

1 tablespoon (15 mL) tamari

1 bunch flat-leaf or curly parsley, chopped and divided

TIP: Substitute parsnips or sweet potato for some of the potatoes for variety, a different colour (if substituting sweet potato), and a different flavour.

NUTRITIONAL INFORMATION This dish is a good source of molybdenum, folate, fibre, manganese, iron, protein, phosphorus, copper, thiamine, and potassium.

1. Place the lentils in a medium saucepan, cover with water, and add the kombu. Bring to a boil and then reduce the heat to low. Simmer for 45 minutes or until soft. Discard the kombu, drain the lentils, and set aside.

2. While the lentils are cooking, fill another medium saucepan with water and bring to a boil. Scrub the potatoes and chop them into medium chunks. Add to the boiling water and cook until fork-tender. Drain and mash with the butter and milk.

3. Heat the olive oil in a medium saucepan over medium heat and sauté the onion and garlic until translucent. Add the carrot and cook for 5 minutes. Add the mushrooms and peas and sauté for 2 minutes longer. Stir in the tomato sauce, tamari, half of the parsley, and the cooked lentils. Cook for a few minutes longer and remove from the heat.

4. Preheat the oven to 375°F (190°C).

5. Pour the lentil mixture into a medium oven-proof dish or muffin tin (if making individual servings) and top with mashed potatoes. Sprinkle with the remaining parsley. Bake for 30 minutes or until the potato is golden brown. Let cool for a few minutes and serve.

6. Store the shepherd's pie in an airtight container in the fridge for up to 3 days or in the freezer for up to 1 month.

SWEET POTATO AND COCONUT SOUP MAKES ABOUT 6 CUPS (1.5 L)

DAIRY-FREE • EGG-FREE • GLUTEN-FREE • NUT-FREE • VEGAN • VEGETARIAN • WHEAT-FREE

This appetizing soup, bursting with flavour and vitamin C, makes a lovely accompaniment to the Bean and Veggie Kamut Quesadillas (page 220) or the Chicken Souvlaki (page 273). It can be served as a main meal with whole-grain bread or by adding in cooked brown rice.

4 cups (1 L) Meat Broth (page 129) or
  Vegetable Broth (page 130)
2 sweet potatoes, peeled and chopped
½ cup (125 mL) red lentils, rinsed well
1 yellow onion, chopped
1 kale leaf, chopped
1 clove garlic, chopped
2 teaspoons (10 mL) ground cumin
1½ teaspoons (7 mL) ground coriander
1½ teaspoons (7 mL) chopped fresh ginger
1 can (14 ounces/398 mL) canned coconut milk
1 tablespoon (15 mL) chopped fresh cilantro

1. Add the broth, sweet potato, lentils, onion, kale, garlic, cumin, coriander, and ginger to a large pot and bring to a boil. Reduce the heat to low and simmer, uncovered, until the sweet potato is fork-tender, about 20 minutes.
2. Stir in the coconut milk and cilantro and purée until smooth.
3. Store the soup in an airtight container in the fridge for up to 3 days or in the freezer for up to 2 months.

NUTRITIONAL INFORMATION This soup is a good source of beta carotene, fibre, potassium, manganese, and vitamins C and E.

SAVOURY AMARANTH WITH VEGETABLES SERVES 6

DAIRY-FREE • EGG-FREE • GLUTEN-FREE • NUT-FREE • VEGAN • VEGETARIAN • WHEAT-FREE

This is a nutritious twist on the standard rice stir-fry. Amaranth is packed full of calcium and protein and is a delicious alternative to rice or quinoa.

1 cup (250 mL) amaranth

2 cups (500 mL) Meat Broth (page 129) or
   Vegetable Broth (page 130)

2 teaspoons (10 mL) pure maple syrup

2 teaspoons (10 mL) virgin coconut oil

½ yellow onion, finely chopped

½ cup (125 mL) chopped broccoli

½ cup (125 mL) chopped cremini mushrooms

½ sweet red pepper, chopped

1 clove garlic, chopped

2 teaspoons (10 mL) sesame oil

1 teaspoon (5 mL) tamari

1. Heat a dry frying pan over medium heat. Pour in the amaranth and toast until most of it pops. Set aside.

2. In a medium pot, combine the broth and maple syrup and bring to a boil. Add the amaranth and simmer until all the liquid has been absorbed, about 7 to 10 minutes.

3. Heat the coconut oil in a skillet over medium heat and add the onion. Cook until the onion is translucent. Add the broccoli, mushrooms, red pepper, and garlic and stir-fry for about 5 minutes or until soft. Stir in the amaranth and cook for about 2 minutes longer. Toss with the sesame oil and tamari and serve.

4. Store in an airtight container in the fridge for up to 3 days or in the freezer for up to 1 month.

NUTRITIONAL INFORMATION This dish is a good source of folic acid, calcium, protein, vitamin C, and vitamin E.

SUPER BURGERS, MEATBALLS, OR MEATLOAF SERVES 6

MAKES ABOUT 3 MINI MEATLOAVES OR 12 MEATBALLS OR MINI BURGERS

DAIRY-FREE • GLUTEN-FREE • NUT-FREE • WHEAT-FREE

This is the perfect place to hide a lot of vegetables. Use a variety of vegetables, especially those you wouldn't normally serve on their own.

1½ pounds (675 g) organic ground chicken, turkey, or grass-fed beef

2½ cups (625 mL) mixed vegetables, finely chopped (see Tip)

1 cup (250 mL) gluten-free breadcrumbs

1 yellow onion, diced

3 cloves garlic, minced

1 egg, beaten

Pinch each of salt and pepper

TIP: **1.** Mixed vegetables can include 3 or 4 of the following options: zucchini, kale, red or yellow pepper, broccoli, carrot, green beans, green peas, corn, parsley, cilantro, and Swiss chard. **2.** For an egg-free meal, omit the egg and reduce the amount of breadcrumbs to ½ cup (125 mL).

NUTRITIONAL INFORMATION These dishes are a good source of protein, fibre, and nutrients.

1. Combine all the ingredients in a large bowl and mix thoroughly with your hands. The texture should be sticky, and the mixture should hold its shape. Form into burger shapes or meatballs or pat into mini loaf pans.

2. For burgers, heat a barbecue to medium heat. Shape into patties between 2 inches (5 cm) and 4 inches (10 cm) inches in diameter and ½ inch (1.5 cm) thick. Barbecue for 5 minutes on each side, or until internal temperature reaches 165°F (74°C). Burgers can also be pan-fried for 15 minutes until golden brown on both sides and cooked through.

3. For meatballs, heat the oven to 350°F (180°C). Cook on a parchment-lined baking sheet for 15 to 20 minutes or until internal temperature reaches 165°F (74°C). Meatballs can also be pan-fried for 15 minutes until golden brown and cooked through.

4. For meatloaves, heat the oven to 350°F (180°C). Bake for approximately 30 minutes or until internal temperature reaches 165°F (74°C).

5. Burgers can be frozen raw by placing individual patties on a parchment-lined baking sheet. Once frozen, transfer the patties to a resealable plastic freezer bag for storage. Store cooked burgers, meatloaves, or meatballs in an airtight container in the fridge for up to 3 days or in the freezer for up to 1 month.

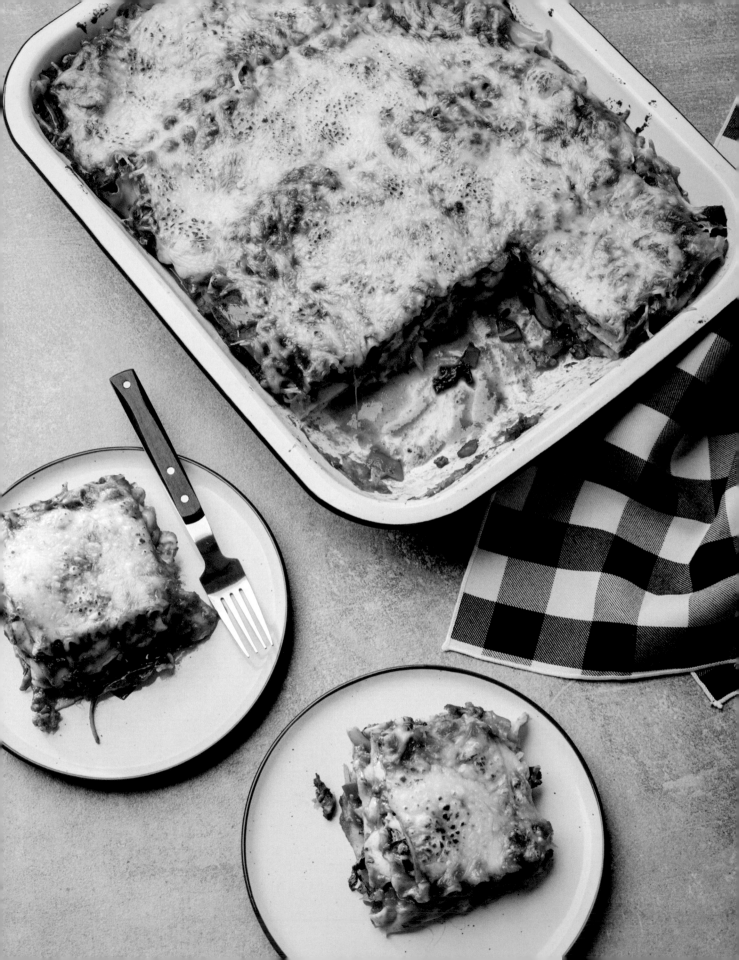

THE ULTIMATE LASAGNA MAKES 3 MINI LASAGNAS OR 1 LARGE LASAGNA

EGG-FREE • GLUTEN-FREE • NUT-FREE • WHEAT-FREE

This is a great weekend recipe to make in a large batch and freeze for future meals. The sauce is another good place to sneak in veggies.

6 to 8 sheets rice or kamut lasagna noodles

2 tablespoons (30 mL) extra virgin olive oil, divided

1 small onion, chopped

1 to 2 cloves garlic, chopped

1 pound (450 g) organic ground chicken (dark meat)

1 jar (24 ounces/710 mL) tomato sauce

½ cup (125 mL) filtered water

1 sweet red or yellow pepper, chopped

2 carrots, chopped

½ cup (125 mL) chopped button or shiitake mushrooms

2 tablespoons (30 mL) chopped fresh flat-leaf or curly parsley

1 tablespoon (15 mL) Italian seasoning

Handful of baby spinach leaves, washed

1½ cups (375 mL) shredded organic mozzarella cheese

TIP: 1. Substitute organic ground turkey (dark meat) or grass-fed ground beef for the chicken for more nutrients and taste. **2.** Canned tomato sauce may contain bisphenol A (BPA), a chemical known for its link to a number of health issues. Use jarred tomato sauce as a safer alternative.

NUTRITIONAL INFORMATION This is a nutrient-rich meal containing antioxidants, calcium, magnesium, iron, zinc, and vitamin C. It's also a balanced meal of protein, carbohydrate, and vegetables.

1. Add the lasagna noodles to a large pot of boiling water and cook until tender, taking care not to overcook, as they may fall apart. Drain noodles, drizzle with 1 tablespoon (15 mL) of the olive oil (so they don't stick together), and place on a parchment-lined baking sheet. Cover with a clean, damp kitchen towel.

2. Heat the remaining 1 tablespoon (15 mL) olive oil in a large skillet. Add the onion and garlic and cook until translucent. Mix in the ground chicken and cook until browned. Stir in the tomato sauce, water, red pepper, carrot, mushrooms, parsley, and Italian seasoning. Cook for about 20 minutes or until the carrots are soft.

3. Assemble the lasagna in three 8- × 4-inch (1.5 L) loaf pans or one 13- × 9-inch (3.5 L) baking dish. Spread 1 to 2 tablespoons (15 to 30 mL) of sauce in the bottom of each pan or baking dish, then layer the noodles, sauce, spinach, and cheese, repeating layers until the pans or dish is full.

4. Heat the oven to 350°F (180°C). Bake for about 30 to 45 minutes or until the cheese is golden and the sauce is bubbling at the edges.

5. Serve with Winter Sunshine Salad (page 304) or freeze, covered, for up to 1 month.

6. To prepare lasagna from frozen, defrost overnight in the fridge, then bake at 350°F (180°C) for 30 to 45 minutes (depending on size) until heated through.

BEAN AND VEGGIE KAMUT QUESADILLAS MAKES 3 TO 4 QUESADILLAS

EGG-FREE • GLUTEN-FREE • NUT-FREE • VEGETARIAN • WHEAT-FREE

These are a crowd pleaser! Make a large batch to take to a picnic or stash some in your bag on a day out. They taste great cold. Feel free to substitute any of your toddler's favourite veggies. All measurements are estimated—add more of whatever you like.

1 cup (250 mL) adzuki, kidney, and/or cannellini beans, drained and rinsed

½ sweet red pepper, diced

½ cup (125 mL) fresh or frozen corn

½ cup (125 mL) finely chopped broccoli

½ cup (125 mL) chopped cooked chicken (optional)

6 kamut whole grain or corn wraps

1 cup (250 mL) shredded goat's milk or organic dairy mozzarella cheese

For serving
Salsa
Guacamole

1. In a medium bowl, combine the beans, red pepper, corn, broccoli, and chicken (if using).

2. Heat a large skillet over medium heat. Place a wrap in the skillet and sprinkle with some cheese and then the bean mixture. Sprinkle with a little more cheese and top with another wrap. Press down firmly with your hands or a spatula and cook until crisp. Flip and cook until the other side of the wrap is crisp, the filling is heated through, and the cheese has melted. Serve with salsa or guacamole.

3. Store the quesadillas in an airtight container in the fridge for up to 3 days.

NUTRITIONAL INFORMATION These quesadillas contain fibre, vitamin C, calcium, protein, and beta carotene.

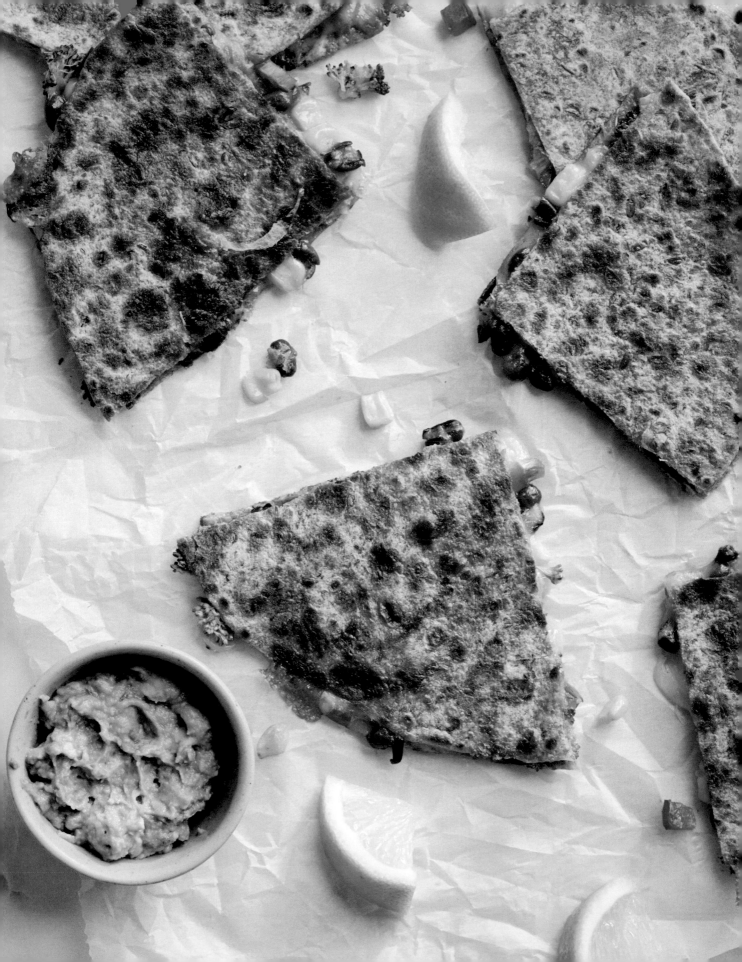

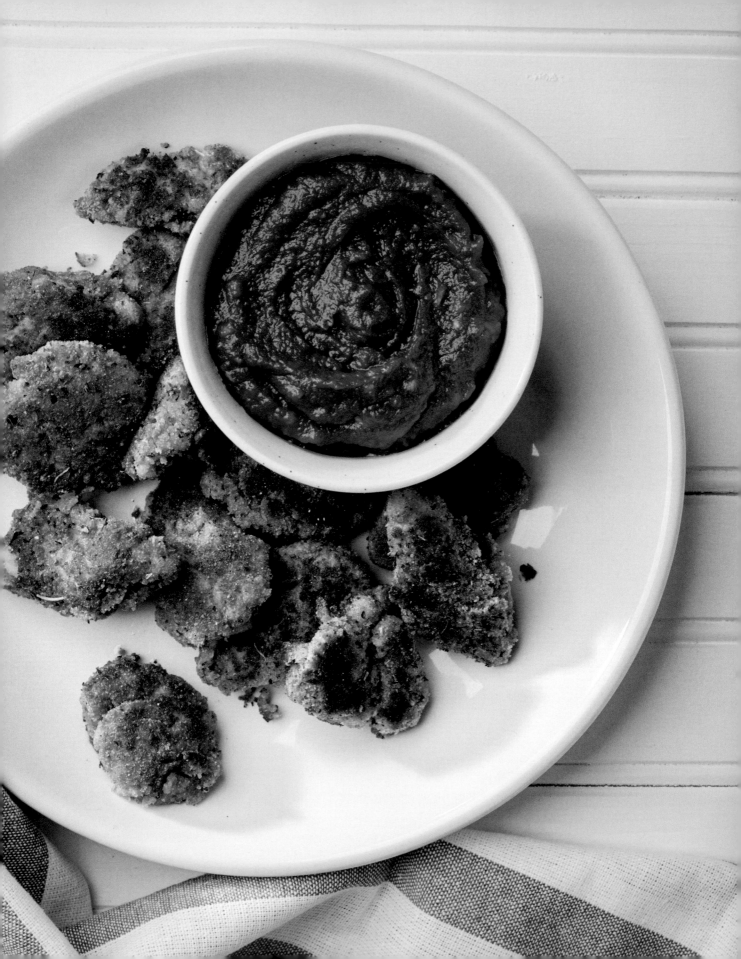

CRISPY CHICKEN NIBBLES SERVES 2 TO 3

DAIRY-FREE • GLUTEN-FREE • NUT-FREE

These are the perfect way to offer chicken to those who aren't too sure about the texture. The dry breadcrumbs on the outside work well for some toddlers and kids, and they are much healthier than store-bought options. My Apple Butter Dip (page 208) is a great alternative to ketchup or plum sauce and can be made ahead or while the chicken is cooking. Chicken thighs are more moist and higher in iron, but you can substitute chicken breasts if you like.

2 skinless, boneless chicken thighs

1 cup (250 mL) gluten-free breadcrumbs

1 to 2 teaspoons (5 to 10 mL) mixed dried herbs (basil, oregano, thyme)

1 teaspoon (5 mL) garlic powder

2 eggs

½ cup (125 mL) whole-grain, rice, or gluten-free flour

Apple Butter Dip (page 208), for serving

1. Cut the chicken into strips or small pieces.
2. Combine the breadcrumbs, herbs, and garlic powder in a bowl. Whisk the eggs in a shallow dish and place the flour in another shallow dish. Coat a chicken piece in flour, then dip into the egg, coating evenly and shaking off excess. Press the chicken into the breadcrumb mixture to coat. Transfer to a clean plate and repeat with the remaining chicken.
3. Heat a nonstick frying pan over medium heat. Cook the chicken for about 7 to 15 minutes (depending on size), turning once, until golden brown and cooked through.
4. Serve with Apple Butter Dip and Lemony Green Beans (page 307). Store the cooked chicken in an airtight container in the fridge for up to 3 days or in the freezer for up to 1 month.

NUTRITIONAL INFORMATION Chicken is an excellent source of protein, and the dark meat is a good source of iron. The breadcrumbs add fibre to the dish as well.

SPROUT RIGHT DIVINE COOKIES MAKES 18 TO 24 COOKIES

GLUTEN-FREE • NUT-FREE • VEGETARIAN • WHEAT-FREE

Nobody will guess there's no refined sugar in these cookies—they're truly divine! They are similar to my favourite cookie, shortbread, but with less sugar and gluten-free. Chopped nuts can be used in place of the coconut, and apple butter can be used in place of the apricot or blueberry fruit spread. Play with different combinations to see which one you like best!

1 cup (250 mL) unsalted butter, room temperature

2½ teaspoons (12 mL) pure vanilla extract

1 egg

¼ cup + 2½ tablespoons (100 mL) pure maple syrup

1½ cups (375 mL) brown rice flour

¼ cup (60 mL) potato starch

¼ cup (60 mL) tapioca starch

¾ teaspoon (4 mL) baking powder

½ teaspoon (2 mL) salt

¼ teaspoon (1 mL) xanthan gum

Shredded unsweetened coconut (optional)

Unsweetened apricot or blueberry fruit spread

1. Preheat the oven to 325ºF (160ºC). Line a baking sheet with parchment paper.

2. In a stand mixer or using a hand mixer, beat the butter, vanilla, and egg. Pour in the maple syrup and beat for 3 minutes longer. The mixture will look curdled. Add the flour, potato starch, tapioca starch, baking powder, salt, and xanthan gum and mix thoroughly. If possible, let the batter stand for 10 minutes at room temperature. This will give time for the gluten-free flour and xanthan gum to bind.

3. Drop the dough by the spoonful onto the prepared baking sheet, or form into balls and roll each ball in the shredded coconut (if using). Use your finger to make an indentation in the centre of each ball and fill with fruit spread.

4. Bake for 15 to 18 minutes or until golden brown around the edges. Remove from the oven, let stand 2 minutes, then transfer to a rack to cool.

5. Store the cookies in an airtight container at room temperature for up to 3 days or in the freezer for up to 1 month.

NUTRITIONAL INFORMATION These healthy cookies are made without gluten or refined sugar and contain protein, iron, and potassium.

SNEAKY LITTLE MUFFINS MAKES ABOUT 36 MINI MUFFINS

GLUTEN-FREE • NUT-FREE • VEGETARIAN • WHEAT-FREE

These muffins make tasty snacks. I like to freeze a batch to defrost later to accompany lunch or have as a snack for car rides. I use silicone mini muffin trays to make these so that I don't need to line the trays with paper.

2 overripe medium bananas

2 eggs

1 cup (250 mL) grated carrots

½ cup (125 mL) pure maple syrup

½ cup (125 mL) rice milk

6 tablespoons (90 mL) melted butter (salted or unsalted)

¼ cup (60 mL) grated zucchini

⅓ cup (75 mL) ground chia seeds

1¾ cups (425 mL) brown rice flour

¼ cup (60 mL) tapioca starch

2 teaspoons (10 mL) baking powder

1 teaspoon (5 mL) baking soda

1 teaspoon (5 mL) ground cinnamon

1. Preheat the oven to 325°F (160°C). Lightly grease 36 mini muffin cups or line them with paper liners.

2. Beat the bananas in a stand mixer or in a medium bowl using a hand mixer. Beat in the eggs. Add the carrot, maple syrup, rice milk, butter, zucchini, and chia seeds. Combine until the consistency is uniform, then let sit for 5 minutes.

3. In a small bowl, combine the rice flour, tapioca starch, baking powder, baking soda, and cinnamon. Add the dry ingredients to the wet ingredients and mix thoroughly.

4. Fill the muffin cups three-quarters full and bake for about 25 minutes or until the muffins are golden and spring back lightly when touched.

NUTRITIONAL INFORMATION These muffins are a healthy gluten-free, refined sugar–free, dairy-free snack containing beta carotene, potassium, fibre, protein, and trace minerals.

APPLE CRUMBLE SERVES 6 TO 8

EGG-FREE • GLUTEN-FREE • VEGAN • VEGETARIAN • WHEAT-FREE

This recipe is based on my mom's apple crumble. I've made it healthier while keeping it scrumptious. It is an excellent meal served with Greek yogurt, as a snack, or as dessert.

Fruit Filling

3 cups (750 mL) sliced fresh fruit (apples, peaches, pears, or a combination)

1 cup (250 mL) fresh or frozen wild blueberries or other berries

¼ cup (60 mL) pure fruit juice, such as apple juice

1 teaspoon (5 mL) ground cinnamon

Crumble Topping

1½ cups (375 mL) old-fashioned rolled oats

¼ cup (60 mL) pure maple syrup

¼ cup (60 mL) sunflower seeds, chopped

¼ cup (60 mL) walnuts, chopped (optional)

¼ cup (60 mL) unsalted butter or virgin coconut oil

1 teaspoon (5 mL) ground cinnamon

1. Preheat the oven to 350°F (180°C).

2. In a medium bowl, toss the sliced fruit, blueberries, fruit juice, and cinnamon.

3. In another medium bowl, mix the oats, maple syrup, sunflower seeds, walnuts (if using), butter, and cinnamon. Combine by squeezing the ingredients between your fingers to create a soft, coarse crumble.

4. Spoon the fruit mixture and its liquid into a 9-inch (23 cm) pie plate. Top with the crumble mixture. Bake for 35 to 45 minutes or until the fruit is fork-tender, the filling is bubbling and thickened, and the topping is golden brown. Cool slightly on a wire rack before serving warm or at room temperature.

5. Store in an airtight container in the fridge for up to 3 days or in the freezer before or after cooking for up to 1 month.

NUTRITIONAL INFORMATION This crumble is rich in vitamin C, fibre, antioxidants, essential fatty acids, trace minerals, and complex carbohydrates.

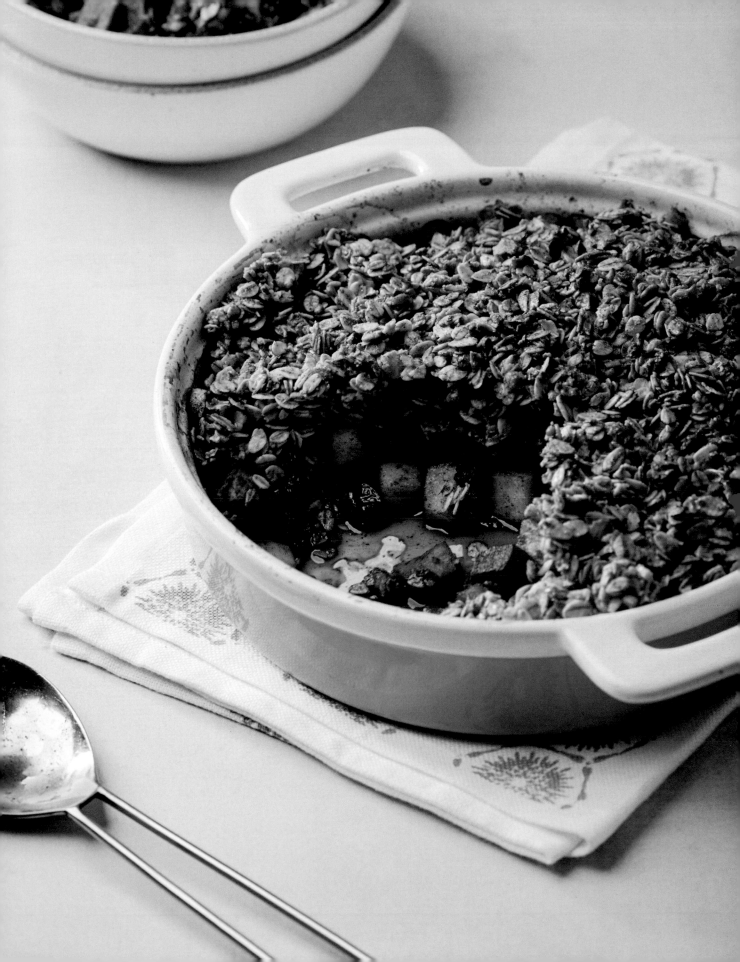

SINLESS CHOCOLATE ALMOND BROWNIES MAKES 16 BROWNIES

GLUTEN-FREE • NUT-FREE • VEGETARIAN • WHEAT-FREE

With dark chocolate, gluten-free flour, natural alternatives to sugar, and even goat's milk butter (you can also use dairy butter), this unique recipe will ease your guilt and offer some power-packed nutrition as well. Although not as sweet as what you might be accustomed to, these brownies are quite addictive! You can easily substitute unsalted butter for the goat's milk butter and cane sugar for the brown rice syrup.

3 ounces (90 g) dark chocolate (at least 70% cocoa solids)

2 tablespoons (30 mL) goat's milk or unsalted butter

½ cup (125 mL) brown rice syrup or barley malt syrup

2 large eggs

1 teaspoon (5 mL) pure vanilla extract

½ cup (125 mL) gluten-free flour mix (Bob's Red Mill)

½ cup (125 mL) chopped raw almonds (optional)

1. Preheat the oven to 350°F (180°C). Grease and then line an 8-inch (2 L) square baking pan or glass dish with parchment paper.

2. Melt the chocolate and butter in a medium saucepan over low heat. Stir in the brown rice syrup and remove from the heat. Whisk in the eggs one at a time and add the vanilla. Stir in the flour and almonds (if using).

3. Pour the mixture into the prepared baking pan and spread evenly to the corners. Bake for 20 to 25 minutes or until just set. Remove from the oven and let cool for 5 minutes before removing the brownies from the pan. Allow to cool completely on a wire rack and cut into squares.

4. Store the brownies in an airtight container at room temperature for up to 3 days (if they last that long!) or in the freezer for up to 1 month.

NUTRITIONAL INFORMATION Dark chocolate is high in magnesium and contains an abundance of antioxidants. Almonds are high in calcium, magnesium, vitamin E, and fibre.

ORGANIC RICE CRISP SURPRISE SQUARES

MAKES ABOUT 48 SMALL SQUARES OR 24 LARGE SQUARES

DAIRY-FREE • EGG-FREE • GLUTEN-FREE • NUT-FREE • VEGAN • VEGETARIAN • WHEAT-FREE

These are an incredibly delicious and healthy version of the blue-wrapper Rice Krispies squares. Packed with good fats, protein, and fibre, they are hard to resist. This recipe can be made school safe by omitting the almond butter.

½ cup (125 mL) brown rice syrup

2 tablespoons (30 mL) blackstrap molasses

¼ cup (60 mL) almond butter or pumpkin seed butter

2 tablespoons (30 mL) tahini

2 tablespoons (30 mL) sunflower seed butter

1 teaspoon (5 mL) pure vanilla extract

½ box (5 ounces/150 g) MadeGood or other rice crisp cereal

⅛ cup (30 mL) sunflower seeds

⅛ cup (30 mL) pumpkin seeds

1. Heat the rice syrup, molasses, almond butter, tahini, sunflower seed butter, and vanilla in a medium saucepan over medium-low heat until well combined and almost runny. Remove from the heat.

2. Add the rice crisp cereal, sunflower seeds, and pumpkin seeds and quickly stir well to coat. Evenly divide the mixture between two 8-inch (2 L) square baking dishes, press evenly into corners, and let cool. Once cooled, cut into squares.

3. Store the squares in an airtight container or airtight bag at room temperature for up to 1 week.

NUTRITIONAL INFORMATION These squares are a good source of vitamin E, calcium, zinc, vitamin B1, manganese, magnesium, copper, selenium, phosphorus, vitamin B5, and folate.

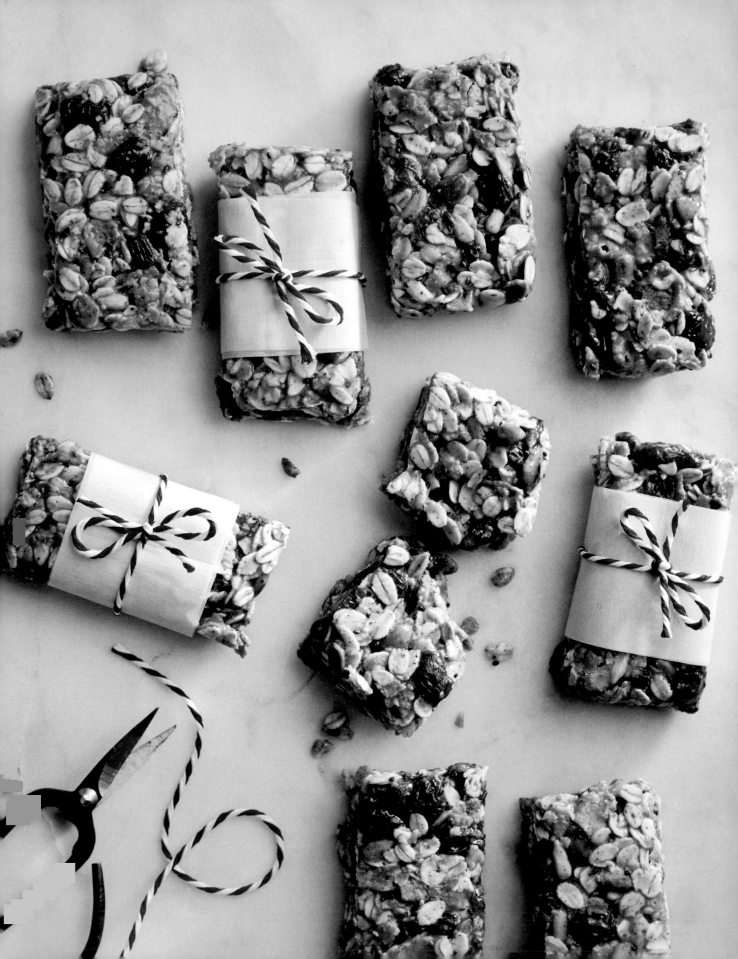

GO FASTER GRANOLA BARS MAKES 16 BARS

DAIRY-FREE • EGG-FREE • GLUTEN-FREE • NUT-FREE • VEGAN • VEGETARIAN • WHEAT-FREE

This recipe is now legendary at Sprout Right! These wholesome granola bars are packed with slow-releasing carbohydrates and healthy fats to keep your toddler and family going longer. Substitute sunflower seed butter for the nut butter to make them safe for school and those with allergies. This will likely become a staple recipe in your home, too!

1 cup (250 mL) flake cereal such as Nature's Path Heritage Flakes, Millet Rice Flakes, or Corn Flakes

1 cup (250 mL) old-fashioned rolled oats

¾ cup (175 mL) dried fruit (Thompson raisins or sultanas, chopped dates, unsulphured apricots)

¼ cup (60 mL) sunflower, pumpkin, or sesame seeds

¼ cup (60 mL) chopped almonds (optional)

½ cup (125 mL) brown rice or barley malt syrup

2 tablespoons (30 mL) coconut butter or unsalted butter

¼ cup (60 mL) almond, pumpkin seed, or sesame seed butter

1. Combine the cereal, oats, dried fruit, seeds, and almonds in a bowl.
2. In a large saucepan, gently heat the brown rice syrup, coconut butter, and almond butter until melted and smooth. Remove from the heat, add the dry ingredients, and quickly stir to coat. Press into an 8-inch (2 L) square pan.
3. Refrigerate for at least 1 hour and cut into squares.
4. Store the bars in an airtight container at room temperature for up to 5 days or in the freezer for up to 2 weeks.

NUTRITIONAL INFORMATION These bars are a good source of vitamin E, calcium, zinc, vitamin B1, manganese, magnesium, protein, copper, selenium, phosphorus, vitamin B5, and folate.

NO-MESS FRUITY ICE POPS

MAKES ABOUT 8 ICE POPS

DAIRY-FREE • EGG-FREE • GLUTEN-FREE •
NUT-FREE • VEGAN • VEGETARIAN • WHEAT-FREE

These ice pops are a refreshing summer treat without sugar and loaded with nutrients that kids will love! Add apple sauce if you have it to make more of the fruit mixture.

4 cups (1 L) fresh fruit (see Tip)
½ cup (125 mL) unsweetened applesauce
 (optional)

1. Blend the fresh fruit in a blender or food processor until smooth. Add applesause, if using, and blend again to combine.
2. Pour the purée into ice pop moulds and freeze for up to 1 month.

TIP: Banana, peach, pear, blueberry, and mango are a good combination, but any fruit will work well.

NUTRITIONAL INFORMATION These ice pops are a good source of fibre, antioxidants, and vitamin C.

FRUITY FROZEN YOGURT

MAKES ABOUT 2 CUPS (500 ML)

EGG-FREE • GLUTEN-FREE • NUT-FREE •
VEGETARIAN • WHEAT-FREE

Your kids will think they're being spoiled when they eat this! It's a delightfully healthy yet tasty treat.

1 cup (250 mL) full-fat plain or Greek yogurt
2½ cups (625 mL) fresh fruit (see Tip)
½ ripe avocado, pitted and peeled (optional)
3 tablespoons (45 mL) pure maple syrup or liquid
 pure honey

1. Divide the yogurt among the cells of an ice cube tray and freeze.
2. Spread the fruit mixture evenly on a baking sheet lined with parchment paper and freeze.
3. Once frozen, let the yogurt soften slightly out of the freezer, about 3 to 5 minutes. Purée the yogurt, frozen fruit, avocado (if using), and maple syrup in a food processor until smooth.
4. Serve immediately or store in an airtight container in the freezer for up to 1 week. Once the fruity yogurt has been frozen, let it thaw slightly before serving, as it will be solid.

TIP: Be sure to include ripe banana as part of your fresh fruit combination for its sweetness and creamy texture.

NUTRITIONAL INFORMATION This frozen yogurt is a good source of calcium, phosphorus, vitamin B2, protein, vitamin B12, potassium, molybdenum, zinc, and pantothenic acid.

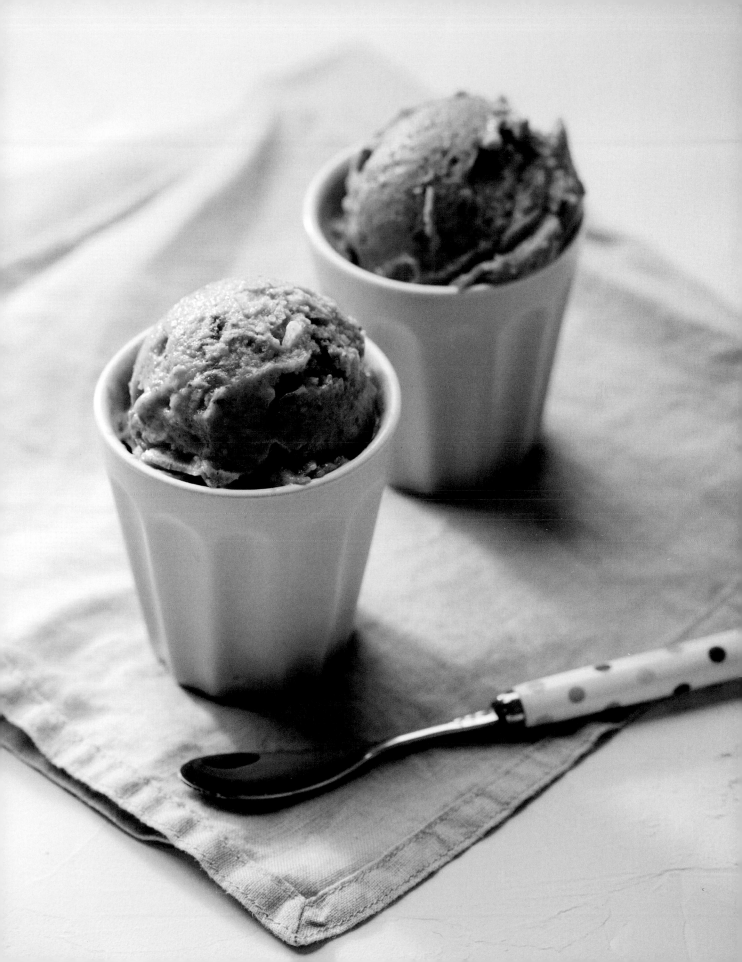

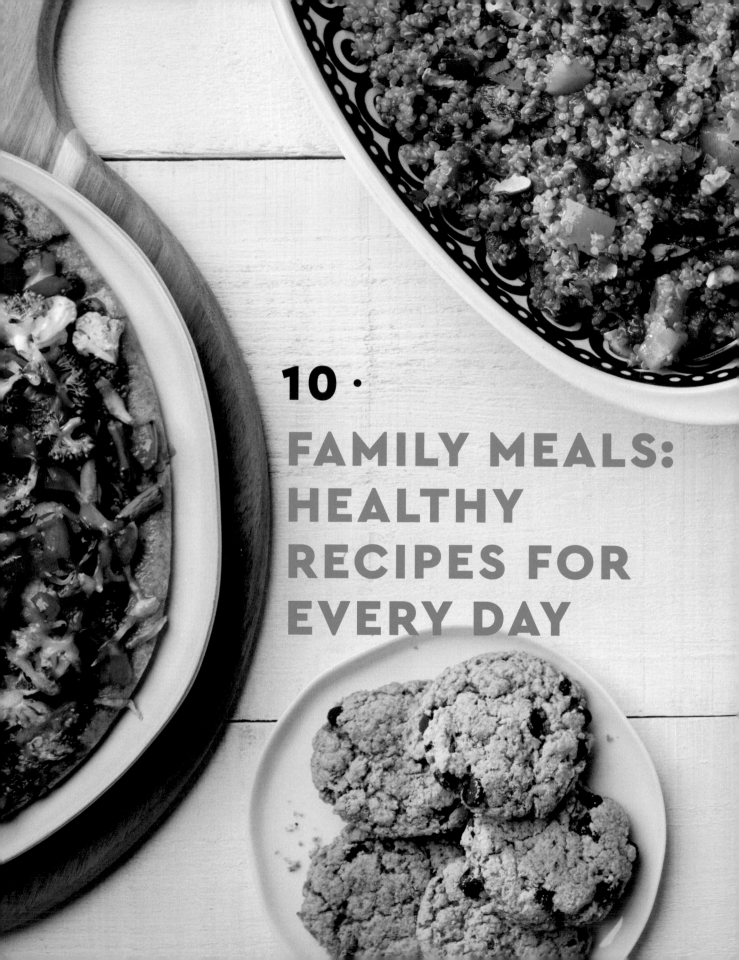

10 ·

FAMILY MEALS: HEALTHY RECIPES FOR EVERY DAY

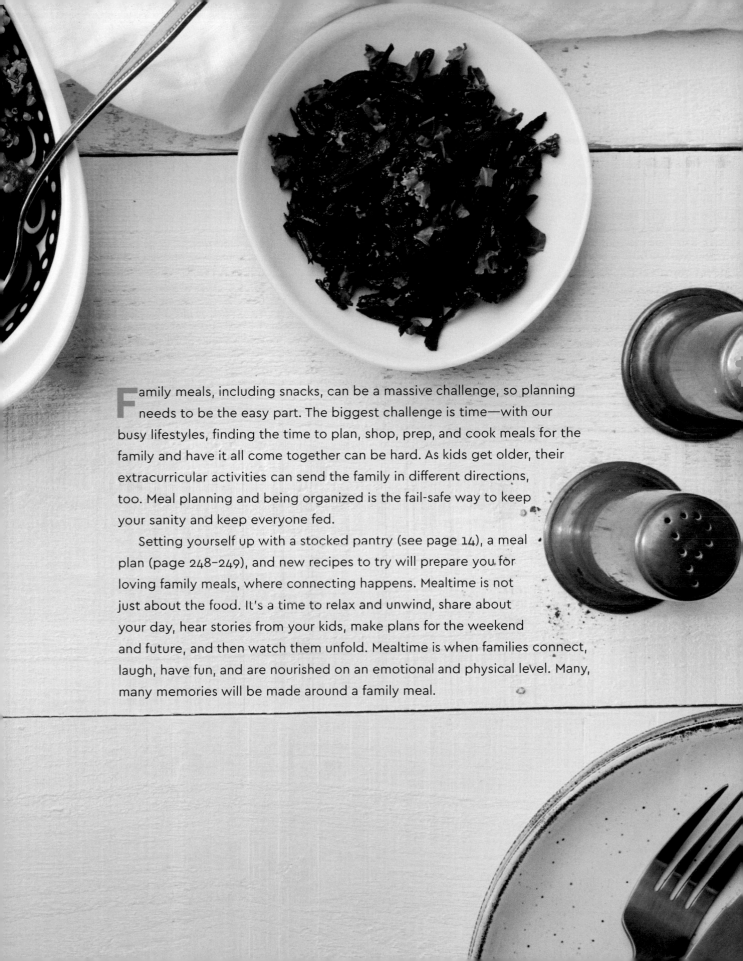

Family meals, including snacks, can be a massive challenge, so planning needs to be the easy part. The biggest challenge is time—with our busy lifestyles, finding the time to plan, shop, prep, and cook meals for the family and have it all come together can be hard. As kids get older, their extracurricular activities can send the family in different directions, too. Meal planning and being organized is the fail-safe way to keep your sanity and keep everyone fed.

Setting yourself up with a stocked pantry (see page 14), a meal plan (page 248–249), and new recipes to try will prepare you for loving family meals, where connecting happens. Mealtime is not just about the food. It's a time to relax and unwind, share about your day, hear stories from your kids, make plans for the weekend and future, and then watch them unfold. Mealtime is when families connect, laugh, have fun, and are nourished on an emotional and physical level. Many, many memories will be made around a family meal.

PLANT-BASED EATING

Eating a plant-heavy diet is always a good idea. I haven't come across many clients who eat enough vegetables or fruit, so a recent push by Health Canada in our country's food guide to eat a more plant-based diet echoes what so many nutritionists, naturopaths, and health-savvy people have being saying for years. A plant-based diet doesn't mean that one that lacks protein. According to Forks Over Knives, a plant-based diet is "a diet based on fruits, vegetables, tubers, whole grains, and legumes; and it excludes or minimizes meat (including chicken and fish), dairy products, and eggs, as well as highly refined foods like bleached flour, refined sugar, and oil."[122] Sounds like an all-around healthy diet.

Although some think that a plant-based diet is essentially vegan, it's really up to you how you decide to create your own plant-based diet. The term *plant-based* is used by Health Canada in the 2019 Canada Food Guide, which does not call for a vegan diet but rather for Canadians to eat more plants.

Some children decide to become vegetarian even if the family is not, and others take it a step further and choose to eat a vegan diet with no animal products at all. Either situation can make for interesting meal prep for the family if you've been meat eaters. This is when understanding proteins and specific nutrients and their sources becomes more important so that deficiencies don't happen as your child continues to grow. Nutritional deficiencies are common for vegans, particularly deficiencies in iron, vitamin B12, and iodine. Growth restriction also may occur if the diet is not optimally providing fats, protein, and overall energy. If anyone in your family is following a plant-based diet and not eating any animal products, as in veganism, then be prepared to supplement with vitamin B12, iron, and iodine.

VEGETARIAN MEALS AND PROTEIN

Proteins provide the building blocks you need to make and maintain your muscles, organs, and immune systems. Amino acids can be thought of as the building blocks of protein. Your body can make some amino acids, but there are eight essential amino acids that your body needs to get from food. For instance, animal protein sources from meat to eggs are complete proteins. Vegetarians and vegans rely on plant sources of protein that offer what's needed by the body, but most individual plant sources are incomplete proteins, and so need to be combined with a variety of other sources of protein to make up a complete protein. It's easily done if a variety of protein sources are eaten—the classic example of this is rice and beans. Rice is low in threonine, and beans are low in methionine and tryptophan. If you combine them at the same meal, you get a delicious dish that has all the essential amino acids. All vegetables also contain protein.

GOOD SOURCES OF PROTEIN

- Beans
- Peas
- Avocado
- Lentils
- Nuts and seeds

- and nut and seed butters
- Soy: tofu, tempeh, edamame, miso, soy milk

- Quinoa*
- Amaranth
- Buckwheat
- Spirulina*
- Hemp seeds*

- Whey, rice, pea, or hemp protein powder*
- Chia (salba)*

*Denotes a complete protein.

Any family member who is vegetarian or vegan needs to combine vegetarian sources of protein in a complementary way to make them complete proteins. Including vegetables with each meal, along with the suggestions below, make this simple to do. Complementing proteins do not need to be eaten at the same meal but should be eaten over the course of a day.

Legumes are beans, peas, and lentils. Combine them with nuts and seeds, whole grains, or corn and you'll be closer to a complex protein that's found in animal foods. Being aware of the amount of protein eaten becomes more important when activity level increases, especially in sports training. Protein is essential for repair of muscles after an activity or workout.

Examples of healthy complete protein combinations are:

- Rice and beans, peas, or lentils
- Beans on whole-grain toast with carrot sticks
- Corn and beans combined
- Hummus and whole wheat pita bread
- Nut or seed butter on whole-grain bread
- Whole-grain or chickpea pasta with sauce including beans

- Bean, pea, and/or lentil soup with whole-grain or seeded crackers or whole-grain bread
- Corn tortillas with refried beans, avocado, and colourful vegetables
- Veggie or plant-based burgers on whole-grain buns served with a side of greens

FERMENTED FOODS

Fermentation is an age-old practice that preserved food when there were no fridges, freezers, or ways to keep produce throughout seasons. In the early days (pre-1950s or so), getting milk from a cow and having it go sour over a week or more was normal. Making sauerkraut from crops of cabbage with salt was as normal as taking food out of a box and putting it in the oven.

I've talked about probiotics throughout this book. It's an area I've focused on in my career, learning from very smart minds about the microbiome and how it affects our health. Taking a probiotic daily is a strong recommendation I make to all of my clients, and eating fermented foods furthers that with more varied strains and benefits. Fermented foods include yogurt, kefir, cottage cheese, cheese, sauerkraut, sourdough, kombucha, pickles, and miso. Fermented foods can be purchased easily, but if you'd like to try making your own, you can find recipes that detail how to make your own yogurt, kombucha, kefir, and sauerkraut on www.sproutright.com. It can be fun for kids to make these foods, as they're a bit like a science experiment, and seeing how commonly eaten foods are made can be fascinating.

Here are a few benefits of fermented foods:

- In the case of dairy, they start the digestion process by using lactose for the proliferation of good bacteria.
- They create billions of beneficial bacteria that, when eaten positively, affect digestive and immune health.
- They maintain the enzymes in food, which gives the pancreas a well-earned break. For instance, sourdough bread is easier to digest than bread made with just yeast.
- They increase vitamin content, as in fermented dairy products, and offer higher levels of B vitamins.
- Fermented foods keep for longer. Fermented cabbage becomes sauerkraut; milk ferments to kefir, yogurt, or cheese; and cucumbers and other vegetables become pickles that keep for longer than fresh.

YOGURT

Can you guess what the most consumed fermented food is? Yogurt.

Fermented from milk and live bacterial culture (such as the probiotic acidophilus), yogurt is well tolerated by those sensitive to most dairy products, especially lactose. Lactose is used or eaten up by the bacteria as they proliferate and turn milk to yogurt.

As you cruise the dairy aisle at the supermarket, there is some stiff competition to make it from the shelf to your cart. Many different types of yogurt—including low-fat and no-fat, Greek, creamy, drinking, bio yogurt, organic, baby, and frozen—can add to the overall confusion about which is best to buy and how the family will like it.

Some yogurts tout their health benefits better than others. When I read the ingredients of some brands, the list seems far too long for a product made from milk and bacteria. Colours, flavouring, sugar (glucose, high-fructose corn syrup, dextrose, and artificial sweeteners), and maybe some fruit on the bottom are most common. Most yogurts look fruity because of added colour, not actual fruit.

Years ago, I remember being asked to spread the word about a new yogurt for babies on the market. At the time, I was doing weekly workshops at Whole Foods Market to a jam-packed classroom of moms and babies. I was the perfect person to help reach the marketing goals for the launch of this new product.

As I do with all products, I read the ingredients label. It contained sugar. I was shocked. A yogurt for babies with sugar in it? In my opinion, that's just wrong. I went back to the company and said that I'd love to share its new product with the loyal attendees of my class and also let them know that it has sugar in it (something I, in no uncertain terms, suggest avoiding for babies and toddlers). After a dialogue with the marketing manager, I found out that during taste tests, babies preferred the product with sugar in it. Fair enough. A business wants sales at the end of the day, but I was so annoyed that a company couldn't take the healthier road and not put sugar in its new product. From then on, I continued to share what I had learned with my classes, although the company withdrew its request for my help to market it. I wonder why!

HYDRATION

Water is essential for life. It gives instant energy, helps to flush toxins out of the body, retains water-soluble nutrients, regulates body temperature, gives moisture and fluidity to lungs and joints, and hydrates the brain and all tissues. With such tempting sweet and filling fluids of juice, coffee, tea, pop, milkshakes, slushies, milk, and others, most head straight to the cooler in the store for refreshment. However, these drinks in fact are *dehydrating*. Sure, they give you an instant boost, but it's short-lived. After drinking any of the above, double up on your water intake so you aren't left low and dry. Your kids need to drink water as their main fluid intake. For so many, one glass of water a day may be a lot, especially when sports drinks or other energy drinks are far more appealing.

Lack of energy, headaches, tiredness, dry skin, muscle cramps, constipation, and wonky blood pressure all may result from dehydration. Not to mention that a 20 percent level of dehydration may lead to death. Not a good situation to be in.

During times of sickness, drinking water is especially important. Whether a cold, virus, or gastrointestinal bug, keeping hydrated at an optimal level is necessary for the nasal passages, lungs, gastrointestinal tract, and all mucous membranes. When dried out, they don't capture or trap the bacteria, virus, or pathogen they'd like to.

Coconut water is another hydrating drink that's very useful during times of sickness. On super-hot days when outdoor soccer, baseball, or other sports are played, coconut water can be more hydrating than regular water. It's a natural sports drink without all the colour, sugar, and flavouring that are marketed to our kids and athletes. Only natural or plain coconut water is naturally sugar-free. Flavoured coconut water will have added sugar.

The best way to tell if you're hydrated is by the colour of your urine. Is it a dark, medium, or light straw colour? When urine is a light straw colour, the body is hydrated. If you or your kids don't pee a lot, you'll also know that there's dehydration. Water goes in, and ideally it comes out within a couple of hours. If there are long periods between urination, that's another sign of dehydration.

HELPING TO IMPROVE FOCUS

In a time and culture that seems designed for multitasking and attention-splitting activities, maintaining focus is a challenge. Distractions like other people, many varieties of screens, social media, email, school, homework, and getting out of doing homework can all suck time and leave the important things at the bottom of the list.

Attention deficit disorder, lack of memory, and poor concentration and focus can be helped by a nutrient-dense diet and staying hydrated. Drinking water can provide instant energy and improve mental alertness. Complex carbohydrates and unrefined foods help to keep blood sugar levels much more even than the highs and lows of sugary and processed foods. Good-quality protein, including eating fish often, and taking a supplement of docosahexaenoic acid (DHA), the brain-boosting omega-3 fat, are also helpful. Check out the Salmon Burgers recipe on page 286.

I've helped many clients and their kids who complain of brain fog or being sluggish in the morning by adjusting their diet to avoid common allergens. Wheat or gluten, dairy, and artificial colours and flavourings are the first to experiment with. Other chemicals can create sensitivities that have speedy reactions of lethargy, poor concentration, hyperactivity, depression, and even confusion. I find that the paradox of food being essential for life and also potentially causing harm to be confusing for those I try to support. The proof comes from a trial of removing such foods and seeing what the results are. Kids can be resistant to losing a usual part of their diet, but explaining why and for how long can ease that resistance. In my experience, the effort of changing the diet helps. Caffeine, chocolate, and sugar all give a short-lived boost to focus, but the crash afterwards could make you feel worse than before you indulged.

IMMUNE BOOSTING FOR KIDS (AND ADULTS)

Can you prevent your kids getting a cold or cough? Maybe not completely, but you can increase the chances of avoiding it turning into a secondary *-itis* like bronchitis, otitis, or sinusitis. Your kids' immune army needs a leg up over what will hit them as they enter through the school gates.

Before I talk about food, remember that lack of sleep makes for a sleepy and weak immune system.

FOODS TO BRACE THE IMMUNE SYSTEM AT LUNCHTIME (AND ANYTIME)

Lunchtime is a great time to keep the nutrients going in. Red, yellow, orange, and green peppers make a sweet side to any sandwich or wrap. They are packed with vitamin C, one of the most important immune-boosting vitamins. Your kids' bones, skin, and heart also benefit from peppers and their powerful antioxidants. Other vitamin C–rich foods include avocado, banana, kiwi, kale, parsley, broccoli, tomato, mango, citrus fruits, black currants, berries, pineapple, cherries, and cantaloupe. Add all of these to lunches at will.

Seaweed is packed with nutrients, trace minerals, and even essential fats. Small packs of seaweed are easily available in stores, so grab some and let the kids try it out. It'll satisfy their need for crunch at lunch. Zinc found in seaweed is what's going to prop up the immune army. Other zinc-rich foods to include are mushrooms, asparagus, oats, wheat germ, brewer's yeast, soybeans, pumpkin and sunflower seeds, herring, eggs, dark meat poultry, and miso (as in soup). My kids would take the small packages of seaweed in their lunch, then add a container of rice and some veggie sticks and smoked salmon and assemble their own sushi at school. It seemed to be a craze for a while! They certainly enjoyed it, and I was happy with their contribution!

Hummus is a sneaky way to get some virus- and bacteria-killing garlic into your kids' lunches. Not that you want to embarrass them with a stinky lunch, but hummus or even garlic bread (made with pressed garlic mixed with butter and spread on bread, then toasted) along with a thermal container full of hot Immune-Boosting Soup (page 297) can give the immune army a boost with each mouthful.

Berries of all kinds offer vitamin C, but also contain flavonoids. These phytonutrients boost vitamin C's effectiveness and help reduce inflammation (think sore throat). All immune complexes are more active in the presence of flavonoids. Their antiviral activity has been studied with more life-threatening viruses than the average cold or cough, so they will be welcome by the body.

Kefir offers probiotics that get to the immune system where it's most vulnerable: the intestines (see recipe on SproutRight.com). Helping overall immunity to beat any type of virus or bacteria, probiotics can also come from plain yogurt. I say *plain* because the addition of sugar negates the beneficial bacteria found in yogurt. Note that most dairy products increase mucus production and are not recommended during diarrhea, so when your child is sick, limit dairy as much as you can. See SproutRight.com for specific recommendations on immune-boosting supplements.

IMMUNE DRAINERS

Avoid high fat, high sugar junk foods, as they can decrease the activity of the immune system. It's also best to avoid too much caffeine (pop, coffee, tea, chocolate), and don't smoke! Smoking can impair your resistance as well as injure the respiratory tract, which makes you more susceptible to the flu.

MANAGING COLDS AND FLUS

Any time of year, colds and flus can hit. They mostly occur in the winter, though. It's just that time of the year when there's an onslaught of sneezes, coughs, sniffles, and all other dreaded mucus-producing bugs.

Whether your kid picks up bacteria or a virus at daycare, at school, or through a sneeze at dance or soccer practice, it's quite likely that it will make the rounds of your whole family. For we parents, that means suffering with a box of tissues on our desk after being off work for one to three days and spending sleepless nights looking after a germy child—plus a stressful catch-up period once your home's patient zero heads back to daycare or school.

I maintain strong boundaries when my kids are sick, and they've learned these over time. Here's a sneak peek at what I do:

STOP ALL SUGAR Any sniffle, headache, aches, or low energy, or an "I'm not feeling well, mom," and my kids know that there will be *no* sugar until they are better. They eat fruit and drink their smoothies but *nothing* with refined sugar in it is allowed. Sugar slows the immune system and its army for hours after it's eaten. If my kids are on the brink of coming down with something or if a virus is in full swing, refined sugar is going to stop their system from doing what it needs to. Fight it, and fight it hard.

ADD GARLIC TO ANYTHING When my youngest was ten months old, I made a purée of avocado, banana, blueberry, and pear; added in raw garlic; and fed it to her daily for a month. She wasn't sick again for ages. I now make my kids eat raw garlic toast that's quickly broiled and add loads of garlic to soup. They know it's coming, so there's no complaining about it.

FEED THEM SOUP Make homemade bone broth from dark meat (see recipe on page 129) or naturally raised chicken, or take some from your store in the freezer. Make the Immune-Boosting Soup on page 297. Your kids will get a bit of carbohydrate from the rice noodles, amino acids (the building blocks of protein) from the protein, easily absorbed minerals, and extra nutrients and anti-inflammatory compounds for all that mucus.

DOSE UP ON IMMUNE BOOSTERS As listed on page 240–241.

REST When they're sick, my kids sleep, bring their duvet and pillow to the couch, and do nothing. They have warm baths with epsom salts and cozy up in their PJs after I've rubbed caster oil on their chests and backs, covering the area where their lungs are. This continues until they or I feel that they're through the sickness enough and won't pass it on when they go back to school.

SCHOOL LUNCHES

This is one of the most asked-for sections in this book. Making lunches day in and day out is one of the most challenging things for parents to really do a great job at. At the beginning of the school year, everyone is ready to pack that bright and shiny new lunch bag. By mid-September, the novelty has worn off and ideas cease to flow or kids start to bring home more than they ate.

One year, my kids kept bringing back their lunches half eaten. Most think that a nutritionist's kids would eat well—and for the most part they do—but when it came to lunch, it was the opposite. Full lunchbox after full lunchbox would come home with crabby kids who couldn't make it to dinner without a meltdown or two. I was losing my mind. So, I decided to pass the responsibility to them. And it worked. A study showed that about 85 percent of kids who participate in preparing a meal are more likely to eat what they've had a hand in making than not. I set guidelines for my kids on what needed to be included in a healthy lunchbox and let them be creative.

WHERE TO START WITH YOUR LUNCH PLANNING

1. Talk to your kids about them taking healthy lunches to school and why it's important.
2. Make a lunch chart or dowload one on SproutRight.com and talk about what's going to be in the lunchbox daily. Creating a chart from scratch can result in a more personal version

designed and agreed on by parents and kids.

3. Shop for or check that you have ample bisphenol A (BPA)–free, leakproof containers. Varied sizes and shapes that fit into the lunchbox or bag are important for a variety of foods, including dips. Have a run-through to ensure that your child can open lids and put them back on. Label everything in case anything is left in the schoolyard (we love Mabel's Labels that never come off).

4. A water bottle that washes easily is essential. Get one that fits inside or hangs off the lunch bag so that it's not left behind in the backpack or locker.

5. Keep a shopping list on the fridge and ask everyone to write down anything that's needed or that you've run out of. Also add special requests.

6. Keep artificial colours and preservatives out of the lunch box. Children with sensitivities, attention deficit disorder, and attention deficit hyperactivity disorder may be more sensitive to processed foods containing additives.

I asked Liza Finlay, a psychotherapist, what her thoughts are about when kids can start to make their own lunches. Here are her recommendations:

> School lunches . . . I don't think of this as something that begins at a certain age, but rather a process that gradually builds until children are able to assume full responsibility. Parents could start by having kids take responsibility for loading and unloading lunch bags from backpacks (also, if the lunch bag is not unpacked, the new lunch is stacked on the counter to be packed by the child as a natural consequence). As early as junior kindergarten, children can pull fruit and a juice box from the fridge and add it to the lunch bag. Gradually, as they grow, they do more, so that by grade 4 they are doing the whole thing.
>
> From the start, encourage cooperation by including the child in decision making. "What would you like in your lunches? Let's make a list together." Be sure to take some time to teach the child how to do new tasks—use the toaster, heat the soup in the microwave, use the can opener. Be there to assist and encourage and say, "Those can openers are tricky and take a bit of practice," but don't take the lunch task back once it's been handed off. That's a recipe for discouragement and entitlement.
>
> Lastly, allow for natural consequences. Everyone forgets their lunch occasionally, but if you run a forgotten lunch to the school every time your child forgets it, there is no reason for them to build the mental muscles of memory, discipline, and strategy.[123]

Wise words that I've followed. I felt as if I were being judged by teachers as they shared some of their own lunches with my kids, but my daughters didn't forget their lunches again!

YOUR HEALTHY LUNCH GUIDE

Sit down and discuss these guidelines so that everyone will be on the same page:

- Limit the amount of processed foods, especially meat that contains nitrates (supermarket lunch meat, ham, smoked meat, roast beef, etc.). Nitrates have been proven to have many adverse health risks, including cancer. Limit processed meat to once a week if you can. This is where leftover chicken or fish comes in very handy.

- Try to switch up the grains you are offering. The most common grain eaten in the Western world is wheat. Try to offer kamut, spelt, rye, or rice-based products as alternatives a few times a week.

- Yogurt can be a fast and easy addition to any lunch as a snack but typically is high in sugar and so a carbohydrate-rich food. Plain Greek yogurt contains more protein, so it makes a perfect addition to lunch (or breakfast) to balance out the carbs. Buy higher fat yogurt pots with fruit rather than low-fat versions, which have added artificial sweeteners or more sugar to help them taste better.

- When choosing any package of crackers or snacks, read the label of what you are buying. If sugar is in the top five ingredients, see if you can do better. If it has artificial colours, leave it on the shelf. Avoid sugary anything, as these snacks really don't offer much nutritional value.

- When buying bread or wraps for fast lunches, try to buy high-fibre options like whole grain and varieties that include flaxseeds (either ground or whole). The carbohydrate or energy releases more slowly and offers a lower glycemic index. By also adding protein to the sandwich or wrap, energy release slows even further.

- If you offer sweets or sugary treats at lunch, which I don't recommend, pack a piece of cheese to eat afterwards to alter the mouth's pH back to acidic to prevent cavities.

Lunches need to have key components. These can help your kids (and you) to know what's essential, and then you can build from there. Combine the essential building blocks listed below for a balanced meal. Ask for input from the family to plan lunches.

PROTEIN Important for growth and development, energy, a healthy immune system, and hormonal balance. Protein is often left out. It helps our energy to stay balanced and not crash after lunch. Some of these options may be on the do-not-bring-to-school list, as a few are common allergens: meat, fish, poultry, dairy products, soy, pulses, beans, eggs, legumes, millet, amaranth, quinoa, and seeds.

CARBOHYDRATE Needed for energy, fibre, vitamins, and minerals. Carbohydrate gives energy; how fast that energy is released will depend on the kind of carbohydrate, whether refined or not. The more sugary and refined the carbohydrate is, the faster the energy will release . . . and then crash. The more you can include whole grains, whole foods, and vegetables or fruits in their natural form, the better and more balanced your child will feel. Options to include are grains and cereals (bread, pasta, oats, wheat, and brown rice), vegetables, fruits, beans, and pulses.

FAT Both saturated and essential fats are important, but saturated fats are easier to get in an everyday diet. Omega-3 and omega-6 fatty acids take more thought to include but are worth the effort, as they are important for brain, nerve, and eye development; alertness; IQ; energy; skin condition; and heart function. Omega-3 and DHA help improve memory, ease hyperactivity, and aid concentration, and can help ease depression. Options to include are tuna, herring, mackerel, sardines, salmon, cod liver oil, walnuts, chia, and flaxseeds. Omega-6 helps increase metabolism, stamina, and energy and alleviates dry skin. Options to include are flaxseeds and sunflower, pumpkin, and sesame seeds and their oils.

FRUIT Fruit can be a sweet ending or part of lunch, like on skewers or toothpicks. All fruit provides essential fibre, vitamins, minerals, antioxidants, and phytonutrients. Lower glycemic index or slow energy-releasing fruits include apple, pear, plums, cantaloupe, mango, orange or clementine/mandarin, strawberries, blueberries, raspberries, and blackberries.

VEGETABLES The almighty vegetable. These are often the most difficult to get into kids, as important as they are. All vegetables provide fibre, vitamins, minerals, and phytonutrients. Options to include are carrots (baby, sticks, grated, or whole), green beans, red or green cabbage, broccoli, celery, sweet potato, white potato with skin, squash, mushrooms, cucumber, tomato, asparagus spears, and cauliflower. For those who don't like raw, send steamed or roasted vegetables.

FLUID Yes, there are water fountains in all schools, but having a measurement of intake is very handy, especially in the case of constipation. Also, not having to drink from the germ-infested water fountain spout could benefit your whole family. Fluid is needed for hydration, energy, and stamina. Water is best, but you can also offer diluted juice: one-third juice and two-thirds water. Diluted juice can hydrate, whereas undiluted juice can be dehydrating. Although they are hugely popular and convenient, avoid juice boxes. Coconut water or herb tea in a thermos also works for some kids. Avoid any tea with caffeine.

LUNCH OPTIONS

I do love dinner turned to lunch the next day, whenever possible. If you need new ideas to add to your weekly meal plan, use any of the ones listed below, write out a meal plan on the weekend, and then everyone will know what's coming.

In a thermal container:

- Veggie-Packed Chili (page 211)
- Gnocchi with tuna or ground beef or turkey and tomato sauce
- Lentil Shepherd's Pie (page 214)
- Ravioli (meat or cheese filled) with kale and oregano pesto
- Tortellini (meat or cheese filled) with fresh tomato and basil sauce
- Baked Butternut Squash and Garlic Risotto (page 264)
- Rice stir-fry with leftover meat or fish and diced colourful vegetables

- Veggie Pesto Pizza (page 212)
- The Ultimate Lasagna (page 219)
- Soup such as Corn, Coconut, and Ginger Soup (page 295), Immune-Boosting Soup (page 297), or Sweet Potato and Coconut Soup (page 215);
- Curried Quinoa Salad with Apricots (page 300)

- Bow tie or spiral noodles with grated Parmesan, fresh basil, chopped baby tomatoes, and leftover diced chicken or sausage
- Mini Frittata (page 257)
- Mini Calzone (page 275)

In a wrap, pita, or sandwich:

- Leftover or sliced chicken with lettuce, cucumber, and tomato
- Leftover or sliced ham or chicken, avocado, and tomato with basil pesto mayo
- Tuna or salmon salad and chopped cucumber or dill pickle
- Grated cheese and cut-up grapes
- Falafel, hummus, and salad
- Grated carrot with cucumber, sunflower or pea sprouts, and hummus
- Brie with cranberry sauce
- Cheddar cheese with sliced apples and sprouts
- Turkey slices with arugula or spinach, apple butter, and mustard

- Mashed hard boiled egg, watercress or chives, and mayonnaise
- Pressed cottage cheese or cream cheese with sweet corn, cucumber, or fruit spread
- Tuna, sweet corn, and a little salad dressing
- Mashed banana and tahini or sunflower seed spread
- Bean Burger (page 206), lettuce, onion, and tomato with yogurt dip
- Sushi (must send with an ice pack to keep fish cool)
- Rainbow Rice Wraps (page 292)
- Roasted Veggie Tagine (page 279)
- Salmon Burgers (page 286)

TOOTHPICK COMBINATIONS

Lunch on a toothpick is such fun to eat. You can put just about anything on a skewer or toothpick to vary what's in the lunchbox. Be sure to discuss not poking any classmates with the toothpick once the food has been eaten.

- Mozzarella or bocconcini cheese, cherry tomato, and basil served with a side of pita and hummus
- Cheddar cheese, apple pieces, and colourful pepper served with a side of pita and tzatziki or hummus
- Feta cheese, grapes, cherry tomatoes, and cube of ham

- Watermelon, feta cheese, and cucumber with Greek yogurt
- Mushroom, chicken, and cooked Brussels sprouts

- Tortellini with tomato and chicken or tofu
- Avocado, smoked salmon, and cubes of bread

SIDES

Sides or accompaniments can round out a meal with anything that's missing from a texture, colour, or taste standpoint.

- Seaweed—nori sheets, strips, or crinkles
- Edamame
- Beany Green Dip (page 181)
- Oatcakes (page 318)
- Guacamole and rice chips or pita
- Yummy Carrot Spread (page 180)
- Cream cheese or soft goat's cheese as a dip with low-sodium pretzels
- Mary's Gone Crackers Sticks and Twigs
- Cherry tomatoes

- Celery sticks filled with tahini or pumpkin seed or sunflower seed butter
- Brown rice cakes with tahini and honey, apple butter, or fruit spread
- Dried fruit with seeds and cereal flakes (or any whole-grain cereal)
- Air-popped or coconut oil–popped popcorn
- Baked tortilla chips with Hummus (page 182) and salsa

TREATS AND DESSERT

- Fruit—peel fruit or cut into pieces for your child so it's easier to eat; drizzle lemon juice or cinnamon over it and it won't go brown
- Cottage cheese with pineapple or other fruit
- Greek yogurt with toppings
- Dried fruit—organic and unsulphured apple, apricot, pineapple, mango, raisins, or prunes
- Fruit salad served with a splash of balsamic vinegar

- Mini Blueberry Muffins (page 315), Pumpkin Muffins (page 316), Zucchini Spice Muffins (page 317), or Sneaky Little Muffins (page 225)
- Unsweetened applesauce
- Whole-grain cereal bars
- Go Faster Granola Bars (page 231) made with school-safe seed butter
- Chocolate Chip Cookies (page 311)

MEAL PLANNING FOR YOUR FAMILY

Meal planning is essential for busy families. No matter what the age of the children in the family, knowing in advance what's for dinner, or in your pantry to grab in a flash, takes the stress out of getting a good meal on the table. Five o'clock seems to come around quickly on a day when you don't have anything planned for dinner.

Stocking your pantry (page 14) and keeping up with dry goods and frozen staples saves you from having to shop every few days. When you shop, use the list on your fridge that everyone contributes to and your meal plan. Shop with intention, too. Having a well-planned week of meals means that you are in and out of the supermarket, buying only what you need for the week. This saves not only money, but valuable time spent wandering the aisles looking for inspiration from a package of food!

Although it's fun to try new recipes, making a new dish on a workday isn't always the answer. Try out new ideas and recipes in this book or those you find in favourite books or online on the weekend. During the week, stick to fast and simple recipes that are a hit. New recipes can be added to your weekend meal plan. I recommend batch cooking, not necessarily on the weekend but also during the week, so that no matter what you are making you'll have extra to put in the freezer for another meal. Fast meals that can be reheated may be all you have time for during the week. If you're making a pizza, for instance, have two pizza bases on the go to be topped with leftover chicken and some colourful vegetables. Top them with grated cheese and then one can be cooked and the other frozen for another day. Soups, stews, lasagna, and meatballs all freeze very well and can be used for speedy evening meals.

PLANNING FOR THE WEEK

If you find meal planning daunting, write down what you eat over a week in a meal planning template and then use that information to plot next week's meals and snacks. This takes the pressure off making a weekly plan from scratch, which doesn't take into

Family Seven-Day Meal Plan

Meal	Day 1	Day 2	Day 3	
Breakfast	Seeds of Success Smoothie (page 253) and two Go Faster Granola Bars (page 231)	Overnight French Toast (page 259) with one piece of fruit	Lovely Soaked Muesli (page 165) with fresh grapefruit on the side	
Snack	Finger Food Pancakes (page 178) with Yummy Carrot Spread (page 180)	Celery with almond or sunflower seed butter	Bite-Size Fruit Balls (page 319) and an apple	
Lunch	Sweet Potato and Coconut soup (page 215) with Mary's Gone Crackers	Mini Frittatas (page 257) with a leafy green salad and Salad Dressing (page 304)	Taco Night (page 291) leftovers in a wrap with a green salad and red peppers with Salad Dressing (page 304)	
Snack (to take to work for parents or as after-school snacks for kids)	Fruit and a handful of Hit the Road Trail Mix (page 319)	Go Faster Granola Bar (page 231) and a pear	Zucchini Spice Muffins (page 317) and an apple	
Dinner	Baked Butternut Squash and Garlic Risotto (page 264) with Pesto Fish (page 289) and steamed broccoli	Taco Night (page 291) with all the fixings and Blueberry Maple Ice Cream (page 312)	Golden Grilled Curried Chicken Thighs (page 274) and Quinoa and Corn Salad (page 298) with wilted kale sprinkled with sesame seeds and tamari	

account what and how you usually eat. There will be some consistent nights when you need quick and easy. On other nights, there will be more time. I've seen many families make a meal plan with all new recipes and then by midweek they give up because it's so much work. Using last week as a template will hopefully help you to gradually improve your meal choices and offerings to be more healthy as you try a new recipe or two a week.

If you have a toddler who is at daycare all day, dinner may not be a hugely successful meal, so plan for that when mapping out dinners. Aim for parts of what you are eating to be part of his meal, even if he isn't quite ready for adult food. Again, planning makes for much easier meals.

With some of the ideas I've shared below, plot a week of meals and snacks and see how it works out for you.

You can download a blank meal plan at www.sproutright.com or make your own!

	Day 4	Day 5	Day 6	Day 7
	Chia Pudding (page 259) with blueberries and maple syrup	Sweet Blue Smoothie (page 253) with ½ cup (125 mL) Crunchy Granola (page 263) and milk or Greek yogurt and fruit	Blender Pancakes (page 255) with fresh fruit and scrambled eggs	Overnight French Toast (page 260) with cut-up melon and strawberries on the side
	Raw carrots, peppers, or zucchini with Beany Green Dip (page 181)	Go Faster Granola Bar (page 231) and melon	Apple and plain Greek yogurt and Crunchy Granola (page 263)	Mini Blueberry Muffins (page 315) and an apple
	Wrap with Roasted Veggie Tagine (page 279) and Hummus (page 182)	Veggie Pesto Pizza (with leftover chicken; page 212) with a green salad, red peppers, and cucumber with sprinkled sunflower and sesame seeds and Salad Dressing (page 304)	Corn, Coconut, and Ginger Soup (page 295) with Oatcakes (page 318)	Salmon or Tuna Burgers (page 286) with Winter Sunshine Salad (page 304)
	Sneaky Little Muffins (page 225) and grapes	Bite-Size Fruit Balls (page 319) and carrot sticks	Pure Green Hummus (page 309) and Oatcakes (page 318)	Baby carrots with Hummus (page 182)
	Easy Asian Soup Bowl (page 296) with kiwifruit slices for dessert	Chicken Breasts with Cheesy Garlic Sweet Potatoes (page 270) and Beet and Carrot Slaw with Ginger Sesame Dressing (page 299)	Turkey Meatloaf (see Super Burgers, Meatballs, or Meatloaf page 217) with mashed potato (add a dash of horseradish or grated cheese) and Lemony Green Beans (page 307)	Garlicky Greens and Chickpeas (page 306) with steamed broccoli sprinkled with sesame seeds and Coconut Rice (page 308)

SUPPLEMENTS

Figuring out what supplements to give your children or take yourself can be very confusing. Getting all our nutrients from food would be ideal, but there are times when the diet isn't as healthy as it could be or you or your kids are passing around a cold or flu. Specific immune boosters can be given in supplement form to help break the cycle of everyone in the family being sick. When in a deficient state, it can take a long time to bring the body back up to an optimal level with food alone.

The key players for immune boosting are listed here.

VITAMIN C Protects against infection and increases the production of white blood cells, which fight off infection. It can also shorten the duration and ease the severity of your cold or flu. Vitamin C food sources include citrus fruits, potatoes, green peppers, strawberries, and pineapple. Supplements: My *Take This* Alka C gives high-dose vitamin C as well as minerals. Emergen-C powder is hugely popular and dissolves easily in water, although it has some extra flavouring in it. Physica Energetics' Camu Camu Liposome is incredibly absorbable in low doses.

VITAMIN E Enhances the production of B cells, the immune cells that produce antibodies that destroy bacteria. Vitamin E–rich foods are seeds, vegetable oils, and grains. You can take vitamin E on its own, but it's better taken in a multivitamin or with a complex that includes vitamins A and C.

BETA CAROTENE Enhances the functioning of your immune system by increasing the number of infection-fighting cells. Foods rich in beta carotene include sweet potatoes, carrots, kale, spinach, turnip greens, winter squash, collard greens, cilantro, and fresh thyme. To enhance the availability of the beta carotene in these foods, they should be eaten raw or lightly steamed. Like vitamin E, I'd only recommend taking beta carotene or vitamin A on its own if there are issues with the lungs or other mucous membranes.

ZINC Helps to prevent a weakened immune system. Deficiency can increase susceptibility to infection. However, excessive zinc intake may impair immunity and increase infections. It's one to take in balance with other minerals. Zinc-rich foods include oysters, liver, lean beef, pork, turkey, lamb, lentils, pumpkin and sesame seeds, chickpeas, and yogurt. Supplements: Gammadyn Zn is zinc in a liquid form, one of the most absorbable ways to get it into your kids. Zinc tablets or capsules in an amino acid chelate form are best.

PROBIOTICS One of the best ways I know to boost the immune system is through the gut (since 80 percent of the immune system lives there). Fermented foods and supplements are your best options. Supplements: My *Take This* brand has human strains: BioBoost Adult, BioBoost Kid, and BioBoost Baby. The dosage depends on the situation, such as after taking antibiotics, digestive issues, or prevention and immune boosting.

VITAMIN D Has become more widely recognized for its role in supporting the immune system. The best source of vitamin D is sunshine. It also occurs naturally in fatty fish and fish oils, such as salmon, mackerel, sardines, herring, and cod liver oil, and in liver and egg yolk. Supplements: My *Take This* Sunshine D + K2 is a liposome spray that also contains vitamin K2 to enhance absorption. Cod liver oil is also a source of vitamin D in lower doses than drops or spray.

GARLIC Known for its cold-fighting abilities and ability to target respiratory infections, garlic and it's sulphur-containing compounds, such as allicin and sulphides, are excellent immune boosters. Best eaten raw, although a bit hot, add garlic to anything and everything at any time. Supplements: Allimax capsules are small and easy for kids to take. Designs for Health Allicillin soft gels are also easy for kids and adults.

OMEGA-3 FATS Increase the activity of white blood cells that eat up bacteria, speed up healing, and strengthen resistance to infection in the body. The best sources of these fats are fatty fish (anchovy, sardines, salmon, mackerel, tuna), flaxseed oil and flaxseeds, omega-3 eggs, nuts, and seeds. Supplements: My *Take This* Omega Power is suitable for the whole family and comes in a capsule form that can be chewed by your toddler or given to your baby by making a hole in the capsule and squeezing the oil into her mouth. Genestra, Carlson and NutraSea also make a range of omega-3 fat supplements.

MULTINUTRIENT When your kids are sick and aren't eating, it's good to have almost all of the above going in them. Many store-bought multivitamins—chewable and gummies—are filled with sugar and not very bioavailable nutrients. I prefer liquids or capsules that can be opened if need be, as in many cases absorption can be better. Supplements: My *Take This* Kid Boost and *Take This* Cell Mins liquid multinutrient for kids under eight years of age. Also look for powders including greens that can be mixed into water or juice.

HERBAL SUPPORT There are many herbs that help boost the immune system that are worth knowing about. In my Immune Boosting Packages on SproutRight.com, I recommend echinacea, probiotics, and other herbal boosters like Imu-Gen from Genestra. These have helped many kids get through winter with a reduced incidence of colds and flu. Deep Immune by St. Francis is also an excellent and very popular herbal product.

YOUR SHORT LIST Multinutrient, probiotic, vitamin C, garlic (if needed), herbal support, omega fats, vitamin D and K2, and extra zinc if you feel the rest isn't doing enough. You will want to ask a nutritionist or reach out to us at SproutRight.com to determine the appropriate dosage for various ages. The whole family can take all of the above, and you can just change the dosage for each family member.

RECIPES

BREAKFAST

MAINS

SALADS AND SIDES

SNACKS AND DESSERTS

SEEDS OF SUCCESS SMOOTHIE

MAKES ABOUT 2 CUPS (500 ML)

DAIRY-FREE • EGG-FREE • GLUTEN-FREE • VEGAN •
VEGETARIAN • WHEAT-FREE

Set the family up for a successful day with omega-3 and omega-6 essential fats. The omega-3 fats and fibre in this smoothie give the brain a boost, providing essential nutrients that help to sustain energy. Use more or less dried fruit depending on how sweet you like your smoothies.

1 tablespoon (15 mL) pumpkin seeds

1 tablespoon (15 mL) sesame seeds

1 tablespoon (15 mL) flaxseeds

1 tablespoon (15 mL) raw unsalted sunflower seeds

2 tablespoons (30 mL) raw almonds

1 to 1½ cups (250 to 375 mL) fresh, frozen, or dried cranberries or cherries, pitted

¾ cup (175 mL) filtered water, plus more for blending

2 teaspoons (10 mL) raw unpasteurized honey or pure maple syrup

1. Soak the pumpkin seeds, sesame seeds, flaxseeds, sunflower seeds, almonds, and dried fruit (if using dried) in the water for 24 hours.
2. Drain and rinse the mixture. In a high-speed blender, blend until smooth, adding up to an additional 1 cup (250 mL) water as needed.
3. Add the fruit (if using fresh or frozen) and honey and blend on high until completely smooth. Serve the smoothie cold.

NUTRITIONAL INFORMATION This smoothie will help keep your digestive system working with loads of fibre! It's a good source of vitamin A, vitamin C, magnesium, and omega-3 fatty acids.

SWEET BLUE SMOOTHIE

MAKES ABOUT 2 CUPS (500 ML)

DAIRY-FREE • EGG-FREE • GLUTEN-FREE •
NUT-FREE • VEGETARIAN • WHEAT-FREE

Smoothies are a fantastic meal, addition to a meal, or snack at any time of day.

1 cup (250 mL) frozen blueberries

1 ripe avocado, pitted and peeled

1 large kale leaf, chopped

¼ cup (60 mL) hemp hearts

1 tablespoon (15 mL) chia seeds

1 tablespoon (15 mL) liquid pure honey

1 tablespoon (15 mL) maca root powder (optional)

½ cup (125 mL) unsweetened almond, coconut, or hemp milk

1. Place the blueberries, avocado, kale, hemp hearts, chia seeds, honey, maca root (if using), and milk in a high-speed blender. Blend on high until completely smooth.
2. Serve the smoothie cold.

NUTRITIONAL INFORMATION This smoothie is a good source of vitamin A, vitamin C, magnesium, zinc, and omega-3 fatty acids.

WARMING GREEN DRINK

MAKES ABOUT 2 CUPS (500 ML)

DAIRY-FREE • EGG-FREE • GLUTEN-FREE • NUT-FREE • VEGAN • VEGETARIAN • WHEAT-FREE

Not only do you add warm water to this, but the ginger is warming for your whole body. Protein keeps your energy stable and keeps you full for longer. The water can be replaced with warmed unsweetened almond milk for additional flavour and nutrients.

1 very ripe pear
2 large handfuls of baby spinach or baby kale
¼ avocado, pitted and peeled
1 teaspoon (5 mL) dried ground ginger
Juice of 1 lemon
1 scoop plant-based protein powder
½ cup (125 mL) warm water

1. Place the pear, spinach, avocado, ginger, lemon juice, protein powder, and water in a high-speed blender. Blend on high for 1 minute until completely smooth.
2. Serve immediately.

NUTRITIONAL INFORMATION This smoothie is a detoxifying and alkalizing elixir packed with vitamin C, calcium, phosphorus, and potassium.

APPLE CINNAMON BAKED PANCAKES

MAKES 6 PANCAKES

GLUTEN-FREE • VEGETARIAN • WHEAT-FREE

This recipe is a staple in my house. One large baking dish can feed my kids for three out of five weekdays. That makes breakfast easier on those hairy mornings when everyone is tired and running a bit late. Almond flour is incredibly satisfying, and you'll find yourself full for hours.

¼ cup (60 mL) unsalted butter
1 cup (250 mL) almond flour
1 cup (250 mL) unsweetened applesauce
6 eggs
¼ teaspoon (1 mL) sea salt
1 teaspoon (5 mL) ground cinnamon

1. Preheat the oven to 425°F (220°C).
2. Put the butter in a 9- × 13-inch (23 × 33 cm) baking dish and set it in the heated oven to melt.
3. Mix the flour, applesauce, eggs, salt, and cinnamon in a bowl.
4. When the butter is melted, pour the batter into the baking dish and spread evenly into the corners.
5. Return the dish to the oven and bake for 25 minutes until golden.
6. Let cool, then cut into 6 pieces. Serve with fruit spread, jam, or honey.
7. Store the pancakes in an airtight container in the fridge for up to 3 days. Reheat in an oven set at 275°F (135°C) for 10 minutes.

NUTRITIONAL INFORMATION These pancakes are a good source of vitamin A, vitamin D, phosphorus, potassium, selenium, folate, and choline.

BLENDER PANCAKES MAKES ABOUT 12 PANCAKES

DAIRY-FREE • GLUTEN-FREE • VEGETARIAN • WHEAT-FREE

Anything that can be made in a blender is a good thing. This recipe is fast and simple, and you'll have only one appliance to wash. I came across these pancakes one weekend, made a massive batch, and then ate them all week long. They are filling, so you won't need as many as your usual mile-high stack.

2 cups (500 mL) gluten-free old-fashioned rolled oats

1½ cups (375 mL) unsweetened vanilla almond milk

1 large ripe banana, roughly chopped

½ teaspoon (2 mL) ground cinnamon

1 tablespoon (15 mL) raw liquid honey

¼ teaspoon (1 mL) sea salt

1 teaspoon (5 mL) pure vanilla extract

1½ teaspoons (7 mL) baking powder

1 egg

Virgin coconut oil or unsalted butter, for cooking

Toppings (optional)

Sliced fresh fruit: apple, pear, or banana

Fresh berries: blueberry, blackberry, or raspberry

Crofters Fruit Spread

Pure maple syrup

1. Heat the oven to 200°F (100°C) to keep the pancakes warm as you make the rest of the batch.

2. Place the oats, almond milk, banana, cinnamon, honey, salt, vanilla, and baking powder in a blender and blend until smooth. Add the egg and pulse a few times.

3. Heat a skillet or griddle over medium heat and melt 1 to 2 teaspoons (5 to 10 mL) of coconut oil. Pour ¼ cup (60 mL) of the batter into the skillet and cook until the pancake is no longer shiny or wet looking, about 3 to 4 minutes. Flip it over and cook another 2 to 3 minutes. Repeat until the batter is all gone, adding a bit more milk if the batter starts to thicken. Place the cooked pancakes in a heat-proof dish in the oven to keep warm.

4. Serve the pancakes with fruit, berries, fruit spread, and maple syrup, if desired.

5. Store the pancakes in an airtight container in the fridge for up to 3 days. Reheat in an oven set at 275°F (135°C) for 10 minutes. The pancakes can also be stored in the freezer for up to 1 month.

NUTRITIONAL INFORMATION The fibre and protein in these pancakes make them hearty and nutritious.

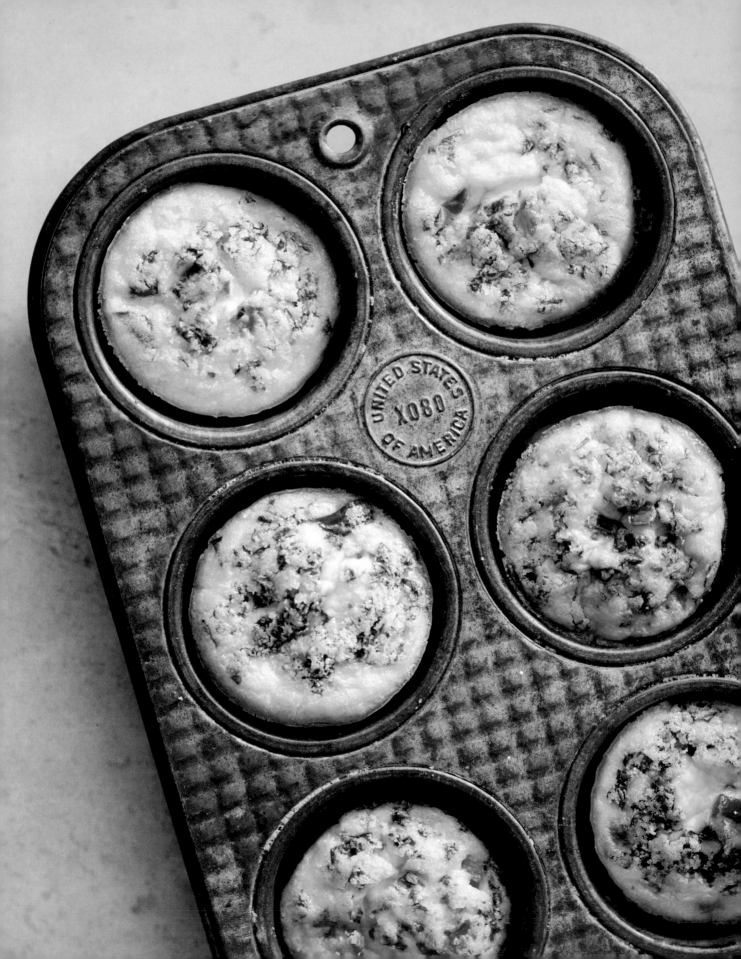

MINI FRITTATAS MAKES 12 FRITTATAS
GLUTEN-FREE • NUT-FREE • WHEAT-FREE

These mini frittatas are fun to make and even more fun to eat. They are the perfect way to get some greens and veggies into your kids (or adults). In addition to being a delicious breakfast, they are an excellent lunchbox staple in our house and now can be in yours, too! Make them for breakfast on the weekend and use them to get you through the first few days of the week with Quinoa and Corn Salad (page 298) on the side.

6 eggs

1½ cups (375 mL) 18% table cream

1 kale leaf, finely chopped

½ large sweet red pepper, diced

½ can (5 ounces/150 g) can wild skinless, boneless pink salmon

1 teaspoon (5 mL) dried basil or fresh basil pesto

Salt

Black pepper

1. Preheat the oven to 350°F (180°C). Grease a 12-cup mini muffin tin (or use silicone).
2. In a large bowl, whisk together the eggs and cream.
3. Stir in the kale, red pepper, salmon, and basil or pesto. Add salt and pepper to taste. Divide the mixture evenly between the 12 mini muffin cups.
4. Bake for 25 to 30 minutes or until the frittatas are firm.
5. Serve immediately or turn out onto a wire cooling rack if using for lunch the next day.
6. Store the frittatas in an airtight container in the fridge for up to 4 days. They are not suitable for freezing.

TIP: For a dairy-free version, substitute canned full-fat coconut milk for the table cream.

NUTRITIONAL INFORMATION These frittatas are a good source of vitamin A, vitamin C, vitamin D, folate, and choline.

EGG AND AVOCADO WRAP SERVES 4

DAIRY-FREE • NUT-FREE • VEGETARIAN

This wrap contains protein, good fats, and greens. It's a win all around, and it only takes a few minutes to make. It's colourful and filling and ticks all the nutrition boxes for a powerhouse breakfast.

4 large eggs

Virgin coconut oil, for cooking

2 handfuls of baby spinach

4 whole-grain wraps

1 ripe avocado, pitted, peeled, and sliced

½ cup (125 mL) salsa

1. Beat the eggs in a small bowl.

2. Heat the coconut oil in a small skillet over medium heat. Pour the eggs into the hot skillet and move them around until they start to cook, then scramble for about 2 minutes. Add the spinach and allow it to wilt slightly from the heat.

3. Remove from the heat. Divide the egg and spinach mixture into 4 portions and spoon each portion onto a whole-grain wrap. Top with a few slices of avocado and salsa. Roll up the wraps and enjoy!

NUTRITIONAL INFORMATION Healthy fats, protein, vitamin K, vitamin A, and folate make this wrap a nutritional powerhouse.

OVERNIGHT OATMEAL

SERVES 4

DAIRY-FREE • EGG-FREE • GLUTEN-FREE •
VEGAN • VEGETARIAN • WHEAT-FREE

Fast and simple and a one-pot wonder! You can make a big batch on Sunday and heat up portions throughout the week. Coconut milk, rice milk, or dairy milk can be substituted for the unsweetened almond milk depending on dietary restrictions and preferences.

---

2 ripe bananas, mashed
1 tablespoon (15 mL) chia seeds
Heaping ⅔ cup (160 mL) old-fashioned rolled oats
1¼ teaspoons (6 mL) ground cinnamon, divided
1⅓ cups (325 mL) unsweetened almond milk
⅓ cup (75 mL) filtered water
Pinch of ground ginger, for garnish (optional)

1. Add the banana, chia seeds, oats, ¼ teaspoon (1 mL) cinnamon, almond milk, and water to a saucepan and stir to combine. Cover and store in the fridge overnight.
2. In the morning, heat the oatmeal over medium heat, stirring frequently, until warmed through and a creamy consistency is achieved. If it thickens too much, add more water or almond milk.
3. To serve, pour the oatmeal into serving bowls and top with the remaining 1 teaspoon (5 mL) of cinnamon or a sprinkle of ginger (if using).

TIP: Substitute half a grated pear for the banana for a different flavour profile.

NUTRITIONAL INFORMATION This oatmeal is high in fibre, protein, and omega-3 fatty acids, which are essential for brain development and health.

CHIA PUDDING

MAKES 1½ CUPS (375 ML)

DAIRY-FREE • EGG-FREE • GLUTEN-FREE •
VEGAN • VEGETARIAN • WHEAT-FREE

Chia seeds are a powerhouse of protein, fibre, calcium, iron, vitamins, and essential fats. It may seem odd to eat seeds and milk, but this is a meal or a snack that will appeal to the whole family. This makes a great breakfast, snack, and lunch addition. Coconut milk or dairy milk can be substituted for the almond milk depending on dietary restrictions and preferences.

⅓ cup (75 mL) white chia seeds
1½ cups (375 mL) unsweetened vanilla almond milk
2 tablespoons (30 mL) pure maple syrup
½ teaspoon (2 mL) pure vanilla extract

For serving (optional)
Fresh blueberries
Fresh strawberries
Fresh raspberries
Fresh grated pear

1. Add the chia seeds, milk, maple syrup, and vanilla to a 16-ounce (475 mL) airtight jar. Secure the lid and shake to combine.
2. Store in the fridge for 1 hour. Shake the mixture again or stir, then return it to the fridge with the lid on and let sit overnight.
3. In the morning, pour about 1 cup (250 mL) of chia pudding into a serving bowl and top with fruit, if desired.

NUTRITIONAL INFORMATION Be sure to drink a lot today, as these seeds are a fantastic source of fibre.

OVERNIGHT FRENCH TOAST SERVES 4 TO 8

NUT-FREE • VEGETARIAN

This is the breakfast that keeps on giving. It can feed a family of four for at least two days, as it reheats easily for the next day's breakfast or a snack. Because the French toast is two layers thick, younger family members may have only an eighth of the pan, so this recipe can feed a family of four with leftovers.

¼ cup (60 mL) pure maple syrup

1 teaspoon (5 mL) ground cinnamon

2 tablespoons (30 mL) butter, melted

8 slices kamut or spelt bread

1 cup (250 mL) fresh or frozen blueberries

4 eggs

1 cup (250 mL) unsweetened almond, coconut, or dairy milk

1 teaspoon (5 mL) pure vanilla extract

Pinch of salt

1. Mix the maple syrup, cinnamon, and melted butter in a small bowl.

2. Pour a third of the maple syrup mixture evenly over the bottom of an 8-inch (20 cm) square pan. Cover with 4 slices of bread.

3. Scatter the blueberries on top of the bread and cover with the remaining 4 slices of bread. Pour the remaining maple syrup mixture overtop.

4. Beat the eggs, milk, vanilla, and salt together in a medium bowl. Pour evenly over the bread and press down lightly. The bread will soak up the liquid, so make sure that the entire top layer of bread is dampened with the egg mixture.

5. Cover and refrigerate overnight or let stand for 2 hours.

6. Preheat the oven to 350°F (180°C). Bake uncovered for 40 to 45 minutes until puffed and golden brown.

7. Store the French toast in an airtight container in the fridge for up to 3 days. Reheat any leftovers in an oven set at 200°F (100°C) for 10 minutes.

NUTRITIONAL INFORMATION This French toast is a good source of vitamin A, vitamin C, vitamin D, calcium, potassium, phosphorus, selenium, choline, and fibre.

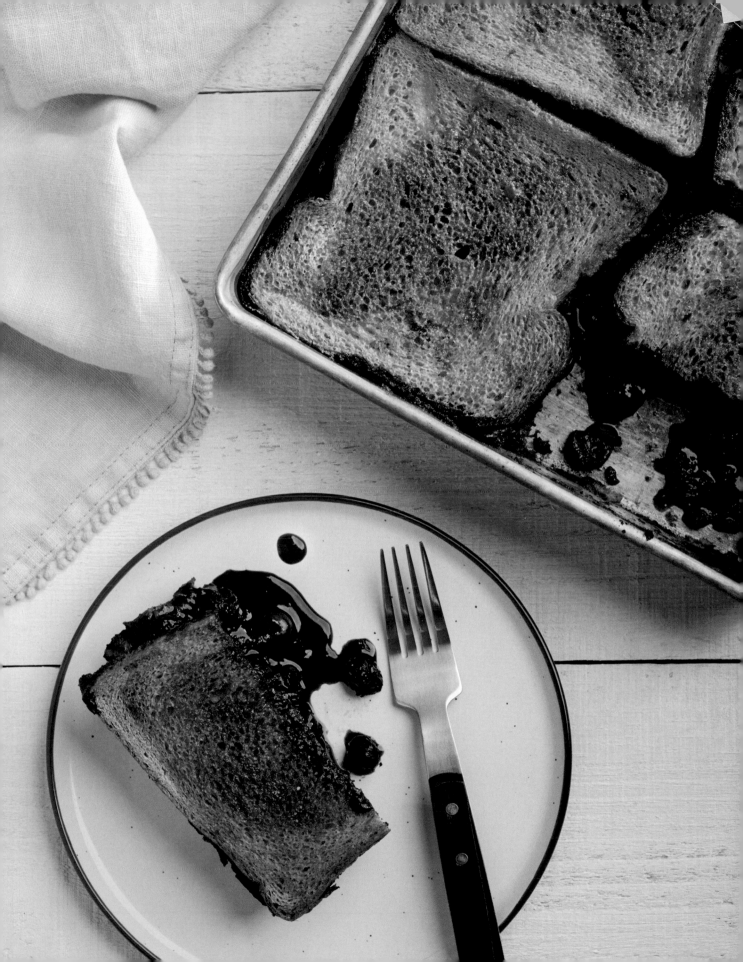

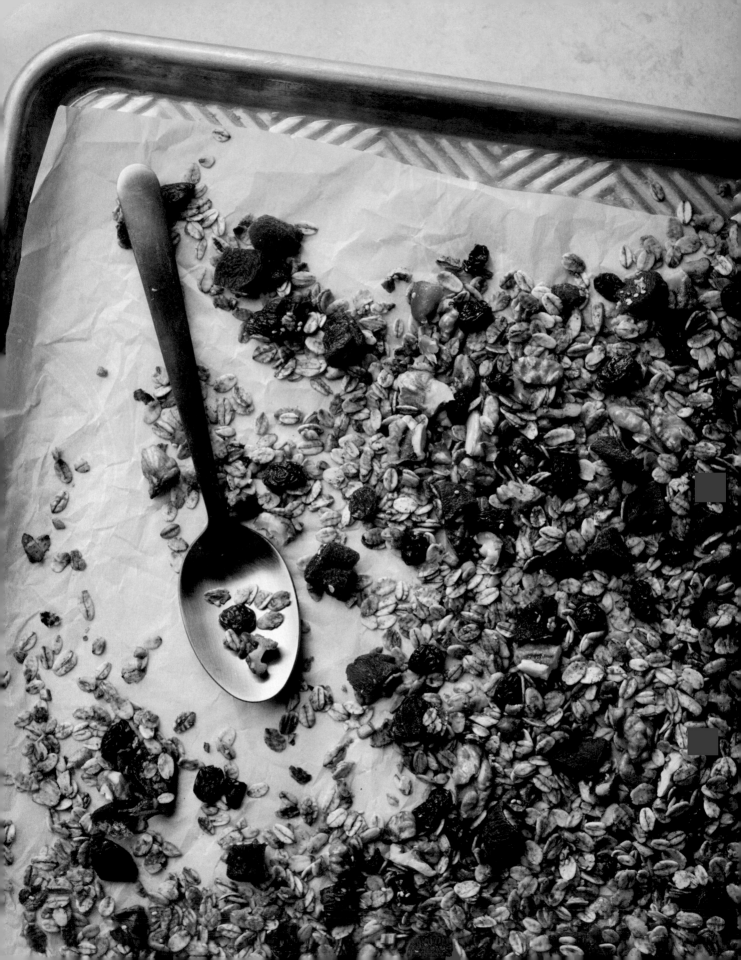

CRUNCHY GRANOLA MAKES ABOUT 3 CUPS (750 ML)

DAIRY-FREE • EGG-FREE • GLUTEN-FREE • VEGAN • VEGETARIAN • WHEAT-FREE

Homemade granola is a delicious breakfast, snack, or addition to Greek yogurt or even Blueberry Maple Ice Cream (page 312). Store-bought options can be high in refined sugar. Using maple syrup is a less refined option. This granola keeps well, so save yourself time and make a double batch.

2 cups (500 mL) old-fashioned rolled oats

1 teaspoon (5 mL) ground cinnamon

2 tablespoons (30 mL) virgin coconut oil or sunflower oil

¼ cup (60 mL) pure maple syrup

¼ cup (60 mL) sunflower seeds, chopped

¼ cup (60 mL) walnuts (or other favourite nuts), chopped

¼ cup (60 mL) chopped dried fruit (Thompson raisins or sultanas, cranberries, apples, unsulphured apricots, and/or dates), soaked for 10 minutes in hot water

1 tablespoon (15 mL) sesame seeds, hemp seeds, or chia seeds

1. Preheat the oven to 350°F (180°C). Line a baking sheet with parchment paper.
2. Add the oats, cinnamon, coconut oil, maple syrup, sunflower seeds, walnuts, soaked fruit, and sesame seeds in a large bowl. Stir to combine.
3. Spread the granola evenly on the prepared baking sheet. Bake for 10 minutes until golden brown, rotating the baking sheet halfway through. If you like crunchier granola, cook for an additional 5 minutes. Remove from the oven and let cool on the baking sheet.
4. Store the granola in an airtight container at room temperature for up to 2 weeks.

TIP: Substitute sunflower or pumpkin seeds for the walnuts for a nut-free version.

NUTRITIONAL INFORMATION This granola is a good source of vitamin C, vitamin B3, calcium, potassium, phosphorus, and folate.

BAKED BUTTERNUT SQUASH AND GARLIC RISOTTO SERVES 6

EGG-FREE • GLUTEN-FREE • NUT-FREE • VEGETARIAN • WHEAT-FREE

Yes, you can bake a risotto. Rather than standing at the stove for a while as you make traditional risotto, try this super-easy baked version. I use my 3-quart (3 L) cast iron pot for this and it comes out beautifully. Feel free to switch up the vegetables. I've also used sweet potato with red onion and prosciutto and it was delicious. To bring more vegetables into this meal, serve with Lemony Green Beans (page 307).

1 medium butternut squash, peeled, seeded and diced

1½ cups (375 mL) arborio rice

2 cloves garlic, finely chopped or minced

4 cups (1 L) meat broth (page 129) or vegetable broth (page 130)

1 yellow onion, finely chopped

1 cup (250 mL) finely grated pecorino cheese

⅓ cup (75 mL) unsalted butter

1 teaspoon (5 mL) sea salt

1 teaspoon (5 mL) freshly ground black pepper

1. Preheat the oven to 350°F (180°C).
2. Add the squash, rice, garlic, broth, and onion to a 3-quart (3 L) baking dish with a lid and stir.
3. Cover and bake for 45 minutes or until most of the stock is absorbed and the rice is al dente.
4. Add the cheese, butter, salt, and pepper. Stir for 3 to 4 minutes or until rice is thick and creamy. Serve.

TIP: Swap the butternut squash for 14 ounces (400 g) mixed mushrooms (shiitake, cremini, brown button), cleaned and sliced.

NUTRITIONAL INFORMATION This risotto is a good source of vitamin A and calcium.

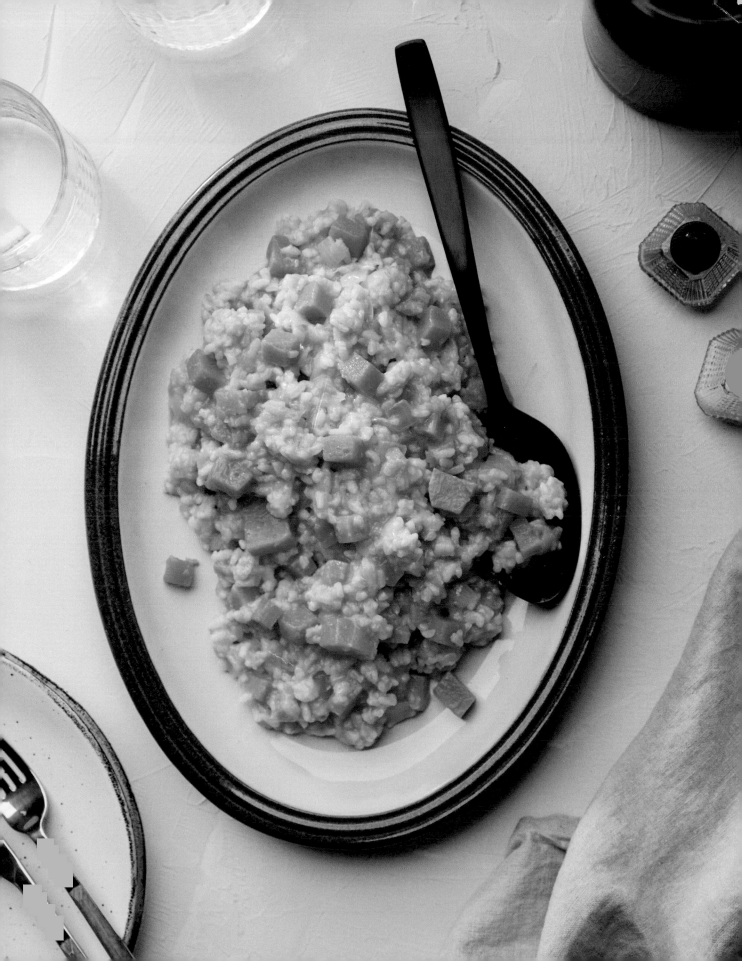

SPROUT RIGHT SPAGHETTI CARBONARA SERVES 4
GLUTEN-FREE • NUT-FREE • WHEAT-FREE

This is a fast, energy-rich dinner that's perfect for all the sports players and watchers in the family. Use coconut milk instead of whipping cream to make this recipe dairy-free, and don't forget to season it well. Save some of the spaghetti cooking water to add when reheating this for tomorrow's lunch.

1 package (12 ounces/340 g) dried rice or kamut spaghetti

4 slices Canadian bacon, cubed

1 head broccoli, cut into small florets

2 egg yolks

¼ cup (60 mL) canned coconut milk or whipping cream

5 to 10 pitted olives, chopped

2 tablespoons (30 mL) capers

⅓ cup (75 mL) grated Parmesan or pecorino cheese

Salt

Black pepper

1. Bring a large pot of salted water to a rolling boil over high heat. Drop the pasta into the water and cook for 10 minutes (follow package instructions for exact timing) or until the noodles are soft with a remaining bit of firmness when bitten.
2. Meanwhile, cook the bacon in a frying pan until crispy, about 7 to 10 minutes. Add the broccoli and cook for an additional 3 minutes.
3. In a small bowl, mix together the egg yolks and coconut milk.
4. Drain the cooked pasta in a colander placed over a large bowl and reserve the pasta water. Return the pasta to the large pot.
5. Pour the egg mixture over the pasta and toss quickly with 2 forks or tongs.
6. Add the bacon and broccoli mixture, olives, capers, and cheese and toss again, adding 1 tablespoon (15 mL) of the reserved pasta water at a time to loosen if noodles stick together. Season with salt and pepper, to taste.
7. Divide among plates or shallow bowls and serve with a leafy green salad with strawberries and Salad Dressing (page 304).

NUTRITIONAL INFORMATION Rice spaghetti is a gluten-free option. This dish is a good source of vitamin D, calcium, choline, and folate.

BROCCOLI AND CHICKEN STIR-FRY SERVES 4
EGG-FREE • GLUTEN-FREE • NUT-FREE • WHEAT-FREE

Broccoli is one of the most nutritious vegetables. This recipe uses broccoli slaw, so it could become a new favourite for anyone who isn't a fan of broccoli, as there are no florets. This makes the perfect next-day lunch, if there are any leftovers.

¼ cup (60 mL) sesame oil

1 bag (12 ounces/340 g) broccoli slaw

½ cup (125 mL) red onion, sliced

8 ounces (225 g) cooked skinless chicken breast, sliced

1 cup (250 mL) thinly sliced or spiralized zucchini

½ cup (125 mL) sweet red pepper, sliced

2 tablespoons (30 mL) tamari sauce

½ cup (125 mL) sesame seeds, for serving

1. Heat the sesame oil in a large skillet over medium heat. Add the broccoli and onion and sauté until just soft, about 2 to 3 minutes.
2. Add the chicken, zucchini, red pepper, and tamari. Toss and cook until the zucchini is soft, but the red pepper is still crisp, and the chicken is warmed through, about 6 to 8 minutes.
3. Divide between 4 plates, top with sesame seeds, and serve.

TIP: To make this dish a plant-based option, use tofu or tempeh instead of chicken.

NUTRITIONAL INFORMATION This is a delicious gluten-free dish that's high in protein and calcium and rich in antioxidants.

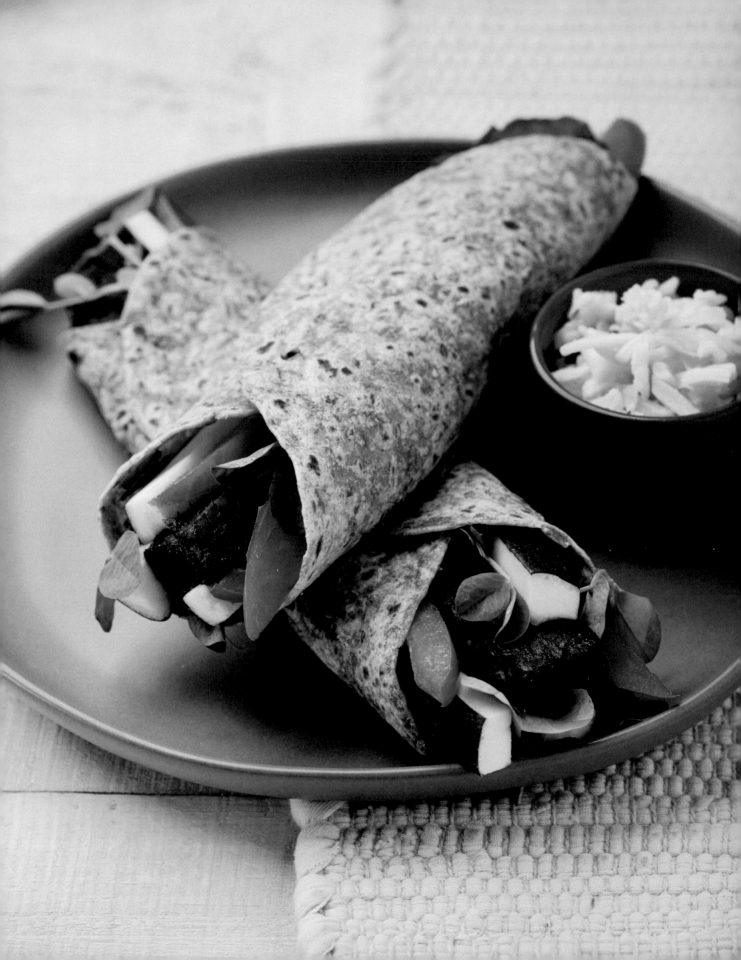

SMOKY TEMPEH WRAP SERVES 4

EGG-FREE • GLUTEN-FREE • NUT-FREE • VEGETARIAN • WHEAT-FREE

Tempeh has more of a nutty texture than tofu and is loved by meat eaters and vegetarians alike. This is quick to cook, and any leftovers can be used for lunch the next day. Using smoked paprika in place of sweet paprika will bring the taste of summertime cooking to the recipe, without the barbecue.

Barbecue Marinade

¼ cup (60 mL) liquid pure honey or pure maple syrup

¼ cup (60 mL) apple butter

¼ cup (60 mL) tamari

1 clove garlic, minced

1 teaspoon (5 mL) smoked paprika

Tempeh Wrap

1 package (9 ounces/250 g) organic tempeh, cut into slices about ¼ inch (5 mm) thick

Olive oil or virgin coconut oil, for brushing

4 corn, kamut, or whole wheat wraps

10 sunflower seed and pea sprouts

¼ cup (60 mL) goat's milk cheddar or medium cheddar, thinly sliced or grated

½ zucchini, cut into matchsticks

½ sweet pepper, thinly sliced

1. To make the marinade, mix the honey, apple butter, tamari, garlic, and paprika in a small bowl.

2. Place the tempeh in a shallow dish and cover with the marinade, turning the tempeh to coat completely. Marinate the tempeh for at least 1 hour or overnight in the fridge.

3. Generously brush a griddle or frying pan with olive oil and heat over high heat.

4. Carefully grill the tempeh for about 4 minutes on each side, occasionally spooning more of the marinade over it.

5. Assemble each wrap by laying the tempeh, sprouts, cheese, zucchini, and peppers down the centre. Fold over the edges, use a toothpick to hold the wrap closed, and serve.

TIP: This can also be made with chicken. Substitute one skinless chicken breast cut into ½-inch (1 cm) strips for the tempeh.

NUTRITIONAL INFORMATION Tempeh is fermented soybeans very high in protein and fibre, and the sprouts offer enzymes, protein, and antioxidants.

CHICKEN BREASTS WITH CHEESY GARLIC SWEET POTATOES SERVES 4

EGG-FREE • GLUTEN-FREE • NUT-FREE • WHEAT-FREE

My kids fight for the crispy sweet potatoes in this dish. When the cheese melts and mixes with the garlic, it's a scrumptious combination alongside the chicken. Serve with steamed greens or my Lemony Green Beans (page 307).

4 medium skinless, boneless chicken breasts

2 tablespoons (30 mL) olive oil, plus a splash for the chicken

1 teaspoon (5 mL) sea salt

1 teaspoon (5 mL) freshly ground black pepper

1 tablespoon (15 mL) coconut oil

2 medium sweet potatoes, peeled and sliced into ¼-inch (5 mm) thick rounds

2 cloves garlic, minced

¼ cup (60 mL) grated pecorino or Parmesan cheese

1. Preheat the oven to 375°F (190°C). Line a baking sheet with parchment paper.
2. Season the chicken with a splash of olive oil and the sea salt and pepper.
3. Heat the coconut oil in a large frying pan over medium heat and sear the outside of the chicken breasts until slightly browned.
4. Put the sliced sweet potato in a large bowl and add the 2 tablespoons (30 mL) olive oil, garlic, and cheese. Toss to coat.
5. Spread the sweet potato evenly on the prepared baking sheet. Place the browned chicken breasts on top of the sweet potato.
6. Bake for 20 to 25 minutes or until the chicken is cooked and the sweet potato is fork-tender and browned at the edges.
7. Divide among 4 plates and serve.

NUTRITIONAL INFORMATION This dish is a good source of calcium and vitamin A.

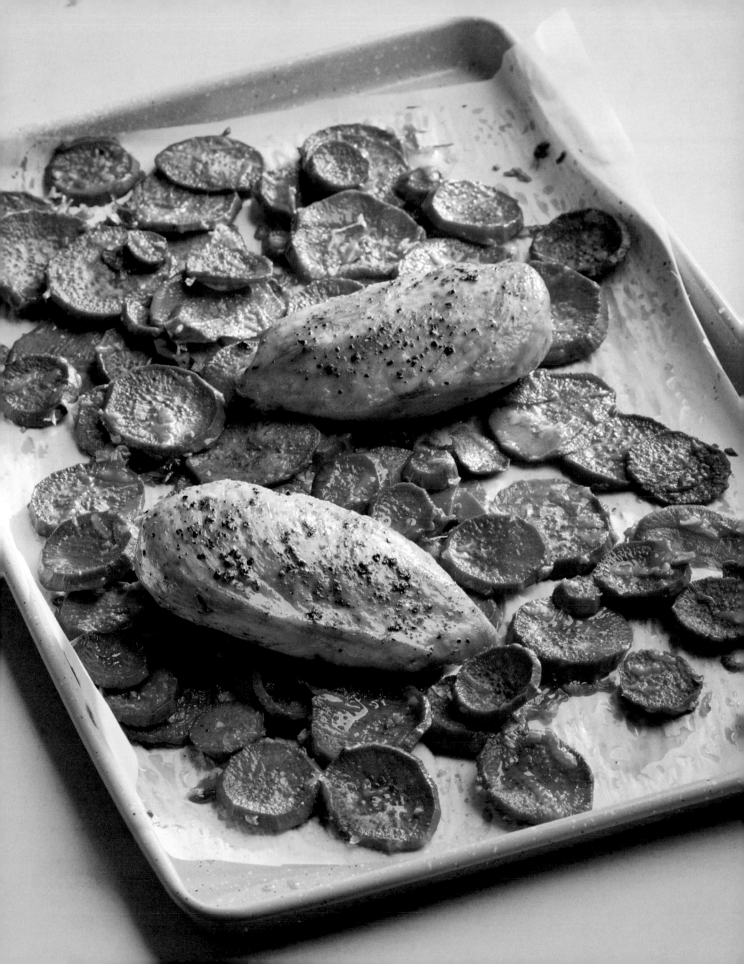

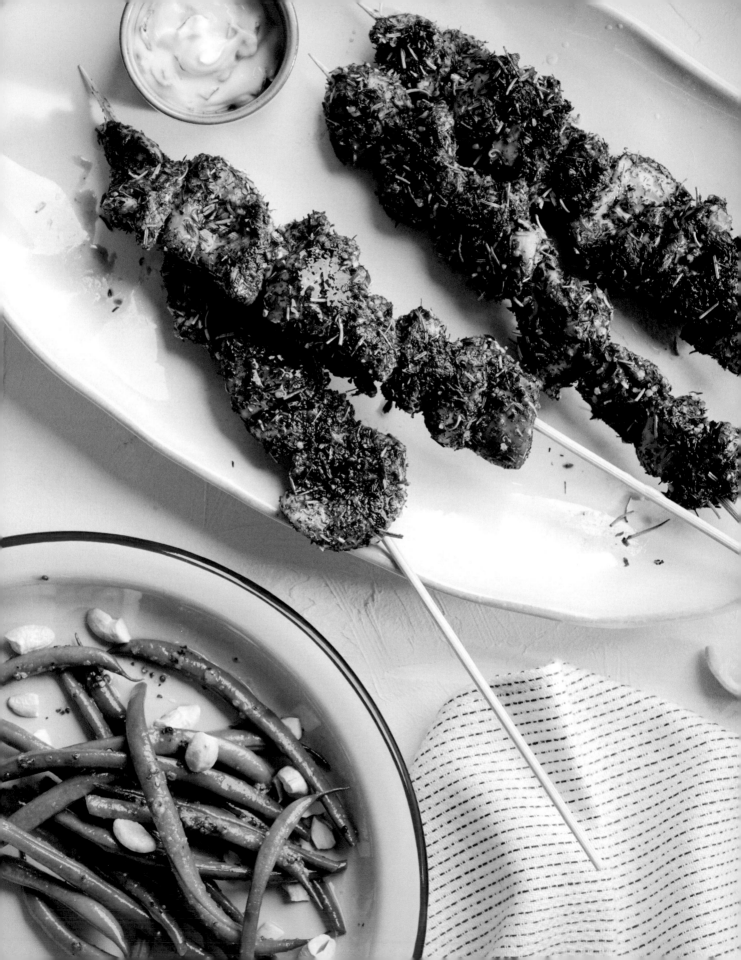

CHICKEN SOUVLAKI SERVES 4

DAIRY-FREE • EGG-FREE • GLUTEN-FREE • NUT-FREE • WHEAT-FREE

I've made this dish for massive parties, small dinners, and everything in between. Skewers are a fun way to eat. A dry rub on any meat is a delicious alternative to a sauce marinade. The herby flavour of this chicken is delicious eaten warm or cold in a salad for lunch or dinner the next day. Serve with Lemony Green Beans (page 307); Wilted Greens with Creamy Miso Sauce (page 280); Corn, Coconut, and Ginger Soup (page 295); or Beet and Carrot Slaw (page 299).

Mediterranean herb rub, makes 1 cup (250 mL)

3 tablespoons (45 mL) dried tarragon

3 tablespoons (45 mL) dried oregano

3 tablespoons (45 mL) dried dill

3 tablespoons (45 mL) dried thyme

3 tablespoons (45 mL) dried rosemary

3 tablespoons (45 mL) coarse sea salt

2 tablespoons (30 mL) lemon pepper

1 tablespoon (15 mL) garlic flakes

Chicken Souvlaki

8 wooden skewers, soaked in water for
    10 minutes

4 chicken breasts or 6 thighs, cubed

1½ tablespoons (22 mL) Mediterranean herb rub

1. Make the Mediterranean herb rub. Combine the tarragon, oregano, dill, thyme, rosemary, salt, lemon pepper, and garlic flakes in a small bowl and stir to mix.

2. Store the leftover rub in an airtight jar away from heat for up to 6 months. You can add it to any meat or fish you're cooking for additional flavour.

3. Make the chicken souvlaki. Place the cubed chicken in a large bowl. Add the Mediterranean herb rub and toss to evenly coat the chicken.

4. Assemble the seasoned chicken on the skewers (not too tightly packed and as flat as possible). Skewers can be assembled the night before, stored in an airtight container, and refrigerated.

5. Grill on an outdoor barbecue over medium heat or broil in the oven for about 6 to 10 minutes on each side until cooked through and slightly browned.

TIP: For a vegetarian option, cube an assortment of vegetables like zucchini, peppers, and onion. Coat the veggies with olive oil and the dry rub, assemble them on the skewers in an alternating pattern, then grill them on the barbecue or cook under the broiler for about 10 minutes, turning regularly.

NUTRITIONAL INFORMATION Chicken is an excellent source of protein, and chicken thighs are higher in iron than chicken breasts. All herbs, dried or fresh, are a great source of antioxidants.

GOLDEN GRILLED CURRIED CHICKEN THIGHS SERVES 4

DAIRY-FREE • EGG-FREE • GLUTEN-FREE • NUT-FREE • WHEAT-FREE

The sweetness and richness of curry makes this an excellent marinade that will have everyone coming back for more. It's a thick marinade, so use a pastry brush to smother your chicken with it. This chicken pairs well with the Quinoa and Corn Salad (page 298), Beet and Carrot Slaw with Ginger Sesame Dressing (page 299), and Winter Sunshine Salad (page 304).

Marinade (makes enough for 7 batches)

3 tablespoons (45 mL) olive oil

3 tablespoons (45 mL) grainy mustard

3 tablespoons (45 mL) pure liquid honey

3 teaspoons (15 mL) curry powder

1½ teaspoons (7 mL) garlic powder

1½ teaspoons (7 mL) ground cinnamon

½ teaspoon (2 mL) salt

¼ cup (60 mL) chopped fresh cilantro (optional)

4 boneless, skinless chicken thighs

1. Preheat the oven to 350°F (180°C). Line a baking sheet with parchment paper.
2. To make the marinade, combine the olive oil, mustard, honey, curry powder, garlic powder, cinnamon, salt, and cilantro (if using) in a small bowl.
3. Add the chicken and 1 to 2 tablespoons (15 to 30 mL) of marinade to a medium bowl and toss to coat. Place the coated chicken pieces on the lined baking sheet.
4. Bake for 15 to 20 minutes or until internal temperature is 165°F (75°C). Serve with steamed broccoli and Quinoa and Corn Salad (page 298).
5. Store the unused marinade in an airtight container in the fridge for up to 4 weeks.

NUTRITIONAL INFORMATION Chicken is high in protein and a good source of iron. All spices are nutrient dense, and cinnamon is very good for blood sugar balance.

MINI CALZONE MAKES 8 CALZONES
EGG-FREE • NUT-FREE

A veggie-packed pizza pocket makes a super-fun change from the usual. Most kids love anything to do with a pizza, and these calzones are no different. Feel free to add any favourites to this recipe, and get your kids involved in making it, too. Pizza dough is a lot of fun to work with!

1 tablespoon (15 mL) extra virgin olive oil

1 yellow onion, finely diced

1 carrot, peeled and diced

1 clove garlic, crushed

¾ cup (175 mL) cooked chicken, diced

½ cup (125 mL) cremini mushrooms, cleaned and diced

½ sweet red or orange pepper, seeded and diced

½ cup (125 mL) baby spinach, washed and roughly chopped

1½ cups (375 mL) tomato sauce

1 teaspoon (5 mL) dried oregano

1 teaspoon (5 mL) dried basil

1 package (1 pound/450 g) whole wheat pizza dough

4 ounces (115 g) mozzarella cheese, shredded

1. Preheat the oven to 400°F (200°C). Line a baking sheet with parchment paper and dust with flour.

2. Heat the olive oil in a medium saucepan or skillet over medium heat. Add the onion and cook until translucent. Add the carrot and cook for 5 minutes longer. Add the garlic, chicken, mushrooms, and pepper and cook for another 5 minutes. Finally, add the baby spinach and stir for 1 minute.

3. Pour the tomato sauce over the vegetable mixture and simmer for 10 minutes. Season with the oregano and basil and remove the pan from the heat.

4. Divide the pizza dough into 8 balls. On a clean surface, roll the dough into 5-inch (12 cm) thin rounds. Evenly spread the filling on one half of each dough round. Scatter the cheese evenly over the filling.

5. Fold the dough over the filling, press the edges together, and crimp to seal with your fingers.

6. Prick a few holes in the dough with a fork and transfer to the prepared baking sheet. Bake for 10 to 12 minutes or until golden brown.

NUTRITIONAL INFORMATION These calzones are a good source of carbohydrate, protein, vitamin C, the antioxidant lycopene, and calcium.

CHICKEN POACHED IN COCONUT CURRY SAUCE SERVES 4

DAIRY-FREE • EGG-FREE • GLUTEN-FREE • NUT-FREE • WHEAT-FREE

I love a one-pot dinner, and this is a staple of mine. Change up the vegetables to your family's taste and make it colourful to tick off many boxes on the "eat a rainbow" chart (see page 4).

3 tablespoons (45 mL) green curry paste

6 boneless, skinless chicken thighs, cubed (about 12 to 14 ounces/340 to 400 g)

2 cups (500 mL) sweet potato, peeled and chopped

2 cups (500 mL) vegetables (bok choy, green beans, sugar snap peas, snow peas, cauliflower, red or yellow peppers), cut into 1-inch (2.5 cm) pieces

2 cups (500 mL) Meat Broth (page 129)

1½ cups (375 mL) canned coconut milk

¼ cup (60 mL) fresh cilantro leaves and stems, chopped

1. Heat the curry paste in a large skillet over medium-high heat. Cook for 1 to 2 minutes until the paste is fragrant.

2. Add the chicken, sweet potato, and vegetables and cook for 3 to 4 minutes.

3. Add the broth and coconut milk and reduce heat to low. Simmer gently for 12 minutes or until chicken is cooked and sweet potato is fork-tender. Be careful not to bring the coconut milk to a boil or it may separate—the flavour will be the same, but the appearance and texture of the sauce will be different.

4. Sprinkle the cilantro over the chicken and serve with long-grain jasmine, basmati, or Coconut Rice (page 308).

TIP: **1.** For a fish version of this dish, poach 12 to 14 ounces (340 to 400 g) cod or haddock pieces in the coconut curry sauce for the last 12 minutes or until cooked through. **2.** For a vegetarian version, replace the chicken with chickpeas, tofu, or tempeh and add to the skillet once the sweet potato is almost fully cooked to fork-tender.

NUTRITIONAL INFORMATION This is a delicious dish you can make with any source of protein that you'd like. It's a good source of vitamin A, vitamin C, and calcium.

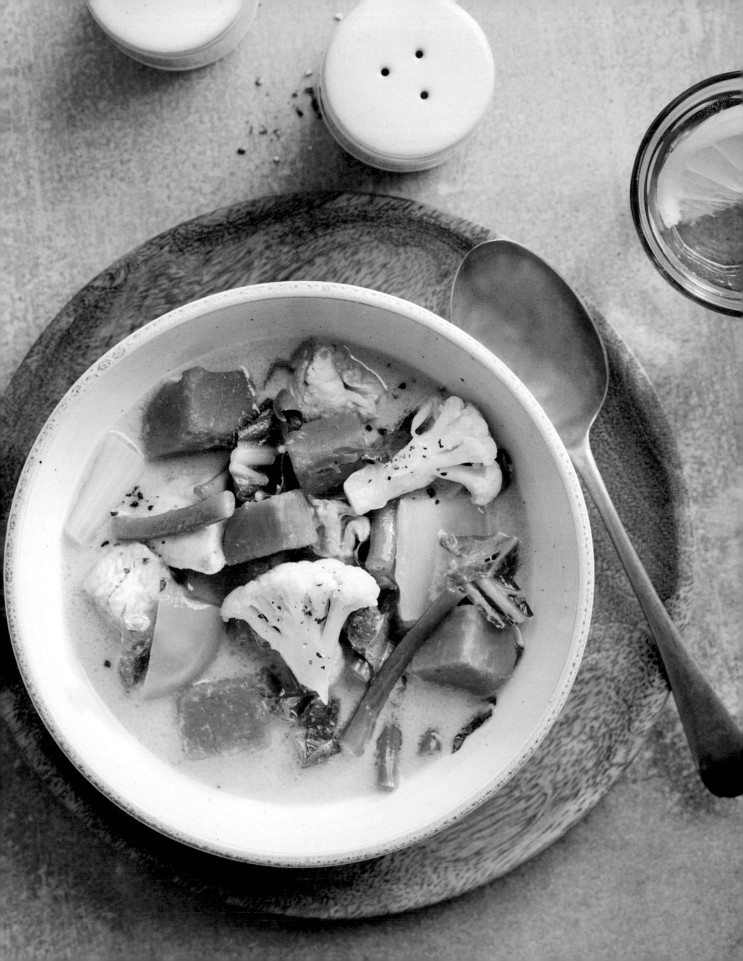

ONE-POT SAUSAGE AND LENTILS SERVES 4 TO 5

DAIRY-FREE • EGG-FREE • GLUTEN-FREE • NUT-FREE • WHEAT-FREE

This one-pot recipe is super-easy and quick to pull off on a busy weeknight and can be prepped the night before so it's ready to go when you get home from work.

1 tablespoon (15 mL) olive oil, divided

12 ounces (340 g) chicken or turkey sausages with no added fillers

1 yellow onion, finely chopped

1 clove garlic, crushed

1 sweet red pepper, diced

1 cup (250 mL) dried French or du Puy lentils, rinsed

1¼ cups (300 mL) Meat Broth (page 129) or Vegetable Broth (page 130)

Mashed potatoes or cooked brown rice, for serving

1. Heat ½ tablespoon (7 mL) olive oil in a medium skillet over medium heat. Add the sausages and cook until browned on all sides, about 15 minutes. Remove the sausages from the pan and set aside.

2. Add the remaining ½ tablespoon (7 mL) olive oil, onion, garlic, and red pepper to the skillet and cook for 5 minutes until softened.

3. Add the lentils, broth, and sausages to the pan. Bring to a boil, then simmer for 20 minutes until the lentils have softened and the sausages are cooked through.

4. Serve with mashed potatoes or brown rice.

NUTRITIONAL INFORMATION This dish is high in immune-boosting onion and garlic, vitamin C, antioxidant-rich peppers, and collagen-rich broth.

ROASTED VEGGIE TAGINE SERVES 4

DAIRY-FREE • EGG-FREE • GLUTEN-FREE • NUT-FREE • VEGETARIAN • WHEAT-FREE

This dish features an explosion of flavours, with the parsnips, all the spices, and the sweetness from the dried fruit. I suggest making a double batch and freezing the leftovers for next week's meal or lunch in appropriate portion sizes. Serve with cooked quinoa or Coconut Rice (page 308) for a protein-rich, plant-based meal. Use raisins as a substitute for dried apricots, if you prefer.

4 medium carrots, cut into chunks

4 small or 3 large parsnips, cut into chunks

1 medium sweet potato, peeled and cubed

3 red onions, cut into wedges

2 sweet red peppers, seeded and cut into chunks

2 tablespoons (30 mL) olive oil, divided

1 teaspoon (5 mL) ground cumin

1 teaspoon (5 mL) sweet paprika

1 teaspoon (5 mL) ground cinnamon

1 teaspoon (5 mL) mild chili powder

1 can (14 ounces/398 mL) diced tomatoes

2 cups (500 mL) filtered water

½ cup (125 mL) soft dried unsulphured apricots, chopped

2 teaspoons (10 mL) liquid pure honey

1. Heat the oven to 375°F (190°C). Line 2 baking sheets with parchment paper.

2. Add the carrot, parsnip, sweet potato, onion, and red pepper to a large bowl. Add 1 tablespoon (15 mL) olive oil and toss to coat.

3. Evenly divide the vegetable mixture between the 2 prepared baking sheets. Bake for 30 minutes until vegetables are fork-tender and beginning to brown.

4. Meanwhile, heat the remaining 1 tablespoon (15 mL) olive oil in a medium skillet over medium heat. Add the cumin, paprika, cinnamon, and chili powder and stir for 1 minute until the spices sizzle and start to smell aromatic.

5. Add the tomatoes, water, apricots, and honey. Simmer for 5 minutes until the sauce has reduced slightly and the apricots are plump. Stir in the roasted vegetables and serve.

NUTRITIONAL INFORMATION This dish is a great source of vitamin A, vitamin C, manganese, and aromatic spices that aid digestion.

WILTED GREENS WITH CREAMY MISO SAUCE SERVES 4 TO 6

DAIRY-FREE • EGG-FREE • GLUTEN-FREE • NUT-FREE • VEGETARIAN • WHEAT-FREE

Sometimes your greens need a lift. This sauce will do that and more! Miso is a tremendously nutritious paste that gives depth of flavour and a hint of saltiness.

¼ cup (60 mL) light-coloured miso, such as white or shiro

½ cup (125 mL) apple cider vinegar

2 tablespoons (30 mL) liquid pure honey

¼ teaspoon (1 mL) minced garlic

2 tablespoons (30 mL) toasted sesame oil

⅓ cup (75 mL) mayonnaise (or more to taste)

Red chili flakes (optional)

1 teaspoon (5 mL) virgin coconut oil

4 cups (1 L) spinach, baby kale, or Swiss chard, roughly torn

1. Place the miso in a medium bowl.

2. Whisk in the cider vinegar, honey, garlic, sesame oil, and mayonnaise and beat until smooth.

3. Add a few chili flakes to taste (if using) and adjust the mayonnaise to taste as well. Set aside.

4. Heat the coconut oil in a skillet over medium heat, add the torn greens, and turn often until wilted.

5. Remove from the heat, pour half of the miso mixture overtop, and check taste. Add more if needed. Serve immediately.

TIP: Substitute ⅓ cup (75 mL) canned coconut milk for the mayonnaise.

NUTRITIONAL INFORMATION These greens are a good source of monounsaturated and polyunsaturated fatty acids.

FISH BAKE WITH MASHED POTATOES SERVES 4 TO 6

EGG-FREE • GLUTEN-FREE • NUT-FREE • WHEAT-FREE

This is a perfect prep-ahead meal or one that you can double up on. Have one batch for dinner tonight and another ready for when you need a quick meal. It's the perfect meal to ensure that your family receives its daily dose of omega fatty acids! Check that your salmon is not genetically modified.

Mashed Potatoes

1½ pounds (675 g) russet potatoes, peeled and cubed

½ pound (225 g) sweet potatoes, peeled and cubed

1 clove garlic

2 teaspoons (10 mL) extra virgin olive oil

¼ cup (60 mL) unsalted butter

½ cup (125 mL) warm milk or the milk used to poach the fish

Salt and pepper

Fish

1 pound (450 g) skinless cod fillet

6 ounces (170 g) wild salmon

Unsweetened almond, coconut, or dairy milk, for poaching

2 teaspoons (10 mL) extra virgin olive oil

1 large yellow onion, chopped

2 cloves garlic, chopped

1 carrot, diced

1½ cups (375 mL) frozen peas

1 cup (250 mL) full-fat canned coconut milk

1 tablespoon (15 mL) Dijon mustard

2 handfuls of fresh baby spinach

2 tablespoons (30 mL) flat-leaf or curly parsley, chopped

1 tablespoon (15 mL) fresh dill, chopped

Salt and pepper

1. Fill a medium pot with water and bring to a boil.

2. Cook the potatoes, along with one whole clove garlic, in boiling water for 15 to 20 minutes until fork-tender. Drain well.

3. While the potatoes are cooking, make the fish. Place the cod and salmon in a frying pan and add the milk until fish are just covered. Poach the fish over medium heat for 8 minutes or until it just flakes.

4. Remove the fish from the poaching liquid and flake into large chunks, removing any bones. Discard the liquid (unless using for the potatoes).

5. Heat the olive oil in a large heavy-based frying pan over medium heat. Sauté the onion for 3 minutes. Add the garlic and carrot and cook for 5 minutes longer.

6. Add the peas and stir as you add the coconut milk and mustard. Cook until heated through. Carefully stir in the spinach, parsley, dill, and poached fish. Season with salt and pepper, to taste.

7. Spoon the mixture into a 9- × 11-inch (23 × 28 cm) oven-safe dish.

8. Preheat the broiler to medium.

9. Place the dish under the broiler for 3 to 5 minutes until the top becomes golden.

10. Make the mashed potatoes. Add the olive oil, butter, and warm milk (or fish-poaching liquid) to the boiled potatoes. Mash until smooth and creamy. Season with salt and pepper, to taste. Spoon the potatoes over the fish and fluff with a fork.

11. Serve with a side salad and Salad Dressing (page 304).

NUTRITIONAL INFORMATION Fish is an excellent source of protein, and salmon is high in essential omega-3 fats.

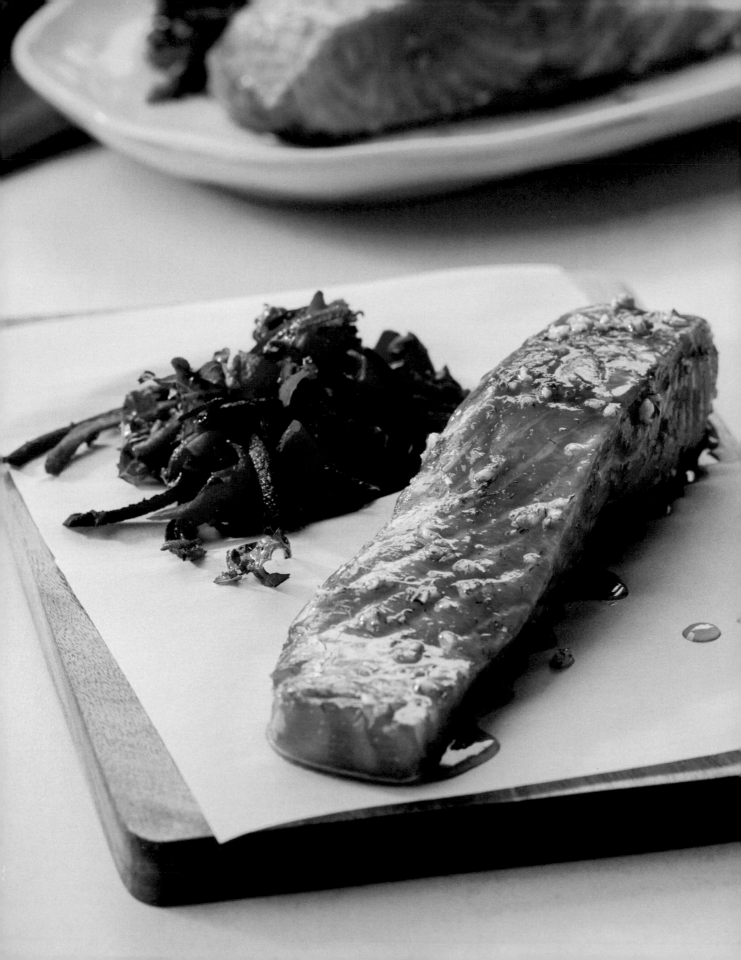

GARLIC MAPLE SALMON SERVES 4

DAIRY-FREE • EGG-FREE • GLUTEN-FREE • NUT-FREE • WHEAT-FREE

Anyone I make this dish for becomes an instant fish lover. Even those who weren't previously convinced. Maple syrup makes everything taste better, and this recipe is no exception. Do check that your salmon is not genetically modified. This is when it's handy to know a fishmonger, so you can ask those questions. For a full meal with a lot of vegetables, serve this salmon with Beet and Carrot Slaw with Ginger Sesame Dressing (page 299) and Lemony Green Beans (page 307).

3 tablespoons (45 mL) pure maple syrup

1 clove garlic, minced

1 teaspoon (5 mL) dried dill

4 (3 ounces/85 g each) organic or wild salmon fillets

1. Preheat the oven to 400°F (200°C). Line a baking sheet with parchment paper.
2. Mix the maple syrup, garlic, and dill in a small bowl.
3. Place the salmon fillets on the prepared baking sheet. Spoon the maple syrup mixture over the fish.
4. Bake for 10 to 15 minutes until the fish flakes easily when tested with a fork. Serve immediately.

TIP: Substitute trout for the salmon for a lighter fish that is still rich in omega-3 fats.

NUTRITIONAL INFORMATION Fatty fish, including salmon and trout, are excellent sources of omega-3 fatty acids.

SUPER SIMPLE BAKED TROUT SERVES 2 TO 4

DAIRY-FREE • EGG-FREE • GLUTEN-FREE • NUT-FREE • WHEAT-FREE

This is a super quick and simple recipe that lets the delicate taste of this fish shine through. It's a good recipe to use to get your toddler familiar with fish. It's also perfect for anyone who loves lemon! Serve with Lemony Green Beans (page 307), Winter Sunshine Salad (page 304), or steamed broccoli.

1 pound (450 g) trout fillet

1 tablespoon (15 mL) fresh lemon juice

1 tablespoon (15 mL) finely chopped red onion

½ teaspoon (2 mL) salt

2 tablespoons (30 mL) chopped fresh herbs
  (cilantro, flat-leaf parsley, dill, or basil)

1. Preheat the oven to 350°F (180°C).
2. Place the fish in a greased, shallow 3-quart (3 L) baking dish.
3. In a small bowl, combine the lemon juice, onion, and salt. Spread the mixture over the fish.
4. Bake, uncovered, for 20 to 25 minutes or until the fish flakes easily with a fork.
5. Sprinkle with herbs and serve with green beans, salad, or broccoli.

NUTRITIONAL INFORMATION Trout is a fatty fish that is high in omega-3 fatty acids and protein.

TUNA MELT SANDWICH SERVES 4

EGG-FREE • NUT-FREE

Some nights, you just need a recipe that's speedy to make and that you know will be well loved. These sandwiches are fast, tasty, and filling. Make them while you have all the ingredients out for the Salmon Burgers (page 286). Serve with Beet and Carrot Slaw with Ginger Sesame Dressing (page 299) or Winter Sunshine Salad (page 304).

2 cans (5 ounces/150 g each) tuna

¼ cup (60 mL) mayonnaise

2 teaspoons (10 mL) Dijon mustard

2 tablespoons (30 mL) chopped flat-leaf or curly parsley

2 teaspoons (10 mL) fresh lemon juice

4 slices sprouted grain bread

4 square slices cheddar or goat's milk cheddar cheese

Toppings (optional)

Lettuce

Sliced tomato

Sliced red onion

1. Preheat the oven to broil.

2. Add the tuna, mayonnaise, mustard, parsley, and lemon juice to a small bowl and mash until well blended. Place slices of bread on a baking sheet, top with equal amounts tuna mixture, and flatten. Cover entirely with cheese.

3. Broil for 5 minutes or until cheese is melted. Serve immediately and top with lettuce, tomato, and red onion as desired. Serve.

NUTRITIONAL INFORMATION Deli meats for sandwiches can be high in sulphites, sulphates, and other preservatives. This tuna sandwich is free from those preservatives and high in omega-3 fatty acids.

SALMON BURGERS SERVES 8

DAIRY-FREE • EGG-FREE • NUT-FREE

These burgers are a staple in my house. My daughters' friends come over and ask me to make these because they love them so much. They are excellent in a lunch the next day, on a bun, or alongside a large spinach salad with Salad Dressing (page 304) or Winter Sunshine Salad (page 304). They're freezer friendly, so make a batch or two!

4 cans (5 ounces/150 g each) skinless, boneless salmon
½ cup (125 mL) green onions, thinly sliced
½ cup (125 mL) old-fashioned rolled oats
⅓ cup (75 mL) chopped fresh parsley or cilantro
¼ cup (60 mL) mayonnaise
¼ cup (60 mL) Dijon mustard
2 eggs, lightly beaten
2 tablespoons (30 mL) fresh lemon juice
1 tablespoon (15 mL) virgin coconut oil
8 whole wheat hamburger buns

Toppings (optional)
Lettuce
Sliced tomatoes
Sliced red onion
Avocado, pitted and peeled

1. Mash the salmon, onion, oats, parsley, mayonnaise, mustard, eggs, and lemon juice together in a large bowl until combined.
2. Form into patties that are about 2 inches (5 cm) in diameter.
3. Heat the coconut oil in a skillet over medium heat and pan-fry the patties for 5 minutes on each side.
4. Serve on a whole wheat bun and top with lettuce, tomato, onion, avocado, and any additional desired toppings.

NUTRITIONAL INFORMATION Salmon is high in protein and omega-3 fats. The oats are a slow-releasing carbohydrate that's a great source of B vitamins and iron. The more colourful toppings you use, the more antioxidants your burger will provide.

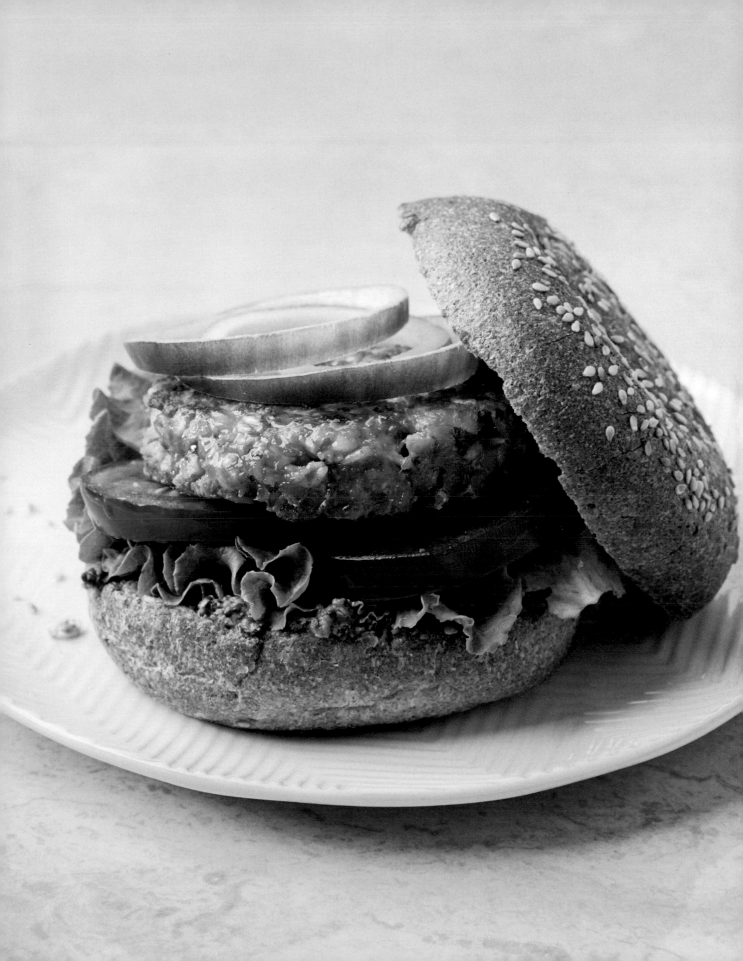

SEARED SALMON WITH BROCCOLI IN BLUEBERRY WALNUT SAUCE

SERVES 4

DAIRY-FREE • EGG-FREE • GLUTEN-FREE • WHEAT-FREE

Sweet meets savoury in this dinner recipe that could turn your whole family into fish lovers! Although salmon works really well in this recipe, feel free to use a white fish like cod, haddock, or halibut instead. Make sure that your salmon is not genetically modified.

4 (4 ounces/115 g each) wild salmon fillets

1 tablespoon (15 mL) chopped fresh rosemary, divided

1 teaspoon (5 mL) sea salt, divided

2 heads broccoli, trimmed

1½ tablespoons (22 mL) extra virgin olive oil, divided

1 small yellow or red onion, diced

3 tablespoons (45 mL) dried blueberries

2 tablespoons (30 mL) walnuts

½ cup (125 mL) filtered water

1. Season the salmon with ½ tablespoon (7 mL) rosemary and ½ teaspoon (2 mL) salt.

2. Cut the broccoli into florets with 2-inch (5 cm) stalks.

3. Heat 1 tablespoon (15 mL) olive oil in a large wide saucepan over medium heat. Add the onion and cook for about 3 to 4 minutes, until translucent.

4. Add the blueberries, walnuts, and the remaining ½ tablespoon (7 mL) rosemary, then toss to coat. Cook for another 3 to 4 minutes, stirring constantly, until the walnuts are fragrant.

5. Add the broccoli, season with the remaining ½ teaspoon (2 mL) salt, and toss to combine. Add the water and bring to a boil. Reduce the heat to maintain a gentle simmer and cook for about 8 to 10 minutes, stirring occasionally, until the water has almost evaporated.

6. Meanwhile, heat the remaining ½ tablespoon (7 mL) olive oil in a large nonstick skillet over medium-high heat. Add the salmon, skin side up, and cook for 5 minutes until golden brown. Turn the salmon over, remove the pan from the heat, and let stand for about 5 minutes until just cooked through.

7. To serve, divide the broccoli among 4 plates. Top with salmon and spoon blueberries, walnuts, and any liquid remaining in the pan over the salmon.

NUTRITIONAL INFORMATION Salmon offers a high amount of protein, omega-3 fatty acids, calcium, and vitamin A.

PESTO FISH SERVES 4

DAIRY-FREE • EGG-FREE • GLUTEN-FREE • WHEAT-FREE

Fish is quick to cook when you're pressed for time, and topping it with pesto takes only a second to do. Save this recipe for one of those nights when everyone is home for just a short period of time before going to their evening activities. Serve with Energizing Green Bean and Carrot Salad (page 302) or Mixed Bean Salad (page 303).

4 (6 ounces/170 g each) salmon, cod, or
   haddock fillets
1 tablespoon (15 mL) olive oil
Salt
Freshly ground black pepper
2 tablespoons (30 mL) pesto

1. Preheat the oven to 375°F (190°C).
Line a baking sheet with parchment paper.
2. Place the fish on the prepared baking sheet. Lightly drizzle with olive oil and season to taste with salt and pepper.
3. Evenly spread a thin layer of pesto over the fish.
4. Bake for 10 to 15 minutes until the fish is cooked through and flakes easily with a fork. Serve immediately.

TIP: There are so many different kinds of pesto. Just about any of them will do here, but my favourites are Sunflower Kitchen's Kale and Oregano Pesto, Basil Pesto, or Sundried Tomato and Olive Pesto.

NUTRITIONAL INFORMATION Fish is a good source of omega-3 fatty acids.

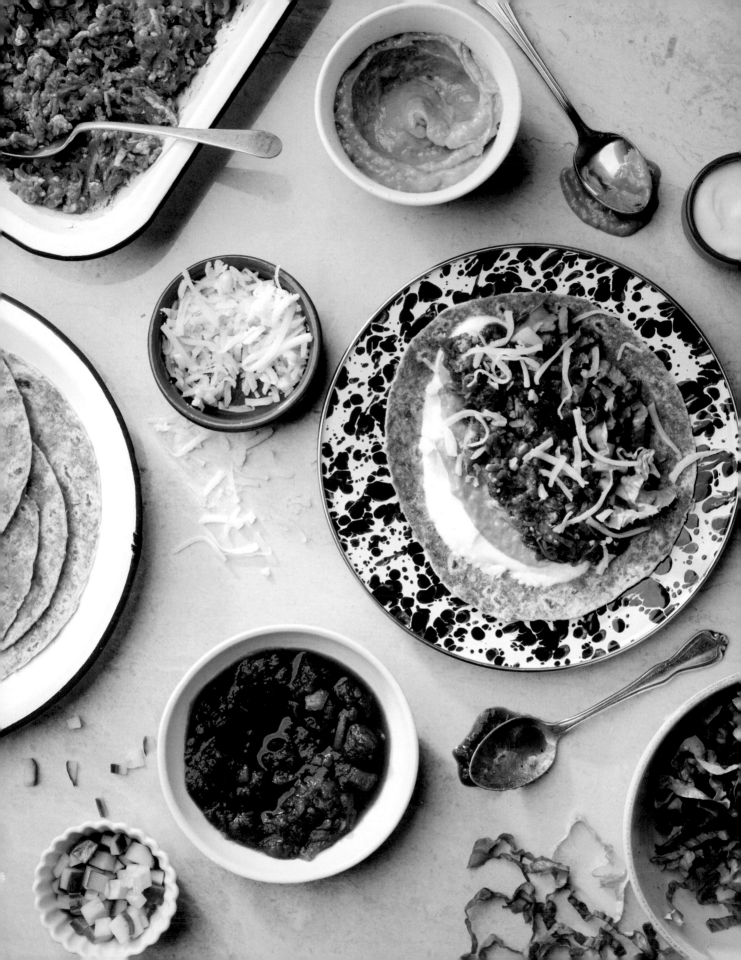

TACO NIGHT SERVES 4

EGG-FREE • GLUTEN-FREE • NUT-FREE • WHEAT-FREE

Tacos are a favourite at my house, especially when we have friends over. I often have to insist that more than one topping go into the tacos, so that there's more than just cheese on top, and my kids have now become pros at getting all toppings into their hard- or soft-shell tacos. Leftovers make a great taco salad for lunch the next day.

2 teaspoons (10 mL) olive oil

1 small yellow onion, grated

2 medium carrots, peeled and grated

1 small zucchini, grated

2 garlic cloves, minced or grated

2 to 3 teaspoons (10 to 15 mL) ground cumin

2 to 3 teaspoons (10 to 15 mL) chili powder

1 pound (450 g) ground turkey, chicken, or
  grass-fed beef

½ cup (125 mL) tomato sauce

½ cup (125 mL) salsa

Salt

Black pepper

12 medium taco shells or soft corn tortillas

Toppings (optional)

Shredded lettuce

Diced cucumber

Shredded cheddar cheese

Shredded mozzarella cheese

Salsa

Guacamole

Greek yogurt or sour cream

1. Heat the olive oil in a heavy large skillet over medium-high heat. Add the onion, carrot, zucchini, and garlic and sauté until soft, about 5 minutes.

2. Add the cumin and chili powder and stir for 1 minute.

3. Add the turkey and cook until browned, breaking it up with the back of a fork if necessary. Spoon off any fat from the meat.

4. Add the tomato sauce and salsa and cook until heated through, stirring occasionally for about 5 minutes. Season with salt and pepper, to taste.

5. Spoon ¼ cup (60 mL) filling into each taco shell or tortilla and roll up. Serve with lettuce, cucumber, cheese, salsa, guacamole, and yogurt or sour cream, if desired.

TIP: Substitute grass-fed ground beef for the ground turkey if desired. To make vegetarian tacos, substitute 2 cans (14 ounces/398 mL each) beans (kidney, adzuki, or pinto), drained and rinsed, for the ground meat. You can also crumble tempeh and cook it like ground beef.

NUTRITIONAL INFORMATION A combination of all the right foods make these tacos high in good-quality proteins, vitamins, and healthy fats.

RAINBOW RICE WRAPS MAKES 4 WRAPS

DAIRY-FREE • EGG-FREE • GLUTEN-FREE • NUT-FREE • VEGAN • VEGETARIAN • WHEAT-FREE

These delicious wraps are best made fresh, so prepare your veggies the night before and assemble in the morning. They are fantastic for kids to make themselves, with a bit of help for the younger ones. Kids tend to eat more of what they make themselves. The freshness of these wraps makes them tastier than you might think. Send them to school in an airtight container. Rice paper wrappers can be found at health food stores and supermarkets. They can be stuffed with just about anything and stick together easily, which is great for small, less dexterous hands.

Half of a 14-ounce (390 g) package vermicelli rice noodles

1 tablespoon (15 mL) tamari, plus more for dipping

2 teaspoons (10 mL) olive oil

4 (each 8½ inches/21 cm long) rice paper wrappers

½ medium carrot, peeled and cut into matchsticks

½ sweet pepper (any colour), seeded and cut into matchsticks

2½ inches (6 cm) English cucumber, cut into matchsticks

4 ounces (115 g) tofu, cut into ½-inch (1 cm) square strips

Handful of sunflower sprouts (optional)

1. Cook the noodles according to the package directions. Drain thoroughly and toss with the tamari and olive oil.

2. Fill a shallow plate with water. Dip one sheet of rice paper into the water and let it soak until it starts to become bendable but still has structure, about 10 seconds. Transfer to a clean working surface (plastic cutting board or plate).

3. Arrange the noodles, carrot, sweet pepper, cucumber, tofu, and sunflower sprouts (if using) across the centre of the rice paper. Begin rolling, tucking the sides in as you roll. Transfer the roll to a platter and repeat with the remaining 3 rice paper wrappers.

4. Serve with tamari on the side for dipping.

TIP: Substitute the same amount of cooked chicken, smoked salmon, or cooked shrimp for the tofu.

NUTRITIONAL INFORMATION These rice wraps are light and a good source of vitamin A, vitamin C, antioxidants, and protein.

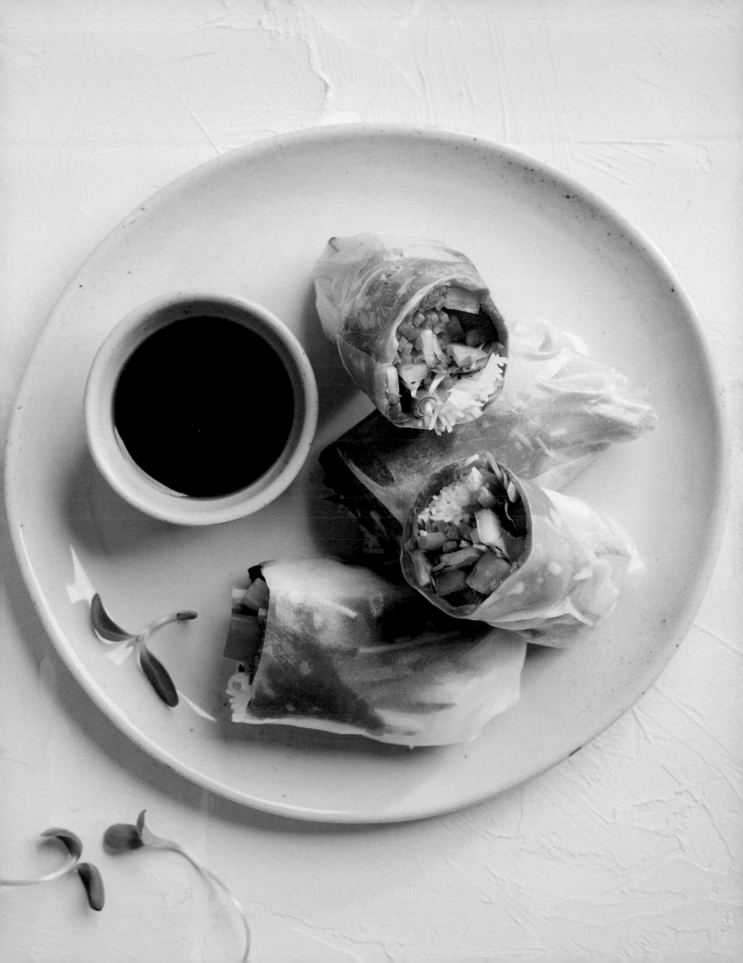

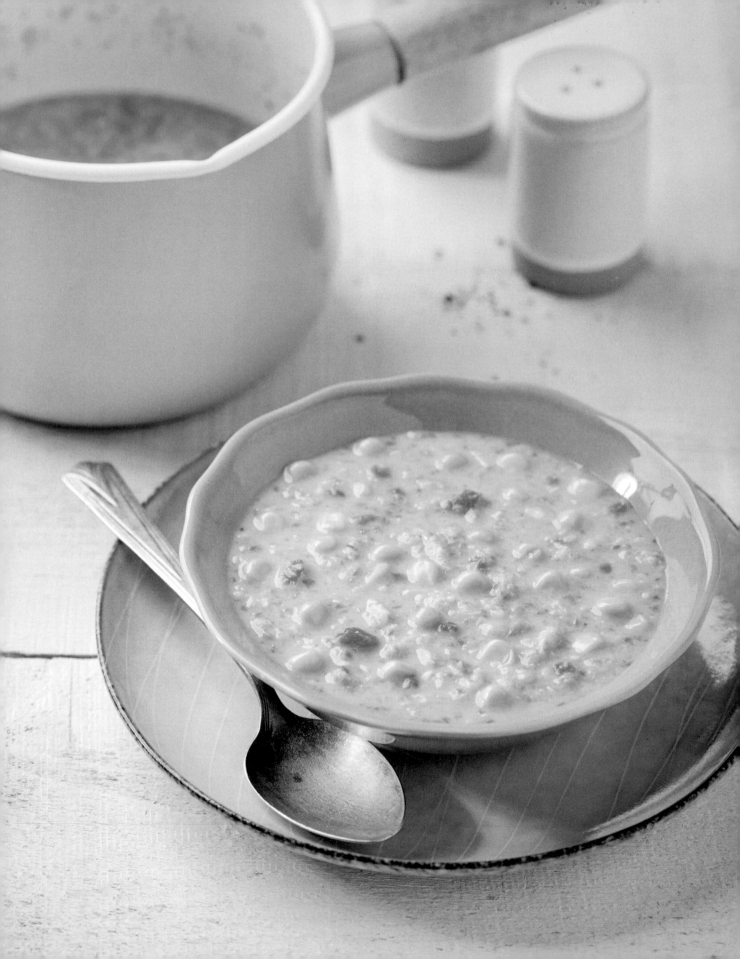

CORN, COCONUT, AND GINGER SOUP MAKES 6 CUPS (1.5 L)

DAIRY-FREE • EGG-FREE • GLUTEN-FREE • NUT-FREE • VEGAN • VEGETARIAN • WHEAT-FREE

This soup was the hit of a soup pilot program I started at my kids' school. It then became a firm favourite at home and is made throughout the winter months. It makes for a speedy dinner and an even faster lunch. It freezes really well, so once you've tried it with your family, make a double batch next time!

1 tablespoon (15 mL) olive oil

3 medium carrots, peeled and diced

1 medium yellow onion, chopped

½ inch (1 cm) piece fresh ginger, peeled and grated

2 cloves garlic, chopped

1 bag (17 ounces/500 g) frozen corn

1⅔ cups (400 mL) Meat Broth (page 129) or Vegetable Broth (page 130)

1⅔ cups (400 mL) canned full-fat coconut milk

Salt

Black pepper

4 whole-grain buns, for serving (optional)

1. Heat the olive oil in a medium saucepan over medium heat.
2. Add the carrot, onion, ginger, and garlic and cook until the onion is translucent.
3. Add the corn, broth, and coconut milk. Simmer for about 15 minutes until the carrot is fork-tender.
4. Remove from the heat and cool slightly. Using a hand-held blender, purée to desired consistency. Season with salt and pepper, to taste.
5. Ladle into bowls and serve with toasted whole-grain buns, if desired.

TIP: For a fast chop, pulse the carrots, onion, and garlic in your food processor.

NUTRITIONAL INFORMATION This is a colourful, antioxidant-rich soup with immune-boosting properties from the garlic, onion, and meat broth (if using). It's also a good source of vitamin A and calcium.

EASY ASIAN SOUP BOWL SERVES 4

DAIRY-FREE • EGG-FREE • GLUTEN-FREE • NUT-FREE • WHEAT-FREE

This is a super-fast recipe. I once made it from start to finish on a TV show, in less than five minutes, which is how long the segment was. If I can do it on TV, you can do it at home!

6 cups (1.5 L) Meat Broth (page 129) or
  Vegetable Broth (page 130)

1 piece kombu seaweed (optional)

1 sweet red pepper, diced

1 clove garlic, sliced or grated

½-inch (1 cm) piece fresh ginger, grated

6 ounces (170 g) rice vermicelli noodles

8 ounces (225 g) raw shrimp, tails removed and
  diced

1 cup (250 mL) snow peas, trimmed

1. Pour the broth into a large pot and bring to a boil over high heat. Reduce the heat to low, add the kombu (if using), and simmer for 10 minutes. Remove the kombu and discard.
2. Add the red pepper, garlic, ginger and noodles and simmer for 3 minutes.
3. Add the shrimp and snow peas and simmer for an additional 3 to 5 minutes or until the shrimp is cooked through.
4. Serve in soup bowls and store leftover soup in an airtight container in the fridge for tomorrow's lunch.

TIP: **1.** Use meat broth in this recipe for a collagen and mineral boost. **2.** Kombu seaweed can be found in health food stores and will increase the nutritional content of your stock, so it is great to use if you have it. **3.** Substitute leftover cooked chicken thigh or tofu for the shrimp.

NUTRITIONAL INFORMATION This soup is nourishing, anti-inflammatory, and alkalizing for your body. It's packed with protein and wonderful minerals like iodine, iron, and calcium from the kombu seaweed.

IMMUNE-BOOSTING SOUP SERVES 4

DAIRY-FREE • EGG-FREE • GLUTEN-FREE • NUT-FREE • WHEAT-FREE

This is a staple in my house. I always have a jar of this in my freezer for when someone has that scratchy-throat or itchy-back-of-the-nose feeling. You can use other noodles like rice spaghetti or wheat noodles instead of the soba if you choose.

8 cups (2 L) Meat Broth (page 129) or Vegetable Broth (page 130)

1 piece kombu seaweed

7 ounces (210 g) 100% soba noodles

1 teaspoon (5 mL) sesame oil

1¼-inch (3 cm) piece fresh ginger, peeled and cut into matchsticks

⅔ cup (150 mL) shiitake or button mushrooms, trimmed and sliced

2 medium carrots, cut into matchsticks

1 clove garlic, minced

4 skinless, boneless chicken thighs, diced

Salt

Freshly ground black pepper

3 tablespoons (45 mL) light-coloured miso, such as white or shiro

4 green onions, trimmed and thinly sliced on the diagonal (optional)

1 teaspoon (5 mL) toasted sesame seeds, for garnish (optional)

1. Pour the broth into a large pot and add the kombu. Bring to a simmer, cover the pot with a lid, and cook gently for 5 to 10 minutes. Remove and discard the kombu.
2. Bring a medium pot of salted water to a rolling boil over high heat. Drop the noodles into the water and cook for 3 to 4 minutes or until they are soft with a remaining bit of firmness when bitten. Drain and immediately toss with sesame oil. Set aside.
3. Add the ginger, mushrooms, carrot, and garlic to the broth and simmer for another 3 to 5 minutes. Add the chicken and cook until opaque throughout, about 15 minutes. Taste and adjust the seasoning with salt and pepper, cover the pot with a lid, and reduce the heat to low. Cook for another 5 minutes.
4. Just before serving, stir in the miso paste (do not boil once miso is mixed in).
5. Divide the soba noodles between 4 bowls and scatter green onion (if using) on top. Ladle the hot soup over the noodles, making sure that you divide the chicken and mushrooms evenly among the bowls.
6. Sprinkle sesame seeds (if using) on top and serve.
7. Store leftover soup in an airtight container in the fridge for up to 3 days or in the freezer for up to 1 month.

NUTRITIONAL INFORMATION This soup is high in immune-boosting nutrients, including antioxidants and protein.

QUINOA AND CORN SALAD MAKES 3 CUPS (750 ML)

EGG-FREE • GLUTEN-FREE • NUT-FREE • VEGETARIAN • WHEAT-FREE

Make ahead and serve on its own or as an accompaniment to dinner or lunch. Add or replace the veggies with other favourites, such as diced green or yellow pepper, peas, or broccoli. Serve with Baked Butternut Squash and Garlic Risotto (page 264), Salmon Burgers (page 286), or Tuna Melt Sandwich (page 285).

2 cups (500 mL) filtered water

1 cup (250 mL) quinoa, rinsed

2½ cups (625 mL) fresh or frozen corn

½ cup (125 mL) feta cheese, crumbled

1 small red onion, diced

¼ cup (60 mL) fresh lemon juice or lime juice

2 tablespoons (30 mL) olive oil

¼ cup (60 mL) chopped fresh cilantro

Salt

Black pepper

1. Bring the water to a boil in a medium saucepan. Add the quinoa and cover. Reduce the heat to low and cook until all the liquid has been absorbed and the quinoa is fluffy.
2. Turn out quinoa into a medium bowl to cool.
3. Defrost the frozen corn or steam fresh corn for 5 minutes until bright yellow. Add to the quinoa along with the cheese, onion, lemon or lime juice, olive oil, and cilantro. Toss to combine. Season with salt and pepper, to taste.
4. Store the salad in an airtight container in the fridge for up to 4 days.

TIP: Substitute Meat Broth (page 129) or Vegetable Broth (page 130) for the water for more nutrients and flavour.

NUTRITIONAL INFORMATION This salad is a good source of vitamin A, vitamin C, vitamin D, folate, and choline.

BEET AND CARROT SLAW WITH GINGER SESAME DRESSING SERVES 4
DAIRY-FREE • EGG-FREE • GLUTEN-FREE • NUT-FREE • VEGETARIAN • WHEAT-FREE

Your taste buds are going to be dancing with this recipe. It's a huge hit, even with those who aren't sure about beets. It is also one of the best dishes I've shared at a backyard barbecue or potluck. This recipe works well with the Tuna Melt Sandwich (page 285), Salmon Burgers (page 286), Chicken Souvlaki (page 273), or Super Simple Baked Trout (page 284). Use a food processor with the grater attachment for speedy prep.

Beet and Carrot Slaw

2 cups (500 mL) grated carrot

1 cup (250 mL) kale, stems removed and finely chopped

1 cup (250 mL) grated red beets

½ sweet red pepper, seeded and diced

1 tablespoon (15 mL) finely chopped red onion

1 tablespoon (15 mL) chopped green onion

Ginger Sesame Dressing

½ cup (125 mL) apple cider vinegar

¼ cup (60 mL) olive oil

1 tablespoon (15 mL) liquid pure honey

1 tablespoon (15 mL) sesame oil

1 tablespoon (15 mL) finely chopped fresh basil

2 teaspoons (10 mL) ground ginger or
   1 tablespoon (15 mL) fresh ginger, peeled and finely chopped

1 teaspoon (5 mL) tamari

1. To make the Beet and Carrot Slaw, combine the carrot, kale, beets, red pepper, red onion, and green onion in a large bowl.

2. To make the Ginger Sesame Dressing, whisk together the apple cider vinegar, olive oil, honey, sesame oil, basil, ginger, and tamari.

3. Pour the dressing over the slaw and toss.

4. Cover and refrigerate for at least 1 hour before serving.

NUTRITIONAL INFORMATION This slaw is a great source of phytonutrients and vitamins, including vitamins A and C.

CURRIED QUINOA SALAD WITH APRICOTS SERVES 6

DAIRY-FREE • EGG-FREE • GLUTEN-FREE • VEGAN • VEGETARIAN • WHEAT-FREE

I have made this recipe so many times, and my family never gets tired of it. It's the best dish to take to a potluck or on a picnic. The curry powder and sweetness from the apricots are a perfect pairing.

2 tablespoons (30 mL) curry powder

¼ cup (60 mL) apple cider vinegar

⅓ cup (75 mL) olive oil

¼ cup (60 mL) fresh orange, pear, or apple juice

1 tablespoon (15 mL) grated fresh ginger

½ teaspoon (2 mL) salt, plus more to taste

2 cups (500 mL) cooked white quinoa

¾ cup (175 mL) dried unsulphured apricots, thinly sliced

½ sweet red pepper, diced

½ sweet yellow pepper, diced

½ cup (125 mL) walnut pieces, toasted

¼ cup (60 mL) fresh cilantro, chopped (optional)

Black pepper

1. Combine the curry powder, apple cider vinegar, olive oil, orange juice, ginger, and salt in a small bowl.
2. In a serving bowl, combine the cooked quinoa, apricots, red and yellow pepper, walnuts, and cilantro (if using). Pour the curry mixture over the salad and gently stir to mix. Add additional salt and pepper, to taste.
3. Refrigerate until ready to serve. Store the salad in an airtight container in the fridge for up to 5 days.

NUTRITIONAL INFORMATION Quinoa is a seed that contains all the essential amino acids, so it is a complete protein. It's a good source of vitamin A, vitamin C, antioxidants, and omega-6 fatty acids.

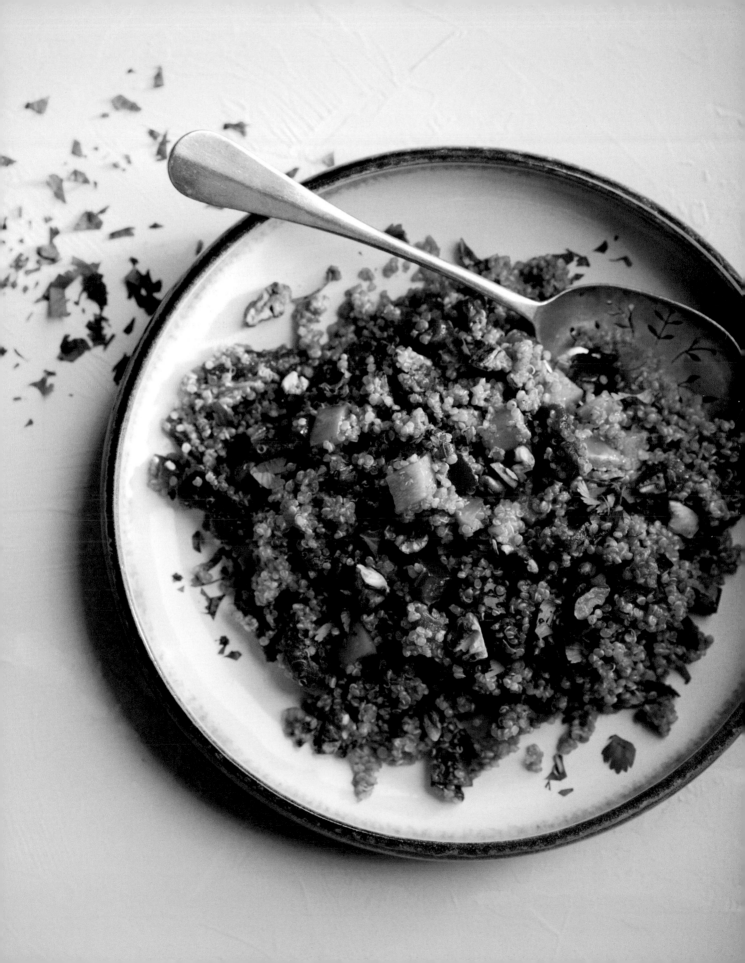

ENERGIZING GREEN BEAN AND CARROT SALAD SERVES 4

DAIRY-FREE • EGG-FREE • GLUTEN-FREE • VEGAN • VEGETARIAN • WHEAT-FREE

If you can't find fresh green beans, try frozen. This recipe also works well with sugar snap peas, snow peas, or yellow beans. It makes a great side dish to Pesto Fish (page 289), Garlic Maple Salmon (page 283), and Mini Calzone (page 275).

1 cup (250 mL) fresh green beans

1 Granny Smith apple, peeled, cored, and diced

1 stalk celery, finely diced

½ medium zucchini, peeled and diced

2 to 3 slices red onion, finely chopped

2 medium carrots, peeled and thinly sliced
  into ribbons

2 tablespoons (30 mL) olive oil

1 tablespoon (15 mL) chia seeds

1 tablespoon (15 mL) sliced almonds

Juice of 1 lemon

1. Trim the ends of the green beans and cut into thirds. If using frozen, defrost in a small amount of hot water for 5 minutes, then drain and cut into thirds.
2. Bring 2 inches (5 cm) of water to a rolling boil in a medium saucepan. Add the green beans to the boiling water and cook for 3 minutes. Drain and rinse with cold water and some ice. Set aside.
3. In a medium bowl, combine the apple, celery, zucchini, and onion.
4. Add the green beans and carrot and stir to combine.
5. In a small bowl, combine the olive oil, chia seeds, almonds, and lemon juice.
6. Drizzle the olive oil mixture over the apple mixture and stir to coat evenly.
7. Store the salad in an airtight container in the fridge for up to 4 days.

NUTRITIONAL INFORMATION This salad aligns well with a "rainbow diet." It's full of phytonutrients, vitamins, fibre, and omega-3 and omega-6 fatty acids.

MIXED BEAN SALAD MAKES 1 TO 1½ CUPS (250 TO 375 ML)

DAIRY-FREE • EGG-FREE • GLUTEN-FREE • NUT-FREE • VEGETARIAN • WHEAT-FREE

Rich in protein and fibre, this bean salad, combined with rice of any kind, makes a complete protein for a plant-based diet. Make this at the beginning of the week and add to main dishes like Golden Grilled Curried Chicken Thighs (page 274), Super Simple Baked Trout (page 284), and Curried Quinoa Salad with Apricots (page 300) for a fully plant-based meal.

2 tablespoons (30 mL) extra virgin olive oil

2 teaspoons (10 mL) apple cider vinegar or white wine vinegar

½ teaspoon (2 mL) Dijon mustard

½ teaspoon (2 mL) liquid pure honey

3 cups (750 mL) mixed beans (chickpeas, adzuki, cannellini, kidney), drained and rinsed

1 sweet red pepper, seeded and diced

1 stalk celery, diced

2 green onions, sliced

2 tablespoons (30 mL) chopped fresh mint

2 tablespoons (30 mL) chopped fresh cilantro

1. In a medium bowl, mix together the olive oil, vinegar, mustard, and honey.

2. Add the, beans, red pepper, celery, onion, mint, and cilantro to the bowl with the dressing. Toss, and serve.

3. Store the salad in an airtight container in the fridge for up to 5 days.

NUTRITIONAL INFORMATION This bean medley is an excellent source of fibre and is high in protein, vitamin A, vitamin C, and flavour!

WINTER SUNSHINE SALAD

SERVES 4

DAIRY-FREE • EGG-FREE • GLUTEN-FREE •
VEGAN • VEGETARIAN • WHEAT-FREE

Citrus fruits taste like sunshine, especially in the cold and dark of winter. This salad can give you a much-needed lift during the darker times of year.

2 red grapefruits
1 tablespoon (15 mL) extra virgin olive oil
1 teaspoon (5 mL) grated fresh ginger
½ teaspoon (2 mL) sea salt
½ small red onion, thinly sliced
2 pears, cored and cubed
1 large ripe avocado
½ head Boston lettuce, leaves separated and
 torn
¼ cup (60 mL) sliced almonds

1. Peel and section the grapefruits over a small bowl, making sure to reserve any juice that falls into the bowl.
2. In a medium bowl, whisk together the olive oil, ginger, salt, and any reserved grapefruit juice.
3. Add the onion, grapefruit, and pear and toss to combine. Cover and refrigerate for at least 1 hour.
4. Just before serving, pit, peel, and slice the avocado.
5. In a serving bowl, add the lettuce and then tip in the fruit mixture and the avocado. Sprinkle the almonds on top and gently toss. Serve immediately.

NUTRITIONAL INFORMATION This salad is a great source of vitamin A, vitamin C, vitamin K, folate, and healthy fats.

SALAD DRESSING

MAKES 1½ CUPS (375 ML)

DAIRY-FREE • EGG-FREE • GLUTEN-FREE •
NUT-FREE • VEGETARIAN • WHEAT-FREE

Homemade salad dressing is so worth the few minutes it takes to throw everything into a jar. There are no extras, thickeners, or flavourings in this. Feel free to change up the mustard to your favourite, and try maple syrup instead of honey.

¾ cup (175 mL) extra virgin olive oil
⅓ cup (75 mL) fresh lemon juice or apple cider
 vinegar
2 tablespoons (30 mL) raw liquid honey
1 tablespoon (15 mL) grainy mustard
Sea salt
Freshly ground black pepper

1. Add the olive oil, lemon juice, honey, and mustard to a jar with a lid. Seal the jar, shake to combine, and season with salt and pepper, to taste.
2. Store the dressing in an airtight container in the fridge for up to 2 weeks. Shake well before each use.

NUTRITIONAL INFORMATION This zesty dressing is a good source of vitamin C.

ASIAN NOODLE SALAD SERVES 4

DAIRY-FREE • EGG-FREE • GLUTEN-FREE • VEGETARIAN • WHEAT-FREE

This recipe takes a bit more prep but is so worth it. The combined ingredients create a taste sensation that could wow guests at your home or friends at a gathering.

¼ cup (60 mL) fresh lime juice

4 to 5 tablespoons (60 to 75 mL) tamari

1½ tablespoons (22 mL) peeled and minced fresh ginger

1 clove garlic, minced

1½ teaspoons (7 mL) liquid pure honey

¼ cup (60 mL) sunflower oil, plus 1 teaspoon (5 mL) more for the noodles

⅓ cup (75 mL) almond butter or smooth peanut butter

½ pound (225 g) thick noodle of choice (soba, rice, linguine)

3 medium carrots, peeled and cut into matchsticks

2 small zucchini, cut into matchsticks

1 sweet red pepper, cut into thin strips

1 bunch green onions or ½ red onion, thinly sliced (optional)

2 to 3 tablespoons (30 to 45 mL) fresh cilantro, chopped

½ teaspoon (2 mL) sea salt

½ teaspoon (2 mL) freshly ground black pepper

Chopped almonds or peanuts, for garnish (optional)

1. Whisk together the lime juice, tamari, ginger, garlic, honey, ¼ cup (60 mL) sunflower oil, and almond butter in a large bowl.

2. Cook the noodles according to the package instructions. Drain the noodles in a colander and rinse under cold water. Return them to the pot and toss with the remaining 1 teaspoon (5 mL) sunflower oil.

3. Add the cooked noodles, carrot, zucchini, red pepper, onion, and cilantro to the bowl. Toss to combine. Season with the salt and pepper.

4. Divide among shallow bowls, top with chopped almonds (if using), and serve at room temperature.

NUTRITIONAL INFORMATION This noodle salad is high in vitamin A and vitamin C, a powerhouse of antioxidants, and great for the immune system.

GARLICKY GREENS AND CHICKPEAS SERVES 4 TO 6

DAIRY-FREE • EGG-FREE • GLUTEN-FREE • NUT-FREE • VEGAN • VEGETARIAN • WHEAT-FREE

This is a lovely dish that can be served as a meatless dinner for the vegetarian or vegan in the family. It also makes a great side dish for Garlic Maple Salmon (page 283), Mini Frittatas (page 257), and Chicken Souvlaki (page 273). Serve with Coconut Rice (page 308).

3 tablespoons (45 mL) olive oil

1 yellow onion, chopped

4 cloves garlic, minced

1 teaspoon (5 mL) ground cumin

½ teaspoon (2 mL) ground cinnamon

10 dried unsulphured apricots, thinly sliced

1 can (12 ounces/340 g) chickpeas

1 tablespoon (15 mL) fresh lemon juice

5 cups (1.25 L) packed baby spinach, chopped

Sea salt

Freshly ground black pepper

Handful of sunflower seeds or pumpkin seeds

Handful of fresh cilantro, chopped

1. Heat the olive oil in a medium saucepan over medium heat. Add the onion and cook, stirring frequently, for 6 to 8 minutes or until soft and translucent.
2. Stir in the garlic, cumin, cinnamon, and apricots and cook for 2 minutes, stirring constantly.
3. Add the chickpeas, including the liquid in the can, and the lemon juice. Bring to a boil and add the spinach. Cover, reduce the heat to low, and simmer for 5 minutes, stirring once.
4. Season with salt and pepper, to taste. Garnish with the seeds and cilantro and serve.
5. Store in an airtight container in the fridge for up to 3 days.

NUTRITIONAL INFORMATION This immune-boosting dish is a great source of antioxidants, fibre, protein, and iron.

LEMONY GREEN BEANS SERVES 6

DAIRY-FREE • EGG-FREE • GLUTEN-FREE • NUT-FREE • VEGETARIAN • WHEAT-FREE

This is a staple go-to recipe in my house. It jazzes up the green beans with fresh flavour and sweetness that the whole family will love. Serve with just about any of the main meals, including Pesto Fish (page 289), Golden Grilled Curried Chicken Thighs (page 274), or Fish Bake with Mashed Potatoes (page 281).

½ cup (125 mL) cashews, sunflower seeds, or pine nuts

1½ tablespoons (22 mL) raw liquid honey

1½ tablespoons (22 mL) Dijon mustard

3 to 4 teaspoons (15 to 20 mL) fresh lemon or lime juice

2 tablespoons (30 mL) filtered water

3 cups (750 mL) green beans, trimmed

1. Mix the nuts or seeds, honey, mustard, and lemon juice in a small bowl.

2. Pour the water into a large frying pan over medium heat.

3. When the pan is warm, add the green beans and stir until bright green. The water will evaporate.

4. Add the nuts or seeds mixture. Gently stir for 3 to 4 minutes until well coated. Serve immediately.

NUTRITIONAL INFORMATION This dish is a good source of calcium and vitamin A.

COCONUT RICE SERVES 4 TO 5

DAIRY-FREE • EGG-FREE • GLUTEN-FREE • NUT-FREE • VEGAN • VEGETARIAN • WHEAT-FREE

Use this recipe for any dish that calls for rice as an accompaniment. Coconut milk and ginger add a gorgeous flavour that will enhance anything this rice is paired with. Serve with Garlic Maple Salmon (page 283), Golden Grilled Curried Chicken Thighs (page 274), Chicken Poached in Coconut Curry Sauce (page 276), or Roasted Veggie Tagine (page 279).

2 cups (500 mL) brown basmati or jasmine rice, rinsed

1 can (12 ounces/340 mL) full-fat coconut milk

2 cups (500 mL) filtered water

1½-inch (4 cm) piece fresh ginger, peeled and grated

Pinch of salt

1. Add the rice, coconut milk, water, ginger, and salt to a medium pot and bring to a boil.

2. Reduce the heat and simmer on low until the liquid has been absorbed and the rice is cooked.

3. Set aside with the lid on for 5 minutes. Fluff with a fork and serve.

4. Store leftover rice in an airtight container in the fridge for up to 3 days.

NUTRITIONAL INFORMATION This creamy rice is a good source of vitamin B1, vitamin B3, and magnesium.

PURE GREEN HUMMUS MAKES 1¼ CUPS (300 ML)

DAIRY-FREE • EGG-FREE • GLUTEN-FREE • NUT-FREE • VEGAN • VEGETARIAN • WHEAT-FREE

This super-healthy hummus has an added protein kick from edamame and cannellini beans, making for a super-tasty, smooth, and delicious dip. Serve with Mary's Gone Crackers, colourful pepper slices, zucchini sticks, or carrot sticks. It tastes better the longer it sits, so make it at least one hour in advance of eating.

1 cup (250 mL) frozen shelled edamame (non-GMO)

½ cup (125 mL) white cannellini beans

¼ cup (60 mL) tahini

¼ cup (60 mL) filtered water

Zest and juice of 1 lemon

3 cloves garlic, smashed

1 teaspoon (5 mL) sea salt

½ teaspoon (2 mL) ground cumin

¼ teaspoon (1 mL) ground coriander

3 tablespoons (45 mL) extra virgin olive oil

1. Add the edamame to a small pot of boiling water over high heat and cook for 4 to 5 minutes, then drain. Alternatively, microwave the edamame in a small bowl, covered, for 2 to 3 minutes.

2. In a food processor, purée the edamame, beans, tahini, water, lemon zest and juice, garlic, salt, cumin, and coriander until smooth.

3. With the motor running, slowly drizzle in the olive oil and continue to blend until combined and smooth.

4. Transfer to a small bowl and refrigerate, covered, until ready to serve. Store the hummus in an airtight container in the fridge for 4 to 5 days.

NUTRITIONAL INFORMATION Edamame are the highest of all beans in protein and are high in fibre, too. This dip is very high in fibre, calcium, and immune-boosting nutrients.

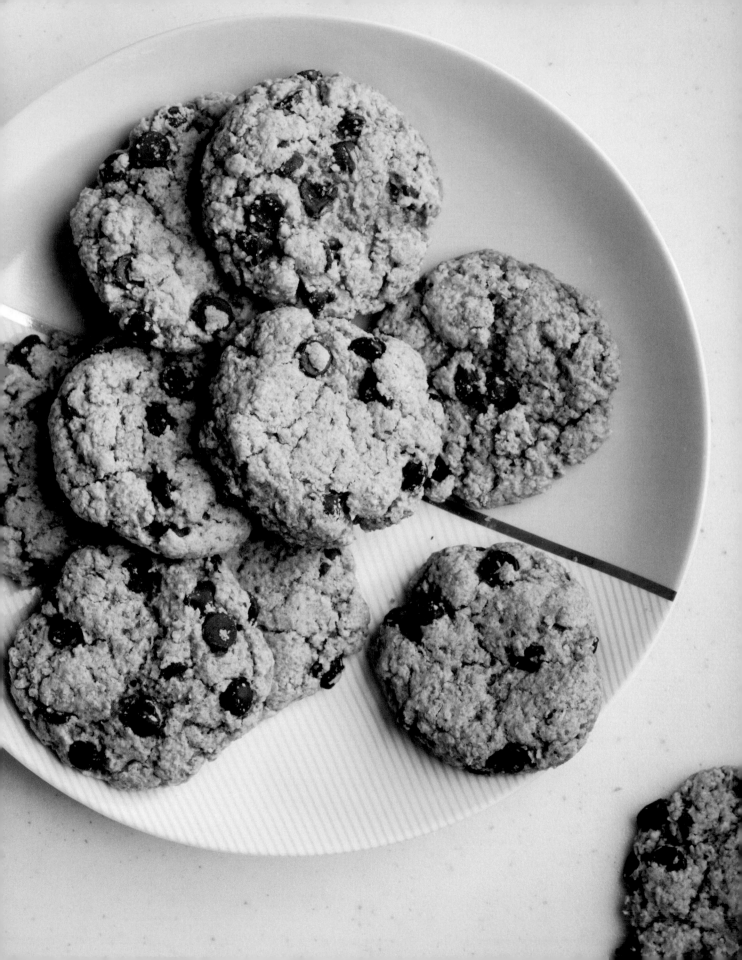

CHOCOLATE CHIP COOKIES MAKES 10 TO 12 COOKIES

DAIRY-FREE • EGG-FREE • GLUTEN-FREE • NUT-FREE • VEGAN • VEGETARIAN • WHEAT-FREE

There are times when only a cookie will do. These oat-based cookies are totally satisfying without being overpoweringly sweet. Try dark chocolate chips—you might be surprised that the cookies are sweet enough without milk chocolate chips. These won't last long, so maybe double the recipe!

1½ cups (375 mL) old-fashioned rolled oats

½ teaspoon (2 mL) baking soda

¼ teaspoon (1 mL) salt

½ cup (125 mL) coconut sugar

2 tablespoons (30 mL) virgin coconut oil or unsalted butter, melted

2 to 3 tablespoons (30 to 45 mL) almond or coconut milk

¼ cup (60 mL) chocolate chips, mini or regular size

1. Preheat the oven to 375°F (190°C). Line a baking sheet with parchment paper.
2. Blend the oats, baking soda, salt, and coconut sugar in a food processor or high-speed blender until the mixture has a flour-like consistency.
3. Add the coconut oil and 2 tablespoons (30 mL) of the milk and pulse until the ingredients form a dough. If too dry and crumbly, slowly add the remaining 1 tablespoon (15 mL) milk. Stir in the chocolate chips.
4. Using a small ice cream scoop or your hands, form the dough into 10 to 12 balls and place them on the prepared baking sheet with 1¼ inches (3 cm) between each ball. Press down on each ball to flatten it a little.
5. Cook for 6 minutes. It's okay that they will look undercooked when you take them out of the oven.
6. Remove from the oven and let sit for 10 minutes before handling. During this time, the cookies will firm up. Once they've cooled, they are ready to serve.

TIP: Use Lily's brand dark chocolate premium baking chips, and coconut oil instead of butter, for a vegan cookie.

NUTRITIONAL INFORMATION These cookies are a good source of magnesium, potassium, folate, fibre, and omega-3 and omega-6 fatty acids.

BLUEBERRY MAPLE ICE CREAM MAKES ABOUT 4 CUPS (1 L)

EGG-FREE • GLUTEN-FREE • NUT-FREE • VEGETARIAN • WHEAT-FREE

This ice cream is without a doubt a favourite in my house, and it beats the long-winded ingredient lists found on store-bought containers. If blueberries aren't your favourite fruit, try replacing them with strawberries, peaches, or blackberries—all are delicious alternatives.

3 cups (750 mL) fresh or frozen blueberries
1 cup (250 mL) whipping cream
¾ cup (175 mL) pure maple syrup

1. Purée the blueberries with a hand blender or food processor. If using frozen blueberries, allow them to thaw a little bit before puréeing them.
2. Add the cream and maple syrup and blend to combine. It's okay if flecks of blueberry remain throughout the cream mixture.
3. Pour into an ice cream maker and leave to churn for 20 minutes or until frozen through.

TIP: If you do not have an ice cream maker, put a medium plastic, glass, or metal bowl in the freezer before you start. Once the ice cream mixture is combined, pour it into the chilled bowl and return to the freezer. Set a timer for 30 minutes, then take the bowl out of the freezer and stir vigorously or use a hand mixer to break up ice crystals. Put back in the freezer for another 30 minutes. Repeat this process another 4 to 6 times until creamy and frozen. The cream can take 2 to 3 hours to become solid. Transfer to an airtight container and store in the freezer for up to 1 week.

NUTRITIONAL INFORMATION This ice cream is a great source of antioxidants, vitamin K, manganese, vitamin C. and fiber. Blueberries are excellent for immunity and brain health.

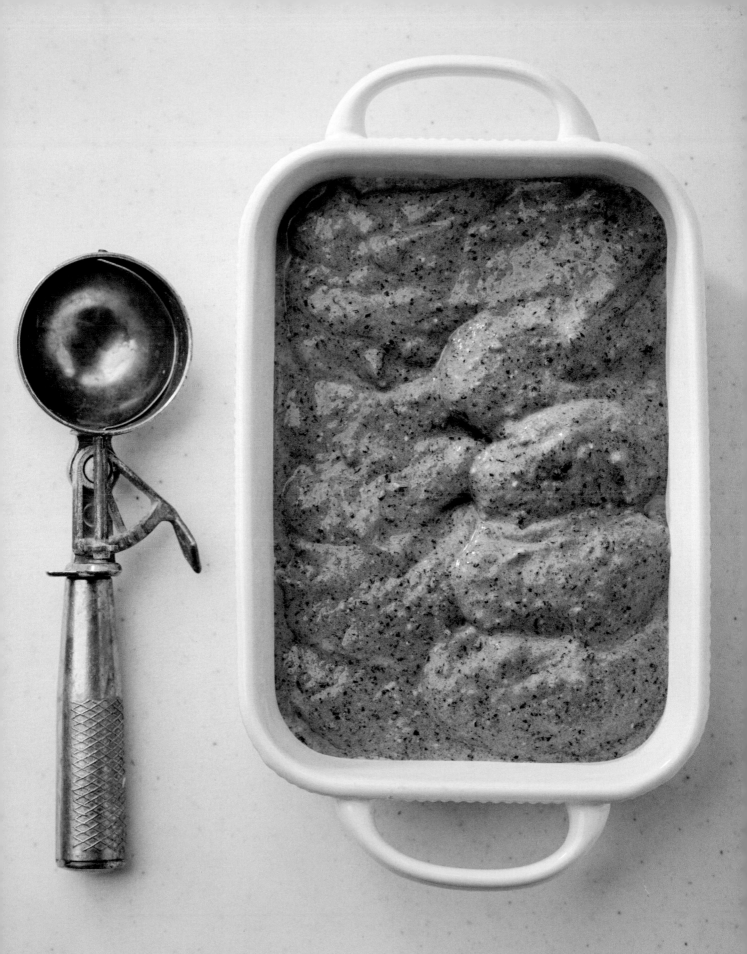

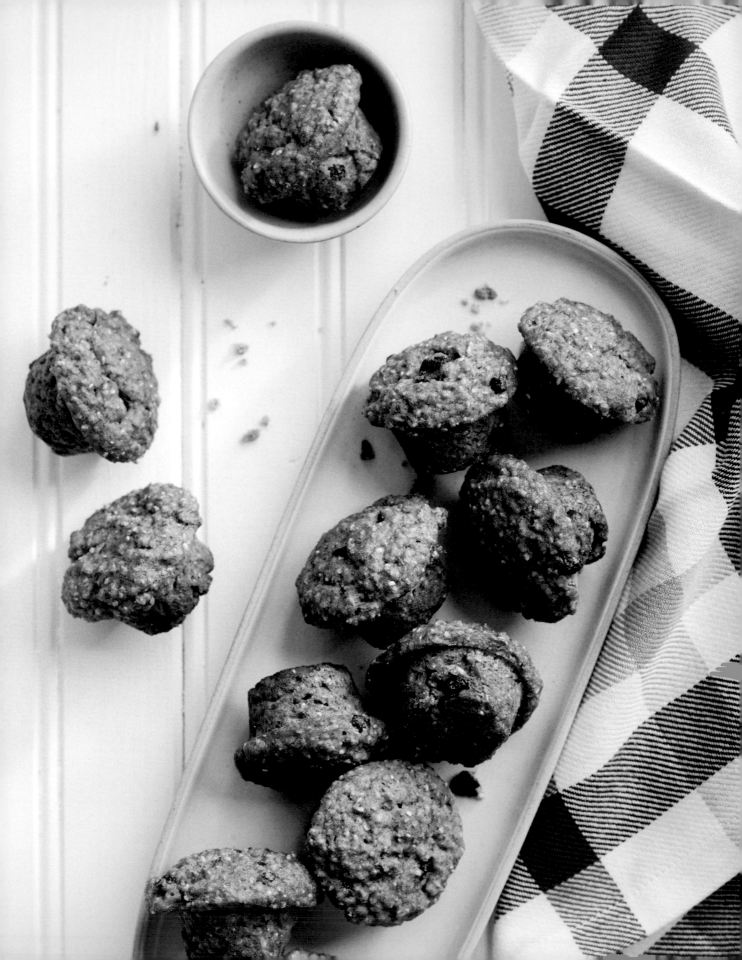

MINI BLUEBERRY MUFFINS MAKES 24 MINI MUFFINS

GLUTEN-FREE • NUT-FREE • VEGETARIAN • WHEAT-FREE

These are satisfying muffins that I love making in mini muffin tins. My kids think they're a treat! Replace the butter with coconut oil for a different flavour and quick energy!

Virgin coconut oil, for greasing the muffin cups

⅔ cup (150 mL) dried blueberries, Thompson raisins, or sultanas

4 ripe bananas

2 eggs

½ cup (125 mL) pure maple syrup

6 tablespoons (90 mL) unsalted butter, melted

⅔ cup (150 mL) chia seeds

1¾ cups (425 mL) brown rice flour

2 teaspoons (10 mL) baking powder

1 teaspoon (5 mL) baking soda

1. Preheat the oven to 300°F (150°C). Lightly grease 24 mini muffin cups with the coconut oil or line with paper liners.

2. Soak the blueberries in a small bowl of boiling water for 10 minutes until plump. Drain.

3. In a medium bowl, mash the bananas. Add the eggs and stir until combined.

4. Add the maple syrup, butter, and chia seeds and let stand for 5 minutes.

5. In another medium bowl, mix the flour, baking powder, and baking soda.

6. Add the drained blueberries and mashed banana mixture to the flour mixture. Stir until well combined.

7. Fill the muffin cups about three-quarters full and bake for 30 minutes until golden brown or until a toothpick comes out clean.

8. Let cool completely in the muffin tin on a wire rack before removing muffins from the tin.

9. Store the muffins in an airtight container at room temperature for up to 3 days or in the freezer for up to 2 weeks.

TIP: You can substitute ¼ cup (60 mL) chopped walnuts for the dried blueberries.

NUTRITIONAL INFORMATION These muffins are a good source of vitamin A, vitamin C, magnesium, potassium, phosphorus, and omega-3 fatty acids.

PUMPKIN MUFFINS MAKES 18 MINI MUFFINS OR 8 REGULAR MUFFINS

GLUTEN-FREE • VEGETARIAN • WHEAT-FREE

Muffins are a staple in many families. If you need to include more vegetables in the diet, this is a great way to do just that! Coconut flour has a moist texture, so makes a quite different muffin than other flours. You can also use ghee or virgin coconut oil instead of butter to change up the fat source.

Coconut oil, for greasing the muffin tins

¼ cup (60 mL) soft unsalted butter

6 eggs

1-inch (2.5 cm) piece fresh ginger,
  peeled and grated

3 tablespoons (45 mL) coconut flour

½ teaspoon (2 mL) sea salt

2 teaspoons (10 mL) ground cinnamon

1 teaspoon (5 mL) pure vanilla extract

2 cups (500 mL) almond flour

1½ cups (375 mL) pure pumpkin purée

¼ cup (60 mL) raw liquid honey

1. Preheat the oven to 375°F (190°C). Grease 1 or 2 muffin tins with the coconut oil or line with paper liners.
2. In a food processor or stand mixer, combine the butter, eggs, ginger, coconut flour, and salt. Blend for about 3 minutes, making sure the coconut flour is well mixed in.
3. Add the cinnamon, vanilla, almond flour, pumpkin, and honey and stir to combine.
4. Fill the muffin cups about three-quarters full. Bake for 18 to 20 minutes for mini muffins or 20 to 25 minutes for regular-size muffins. Remove the muffins from the oven when they are lightly golden brown or when a toothpick inserted in the middle comes out clean. Let cool completely in the muffin tins on a wire rack before removing muffins from the tins.

NUTRITIONAL INFORMATION These muffins are a good source of vitamin A, vitamin D, vitamin K, calcium, magnesium, phosphorus, potassium, folate, and choline.

ZUCCHINI SPICE MUFFINS MAKES 12 MUFFINS

DAIRY-FREE • GLUTEN-FREE • NUT-FREE • VEGETARIAN • WHEAT-FREE

These are the perfect snack for school, as they use coconut flour as the base. Coconut flour is perfect for those who are sensitive to grains or feel sleepy after a wheat-filled lunch.

½ cup (125 mL) unsalted butter or virgin coconut oil

1 teaspoon (5 mL) ground cinnamon

1 teaspoon (5 mL) ground ginger

½ teaspoon (2 mL) baking soda

Scant ⅛ teaspoon (0.5 mL) ground cloves

Scant ⅛ teaspoon (0.5 mL) ground nutmeg

6 eggs

1 teaspoon (5 mL) pure vanilla extract

¾ teaspoon (4 mL) sea salt

½ cup (125 mL) raw liquid honey

¾ cup (175 mL) coconut flour

2 medium zucchinis, grated and squeezed to remove some liquid

1. Preheat the oven to 325°F (160°C). Line a muffin tin with paper liners.

2. Melt the butter or coconut oil in a small saucepan over low heat. Remove from the heat and allow to cool slightly.

3. Meanwhile, combine the cinnamon, ginger, baking soda, cloves, nutmeg, eggs, vanilla, and salt in a large bowl and blend well with a hand mixer.

4. Add the honey and stir to combine.

5. Pour in the melted butter and blend well.

6. Add the coconut flour and blend with a hand mixer or stir vigorously to thoroughly combine all ingredients, making sure there are no lumps.

7. Fold in the grated zucchini.

8. Fill the muffin cups about three-quarters full. Bake for 40 to 50 minutes until set and a toothpick inserted in the middle comes out clean. The cups may be quite full if the zucchini were large.

9. Let cool completely in the muffin tins on a wire rack before removing muffins from the tins. Store the muffins in an airtight container at room temperature for up to 4 days.

NUTRITIONAL INFORMATION These muffins are a good source of vitamin A, vitamin D, vitamin K, calcium, magnesium, phosphorus, potassium, folate, and choline.

OATCAKES MAKES ABOUT 24 OATCAKES

DAIRY-FREE • EGG-FREE • GLUTEN-FREE • NUT-FREE • VEGAN • VEGETARIAN • WHEAT-FREE

Store-bought oatcakes are simple to grab, but homemade are fun to make and enjoy with your kids.

1½ cups (375 mL) finely ground old-fashioned rolled oats
⅛ teaspoon (0.5 mL) baking soda
1 tablespoon (15 mL) sunflower oil
6 tablespoons (90 mL) boiling water

1. Preheat the oven to 350° F (180°C). Line a baking sheet with parchment paper.
2. Mix the oats and baking soda in a medium bowl.
3. Mix the sunflower oil and water in a bowl and slowly add it to the oat mixture, stirring until a doughy consistency is achieved. Let rest for 5 minutes until the liquid is absorbed.
4. On a clean surface lightly dusted with ground oats, roll out the dough into a disc that is ¼ inch (5 mm) thick. Use a glass or cookie cutter to cut out 2-inch (5 cm) rounds.
5. Place the oatcakes on the prepared baking sheet, evenly spaced. Bake for 20 to 25 minutes or until golden brown, rotating the baking sheet halfway through. Transfer the oatcakes to a wire rack and let cool.
6. Store the oatcakes in an airtight container at room temperature for up to 1 week.

NUTRITIONAL INFORMATION These oatcakes are a hybrid between oatmeal porridge and pancakes that is high in fibre, B vitamins, and iron.

BITE-SIZE FRUIT BALLS

MAKES ABOUT 40 MINI BALLS OR 24 MEDIUM BALLS

DAIRY-FREE • EGG-FREE • GLUTEN-FREE •

NUT-FREE • VEGAN • VEGETARIAN • WHEAT-FREE

Anything bite size for kids is loads of fun. These fruit balls are an excellent snack that give tons of energy on top of taste—and they require very few ingredients. Get your kids in the kitchen to help you prepare these. The more they contribute, the more likely they are to eat them!

½ cup (125 mL) unsweetened dried cranberries
½ cup (125 mL) dried unsulphured apricots
½ cup (125 mL) Thompson raisins or sultanas
⅓ cup (75 mL) unsweetened dried coconut
2 tablespoons (30 mL) raw liquid honey or
   brown rice syrup
2 tablespoons (30 mL) fresh apple juice
½ cup (125 mL) finely chopped almonds or
   sesame seeds

1. Add the cranberries, apricots, raisins, and coconut to a food processor and pulse until all ingredients are finely chopped and combined.
2. Add the honey and apple juice and pulse until the mixture clumps together.
3. Roll into balls that are about 1 heaping teaspoon (7 mL) in size for a mini ball or 1 tablespoon (20 mL), then roll each ball in chopped almonds or sesame seeds.

NUTRITIONAL INFORMATION These fun fruit bites are packed with vitamin C.

HIT THE ROAD TRAIL MIX

MAKES 3¼ CUPS (810 ML)

DAIRY-FREE • EGG-FREE • GLUTEN-FREE •

VEGAN • VEGETARIAN • WHEAT-FREE

This homemade trail mix is full of flavour and texture and packs a powerful punch of nutrients.

1 cup (250 mL) dried fruit (cranberries, chopped
   apricots, chopped dates, apples, or a mix)
½ cup (125 mL) Thompson raisins or sultanas
½ cup (125 mL) pumpkin seeds
½ cup (125 mL) sunflower seeds
½ cup (125 mL) raw almonds
½ cup (125 mL) raw walnuts, hazelnuts, or Brazil
   nuts

1. Mix together the dried fruit, raisins, pumpkin seeds, sunflower seeds, almonds, and walnuts.
2. Store the trail mix in an airtight container at room temperature for up to 4 weeks.

NUTRITIONAL INFORMATION This trail mix is high in omega-3 and omega-6 fatty acids, magnesium, vitamin E, manganese, selenium, and protein working simultaneously to support brain, heart, and immune health.

NOTES

1. Brad Plumer, "We've Covered the World in Pesticides. Is That a Problem?" *Washington Post*, August 18, 2013. https://www.washingtonpost.com/news/wonk/wp/2013/08/18/the-world-uses-billions-of-pounds-of-pesticides-each-year-is-that-a-problem/?noredirect=on&utm_term=.ca4382d543ab

2. Pesticide Action Network, "Pesticides: A Public Problem." http://www.whatsonmyfood.org.

3. Copyright © Environmental Working Group, www.ewg.org. Reproduced with permission. https://www.ewg.org/foodnews/dirty-dozen.php

4. Copyright © Environmental Working Group, www.ewg.org. Reproduced with permission. https://www.ewg.org/foodnews/clean-fifteen.php

5. Health Canada, "Prenatal Nutrition Guidelines for Health Professionals—Fish and Omega-3 Fatty Acids." https://www.canada.ca/en/health-canada/services/food-nutrition/reports-publications/nutrition-healthy-eating/prenatal-nutrition-guidelines-health-professionals-fish-omega-3-fatty-acids-2009.html

6. Dr. Nigel Plummer, "The Developmental Origins of Modern Disease—Are We Programmed to Develop Disease in the Womb?" Seroyal Conference May 9–10, 2009 Toronto, ON.

7. Allen SJ et al., "Probiotics in the prevention of eczema: a randomised controlled trial." *Archives of Disease in Childhood* 2014 Nov; 99 (11): 1014–1019.

8. Bruce W. Hollis and Carol L. Wagner, "Nutritional Vitamin D Status during Pregnancy: Reasons for Concern." *Canadian Medical Association Journal* 174, no. 9 (April 25, 2006): 1287–1290.

9. Marja Ala-Houhala, "25-Hydroxyvitamin D Levels during Breast-feeding with or without Maternal or Infantile Supplementation of Vitamin D," *Journal of Pediatric Gastroenterology and Nutrition* 4, no. 2 (1985): 220–226.

10. Public Health Agency of Canada, "Canadian Paediatric Surveillance Program—2003 Results," November 8, 2004. http://www.phac-aspc.gc.ca/publicat/cpsp-pcsp03/page8-eng.php

11. Leanne M. Ward et al., "Vitamin D–Deficiency Rickets among Children in Canada," *Canadian Medical Association Journal* 177, no. 2 (July 17, 2007): 161–166. https://www.ncbi.nlm.nih.gov/pmc/articles/PMC1913133/

12. Shashi Raj et al., "A Prospective Study of Iron Status in Exclusively Breastfed Term Infants Up to 6 Months of Age," *International Breastfeeding Journal* 1, no. 3 (March 2008): 3.

13. Kelly Bonyata, "Is Iron-Supplementation Necessary?" April 10, 2018. https://kellymom.com/nutrition/vitamins/iron/

14. Health Canada, "Iron," June 23, 2009. http://www.hc-sc.gc.ca/dhp-mps/prodnatur/applications/licen-prod/monograph/mono_iron-fer-eng.php

15. Ann Prentice, "Calcium in Pregnancy and Lactation," *Annual Review of Nutrition* 20 (2000): 249–272.

16. Carolee Bateson-Koch, *Allergies: Disease in Disguise* (Burnaby, BC: Alive Books, 1994).

17. EatRight Ontario, "Calcium Sources," 2009. http://www.eatrightontario.ca/en/ViewDocument.aspx?id=203

18. Janet Zand, Robert Rountree, and Rachel Walton, *Smart Medicine for a Healthier Child*, 2nd ed. (New York: Penguin Group, 2003).

19. Dr. Shonna Masse (pediatric dentist) in discussion with the author, June 2009.

20. Dr. Dana Colson (dentist). Interview with the author, May 2009.

21. Dr. Shonna Masse (pediatric dentist) in discussion with the author, June 2009.

22. Dr. Robert Penning (pediatric dentist) in discussion with the author, June 8, 2009.

23. Eleanor Bimla Schwarz et al., "Duration of Lactation and Risk Factors for Maternal Cardiovascular Disease," *Obstetrics & Gynecology* 113, no. 5 (May 2009): 974–982.

24. Lars A. Hanson, *Immunobiology of Human Milk: How Breastfeeding Protects Babies* (Amarillo, TX: Pharmasoft Publishing, 2004), 77.

25. Ibid., 82.

26. Ibid., 93.

27. Zachery T. Lewis and David A. Mills, "Differential Establishment of Bifidobacteria in the Breastfed Infant Gut," *Nestlé Nutrition Institute Workshop Series 2017* 88: 149–159. https://www.ncbi.nlm.nih.gov/pmc/articles/PMC5535791/

28. E. Bezirtzoglou, A. Tsiotsias, and G.W. Welling, "Microbiota Profile in Feces of Breast- and Formula-Fed Newborns by Using Fluorescence In Situ Hybridization (FISH)," *Anaerobe* 17, no. 6 (2011): 478–482. https://www.ncbi.nlm.nih.gov/pubmed/21497661/

29. Clare E. Casey, Anne Smith, and Peifang Zhang, "Microminerals in Human and Animal Milks," in *Handbook of Milk Composition*, ed. Robert G. Jensen (San Diego: Academic Press, 1995), 622–673.

30. Rosine Bishara et al., "Nutrient Composition of Hindmilk Produced by Mothers of Very Low Birth Weight Infants Born at Less Than 28 Weeks' Gestation," *Journal of Human Lactation* 24, no. 2 (2008): 159–167.

31. Mary Frances Picciano, "Vitamins in Milk," in *Handbook of Milk Composition*, 675–687.

32. Timo Saarela, Jorma Kokkenen, and Maila Koivisto, "Macronutrient and Energy Contents of Human Milk Fractions during the First Six Months of Lactation," *Acta Paediatrica* 94 (2005): 1176–1181.

33. Jan Riordan and Kathleen G. Auerbach, *Breastfeeding and Human Lactation* (Boston: Jones and Bartlett, 1993).

34. Margit Hamosh, "Enzymes in Human Milk," in *Handbook of Milk Composition*, 388–427.

35. Bo Lonnerdal and Stephanie Atkinson, "Nitrogenous Components of Milk," in *Handbook of Milk Composition*, 351–368.

36. Hanson, *Immunobiology of Human Milk*, 83.

37. Ibid., 91.

38. Ibid., 91

39. Ibid., 83.

40. W.H. Oddy et al., "Early Infant Feeding and Adiposity Risk: From Infancy to Adulthood," *Annals of Nutrition and Metabolism* 64, no. 3–4 (2014): 262–270. https://www.ncbi.nlm.nih.gov/pubmed/25300269

41. J. Yan et al., "The Association between Breastfeeding and Childhood Obesity: A Meta-analysis," *BMC Public Health* 14 (2014):1267. https://www.ncbi.nlm.nih.gov/pubmed/25495402/

42. Hanson, *Immunobiology of Human Milk*, 97.

43. Dr. Dana Colson (dentist). Interview with the author, May 2009.

44. S.S. Yalçin et al., "The Factors That Affect Milk-to-Serum Ratio for Iron during Early Lactation," *Journal of Pediatric Hematology/Oncology* 31, no. 2 (February 2009): 85–90.

45. Riordan and Auerbach, *Breastfeeding and Human Lactation*.

46. Natalie Rogers (childbirth educator), email message to the author, June 8, 2009.

47. Riordan and Auerbach, *Breastfeeding and Human Lactation*.

48. Ibid.

49. Jack Newman, *Dr. Jack Newman's Guide to Breastfeeding* (Toronto: HarperCollins, 2000).

50. Natalie Rogers (childbirth educator), email message to the author, June 8, 2009.

51. Natalie Rogers (childbirth educator), email message to the author, June 8, 2009.

52. "Infant Formula: The Canadian Study," July 3, 2004. http://www.truthinlabeling.org/formulacopy.html

53. A.C. Ross et al., "The 2011 Report on Dietary Reference Intakes for Calcium and Vitamin D from the Institute of Medicine: What Clinicians Need to Know," *Journal of Clinical Endocrinology & Metabolism* 96 (2011): 53–58.

54. R.I. Mackie, A. Sghir, and H.R. Gaskins, "Developmental Microbial Ecology of the Neonatal Gastrointestinal Tract," *American Journal of Clinical Nutrition* 69 (1999): 1035S–1045S.

55. D.S. Newburg, "Glycobiology of Human Milk," *Biochemistry (Moscow)* 78 (2013): 771–785.

56. A.R. Pacheco et al., "The Impact of the Milk Glycobiome on the Neonate Gut Microbiota," *Annual Review of Animal Biosciences* 3 (2015): 419–445.

57. A.M. Zivkovic et al., "Human Milk Glycobiome and Its Impact on the Infant Gastrointestinal Microbiota," *Proceedings of the National Academy of Sciences of the United States of America* 108, Suppl. 1 (2011): 4653–4658.

58. Jay Highman, Founder Nature's One. Interview with author, May 2009.

59. Beate Lloyd et al., "Formula Tolerance in Postbreastfed and Exclusively Formula-Fed Infants," *Pediatrics* 103, no. 1 (January 1999): e7.

60. W.W.K. Koo et al., "Reduced Bone Mineralization in Infants Fed Palm Olein-Containing Formula: A Randomized, Double-Blinded, Prospective Trial," *Pediatrics* 111 (2003): 1017–1023.

61. O. Hernell et al., "Clinical Benefits of Milk Fat Globule Membranes for Infants and Children," *Journal of Pediatrics* 173 (June 2016): S60–S65.

62. Charlotte Vallaeys, *DHA/ARA: Replacing Mother—Imitating Human Breast Milk in the Laboratory* (Cornucopia, WI: Cornucopia Institute, 2008).

63. K. Kennedy et al., "Double-Blinded, Randomized Trial of a Synthetic Triacylglycerol in Formula-Fed Term Infants: Effects on Stool Biochemistry, Stool Characteristics, and Bone Mineralization," *American Journal of Clinical Nutrition* 70 (1999): 920–927.

64. Catherine L. Witt, "When Are Soy Formulas Appropriate for Infants Younger Than Age 1?", *Medscape*, September 15, 2006. http://www.medscape.com/viewarticle/544436

65. Jeffrey M. Smith, *Genetic Roulette: The Documented Health Risks of Genetically Engineered Foods* (Fairfield, IA: Yes! Books, 2007).

66. Ibid.

67. J.B. Lasekan et al., "Growth of Newborn, Term Infants Fed Soy Formulas for One Year," *Clinical Pediatrics* 38 (1999): 563–571.

68. "NANNYCare Goat Milk Nutrition," 2007. http://www.vitacare.co.uk/ProductInfo.aspx

69. Julia Moskin, "For an All-Organic Formula, Baby, That's Sweet," *New York Times*, May 19, 2008. http://www.nytimes.com/2008/05/19/us/19formula.html?_r=1

70. "Types of Lactose Intolerance," Foodreactions.org, 2005. http://www.foodreactions.org/intolerance/lactose/types.html

71. K. Kennedy et al., "Double-Blinded, Randomized Trial of a Synthetic Triacylglycerol in Formula-Fed Term Infants."

72. Ibid.

73. Ontario Association of Osteopathic Manual Practitioners home page, December 17, 2009. http://www.osteopathyontario.com

74. Tema Stein (pediatric osteopath), in discussion with the author, June 8, 2009.

75. I. Alexandrovich et al., "The Effect of Fennel (*Foeniculum vulgare*) Seed Oil Emulsion in Infantile Colic: A Randomized, Placebo-Controlled Study," *Alternative Therapies in Health and Medicine* 4 (July/August 2003): 58–61.

76. Bastyr Center for Natural Health, "Herbal Combination Relieves Colic in Babies," 2009. http://bastyrcenter. org/content/view/943/&page=

77. Dr. Nigel Plummer, "Choosing the Right Probiotics." Seroya Teleconference, September 24, 2008.

78. Scott H. Sicherer and Hugh A. Sampson, "Food Allergy: A Review and Update on Epidemiology, Pathogenesis, Diagnosis, Prevention, and Management," *Journal of Allergy and Clinical Immunology*, 141, no. 1 (January 2018): 41–58. https://www.sciencedirect.com/science/article/pii/S0091674917317943

79. Ibid.

80. Josef Neu and Jona Rushing, "Cesarean versus Vaginal Delivery: Long Term Infant Outcomes and the Hygiene Hypothesis," *Clinics in Perinatology* 38, no. 2 (June 2011): 321–331. https://www.ncbi.nlm.nih.gov/pmc/articles/PMC3110651/#R33/

81. Amy Langdon, Nathan Crook, and Gautam Dantas, "The Effects of Antibiotics on the Microbiome throughout Development and Alternative Approaches for Therapeutic Modulation," *Genome Medicine* 8 (2016). 39. https://genomemedicine.biomedcentral.com/articles/10.1186/s13073-016-0294-z

82. Susan F. Plummer et al., "Effects of Probiotics on the Composition of the Intestinal Microbiota Following Antibiotic Therapy," *International Journal of Antimicrobial Agents* 26 (2005): 69–74.

83. Chris Keenan, "Top 10 Most Common GMO Foods," The Cornucopia Institute, June 19, 2013. https://www.cornucopia.org/2013/06/top-10-most-common-gmo-foods/?gclid=CjoKCQiA5t7UBRDaARIsAOreQtj-BAw2AvoPRjYf9kQW2doQuHSdy_gfYyapj_XxRNo6nT2p7oE-ugkaArqvEALw_wcB

84. Scott H. Sicherer and Hugh A. Sampson, "Food Allergy: A Review and Update on Epidemiology, Pathogenesis, Diagnosis, Prevention, and Management."

85. "Our History: Alan Brown," The Hospital for Sick Children (SickKids). http://www.sickkids.ca/AboutSickKids/History-and-Milestones/Our-History/Alan-Brown.html

86. G.Y. Du Toit et al., "Early Consumption of Peanuts in Infancy Is Associated with a Low Prevalence of Peanut Allergy," *Journal of Allergy and Clinical Immunology* 122, no. 5 (November 2008): 984–991.

87. L. Mondoulet et al., "Influence of Thermal Processing on the Allergenicity of Peanut Proteins," *Journal of Agricultural and Food Chemistry* 53 (2005): 4547–4553.

88. "Study Finds Delayed Food Introduction Increases Risk of Sensitization," CHILD Study, June 8, 2017. http://childstudy.ca/media/press-releases/study-finds-delayed-food-introduction-increases-risk-of-sensitization/

89. Elissa M. Abrams et al., "Early Solid Food Introduction: Role in Food Allergy Prevention and Implications for Breastfeeding," *Journal of Pediatrics* 184 (May 2017): 13–18. http://www.jpeds.com/article/S0022-3476(17)30163-4/fulltext#s0010

90. F. Sanchez-Valverde et al., "The Impact of Caesarean Delivery and Type of Feeding on Cow's Milk Allergy in Infants and Subsequent Development of Allergic March in Childhood," *Allergy* 64, no. 6 (June 2009): 884–889.

91. Bateson-Koch, *Allergies: Disease in Disguise*, 54.

92. Bateson-Koch, *Allergies: Disease in Disguise*, 157.

93. Maxwell M. Tran et. al., "Study Finds Delayed Food Introduction Increases Risk of Sensitization," *Pediatric Allergy and Immunology* 28 (2017): 471–477.

94. Katherine Anagnosou et al., "Assessing the Efficacy of Oral Immunotherapy for the Desensitisation of Peanut Allergy in Children (STOP II): A Phase 2 Randomised Controlled Trial," *Lancet* 383, no. 9925 (April 12, 2014): 1297–1304. http://www.thelancet.com/journals/lancet/article/PIIS0140–6736%2813%2962301–6/abstract

95. Janet Neilson (homeopath), in discussion with the author, June 8, 2009.

96. "Egg Allergy Diet for Children," Stanford Children's Health. http://www.stanfordchildrens.org/en/topic/default?id=egg-allergy-diet-for-children-90-P01684

97. "Wheat Allergy Diet for Children," Stanford Children's Health. http://www.stanfordchildrens.org/en/topic/default?id=wheat-allergy-diet-for-children-90-P01712

98. "Soy Allergy Diet for Children," Stanford Children's Health. http://www.stanfordchildrens.org/en/topic/default?id=soy-allergy-diet-for-children-90-P01709

99. Riordan and Auerbach, *Breastfeeding and Human Lactation*.

100. Online survey via sproutright.com, weewelcome.ca, facebook/canadianbabies.ca, and meetup.com, June 8, 2009.

101. Tracey Devine ("The Sleep Doula"), in discussion with the author, June 8, 2009.

102. B.J. Morison et al., "How Different Are Baby-Led Weaning and Conventional Complementary Feeding? A Cross-Sectional Study of Infants Aged 6–8 Months," *BMJ Open* 6, no. 5 (2016): e010665.

103. A. Brown, "No Difference in Self-Reported Frequency of Choking between Infants Introduced to Solid Foods Using a Baby-Led Weaning or Traditional Spoon-Feeding Approach," *Journal of Human Nutrition and Dietetics* (2017). Epub ahead of print.

104. "Food Allergies in Children," Johns Hopkins Medicine. https://www.hopkinsmedicine.org/healthlibrary/conditions/adult/pediatrics/food_allergies_in_children_90,P01993

105. Healthy Babies Bright Futures, "Arsenic in 9 Brands of Infant Cereals," December 2017. http://www.healthybabycereals.org/sites/healthybabycereals.org/files/2017–12/HBBF_ArsenicInInfantCerealReport.pdf

106. Consumer Reports, "Arsenic in Your Food," November 2012. https://www.consumerreports.org/cro/magazine/2012/11/arsenic-in-your-food/index.htm

107. "Study Finds Delayed Food Introduction Increases Risk of Sensitization."

108. A.F. Kagalwalla et al., "Identification of Specific Foods Responsible for Inflammation in Children with Eosinophilic Esophagitis Successfully Treated with Empiric Elimination Diet," *Journal of Pediatric Gastroenterology and Nutrition* 53, no. 2 (August 2011): 145–149. https://www.ncbi.nlm.nih.gov/pubmed/21788754/

109. "What Are Food Allergies in Babies?" BabyCenter, September 2015. https://www.babycenter.ca/a555826/what-are-food-allergies-in-babies#ixzz57Uu5PJ4T

110. The Food Allergy and Anaphylaxis Network, "Allergens: Tree Nuts." http://www.foodallergy.org/page/tree-nuts1

111. Valerie Elliot, "Cow&Gate and Farley's Rusks Attacked for Fat, Sugar and Salt Content," *The Times*, May 5, 2009. http://www.timesonline.co.uk/tol/news/uk/health/article6216207.ece

112. Ask Dr. Sears Nutrients in Eggs https://www.askdrsears.com/topics/feeding-eating/family-nutrition/eggs

113. Fernandez ML. "Dietary cholesterol provided by eggs and plasma lipoproteins in healthy populations." *Current Opinion in Clinical Nutrition and Metabolic Care* 9, no. 1 (January 2006): 8–12.

114. *Marketplace*, Dr. Richard Mass interview, aired March 2001 on CBC, http://www.cbc.ca/consumers/market/files/health/leadwater/index.html

115. Ibid.

116. Saima Rafiq et al., "Chemical Composition, Nitrogen Fractions and Amino Acids Profile of Milk from Different Animal Species," *Asian-Australasian Journal of Animal Sciences* 29, no. 7 (July 2016): 1022–1028. https://www.ncbi.nlm.nih.gov/pmc/articles/PMC4932579/

117. "Is Carrageenan Safe?" Weil: Andrew Weil, M.D., November 1, 2016. https://www.drweil.com/diet-nutrition/food-safety/is-carrageenan-safe/

118. Dr. Dana Colson, dentist. Interview with the author, May 2009.

119. Public Health Ontario, "Two-Thirds of Packaged Foods and Drinks in Canada Have Added Sugars," January 12, 2017. https://www.publichealthontario.ca/en/About/Newsroom/Pages/Two-thirds-of-packaged-foods-and-drinks-in-Canada-have-added-sugars.aspx

120. Liza Finlay (phychotherapist) email interview with author. Feburary 26, 2018.

121. Alyson Shafer (psychotherapist, author and parenting expert) email interview with author. March 1, 2018.

122. Naomi Imatome-Yun, "Plant-Based Primer: The Beginner's Guide to Starting a Plant-Based Diet," January 3, 2017. https://www.forksoverknives.com/plant-based-primer-beginners-guide-starting-plant-based-diet/

123. Liza Finlay (psychotherapist) email interview with author. February 26, 2018.

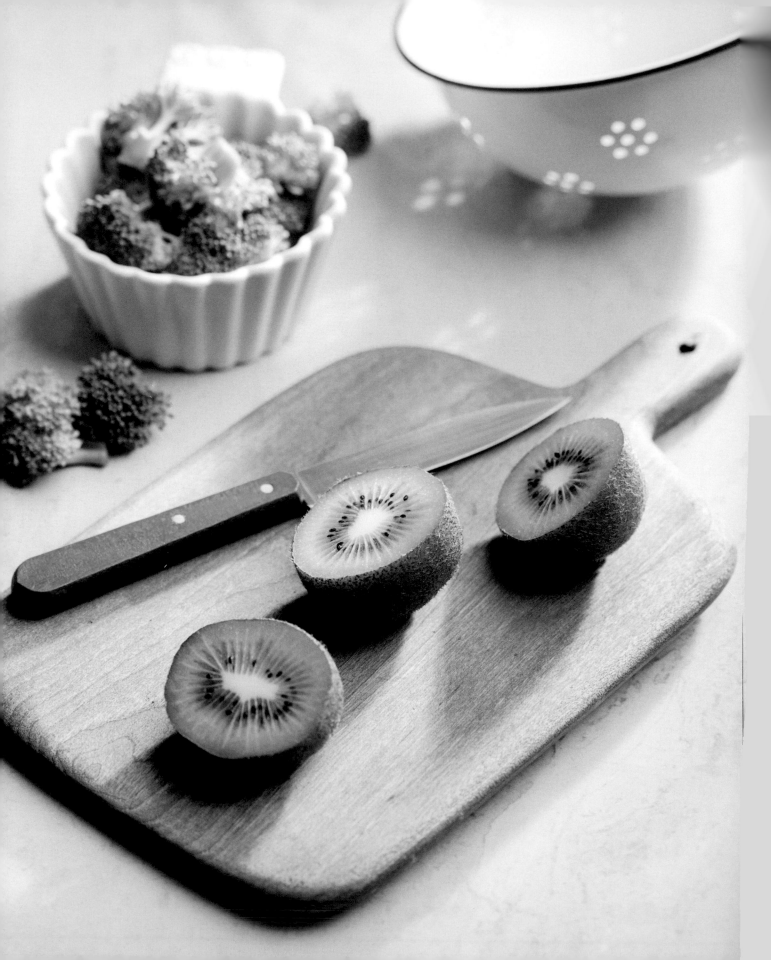

ACKNOWLEDGMENTS

Thank you, thank you, thank you. So many people were involved in helping with this updated edition of my first book. First, thank you to every mom and dad I meet in my workshops, cooking classes, and trade shows, and speak with on the phone. You're why I do what I do, and I feel honoured to support you through such an important time in your lives. To my research team of nutrition students who searched for the most current and up-to-date information and the newest formulas available around the world: Jennifer, Kristine, Hollie, and Tricia. Another thank you to Hollie, Tricia, Kristine, and Monica for your incredible support and the photo shoot. Thank you to Julia from the Institute of Holistic Nutrition for finding me such a great team. Thank you to my assistant Kristin Diehl for taking care of all that I couldn't while writing and editing. A monstrous thank you to the Sprig Creative team—Brendan Fisher and Jennifer Bartoli and their photographer Rob Dann—who organized, styled, and shot all the stunning and vibrant photos in this book. I'm thrilled with how they turned out! A heartfelt thank you to The Sweet Potato in the Junction area of Toronto, which donated all the organic food and ingredients for the photo shoot, for your continued support over the years. You guys really are the best!

Thank you to all the experts who allowed me to pick their clever brains and gain insight into their areas of expertise: psychotherapists Alyson Schafer and Liza Finlay; dentists Dr. Dana Colson, Dr. Shonna Masse, and Dr. Robert Penning; osteopath Tema Stein; The Sleep Doula, Tracey Devine; homeopath Janet Neilson; and childbirth educator Natalie Rogers.

Thank you to the great editorial team at Penguin for the opportunity to write this book: Andrea Magyar, publishing director; Rachel Brown, assistant editor; and Susan Broadhurst, copy editor. After the stars aligned and I wrote the first edition of this book in 2009, this update has given me the opportunity to share more relevant information with readers.

And last, but certainly not least, thank you to my beautiful and super-healthy daughters, Logan and Hadley, for being so patient with all the hours, late nights, and weekends I spent sitting at my laptop, not able to take part in stuff that was going on with you. I know you see me working and wonder at times what it's all about, so thank you for your understanding and patience. I hope one day you'll understand how much you both inspire me to be the best mum I can be. And at all those times when I say no to a sugary or processed food, know that it's because I love you and want you to be the healthiest you can be. Finding a balance between healthy and happy is my wish for you both as a part of your journey throughout your lives. I love you both so very much.

SUBJECT INDEX

Notes: The italic letter *t* following a page number indicates a table or chart. For recipes, see the Recipe Index immediately following the Subject Index.

Dirty Dozen (pesticides), 6
health concerns, 124
introducing, 104, 106, 122
as iron source, 33–34*t*
rainbow eating, 4–5
in school lunches, 245
fruits, dried
for constipation, 80
as finger food, 158–59
preparation, 106
fussiness, 52, 81

gagging, 114, 156, 157
galactooligosaccharides (GOS),
66, 71
garbanzo beans (chickpeas):
cooking, 10*t*
garlic
benefits, 199–200, 242
supplements, 251
gassiness
and breast milk, 52, 53, 81
causes, 81–82
and formula, 66, 81
stinky toots/poo, 82
supportive relief, 82–83
symptoms, 80, 81
genetically modified (GM) foods
and allergies or disorders, 95
soy products, 67, 187
types, 95
ginger, 13
glucose: in formula, 63
gluten: and constipation, 79
goat's milk
about, 189, 189–90*t*
formula, 67
grains
cooking, 9–10, 10*t*
as iron source, 33–34*t*
granulocytes, 86
Great Northern beans: cooking,
10*t*
gripe water, 83

healing: and breast milk, 49
healthy eating
definition, 4
fermented foods, 237–38
plant-based, 236
rainbow eating, 4–5
school lunches, 242–47
upside-down bowl night, 193
vegetarian, 236–37
hemp seed oil, 80
herbs
immune-boosting supplements,
251
introducing, 161
nutrients and uses, 12–13
high-oleic acid oil, 64

homeopathy
for gassiness, 82–83
for teething pain, 41–42
honey: health concerns, 124
hummus, 240–41
hybrid method feeding, 115–16
hydrolyzed formula, 69

ibuprofen, 91
immune cells, 86–87
immune system
and allergies, 93–94
boosting, 240–41
and breast milk, 46–47, 48, 87
and Caesarean birth, 88–89
and cleanliness, 88
development, 87–88
drainers, 89, 99, 241
how it works, 86–87
and intolerances/sensitivities,
97
and nutrients, 89, 198–200
and sugar, 158
of toddlers, 198
and vaginal birth, 46, 87, 88
immunoglobulin A (sigA), 46–47, 48
immunoglobulins, 87, 89
intolerances/sensitivities
common, 98
definition, 97
preventive strategies, 98–99
symptoms, 97–98, 117–18, 193
treatments, 99–100
iron
for babies, 31–33, 43*t*
in breast milk, 47, 49
in cereals, 118–19
and constipation, 78
foods rich in, 161
in formula, 64–65
for mothers, 22, 24, 34, 43*t*
recommended daily allowances,
34*t*
sources, 33–34, 33–34*t*
for toddlers, 199
iron deficiency, 24, 31, 32

Jacob's Cattle beans: cooking, 10*t*
juice
avoiding, 163
as iron source, 33–34*t*
in school lunches, 245
and tooth health, 39, 42

kasha: cooking, 9–10, 10*t*
kefir, 242
kidney beans: cooking, 11*t*
kitchen essentials
foods, 16–17, 247
tools, 18–19

lactation consultants, 46, 50, 53–54,
56, 61, 77
Lactobacillus acidophilus, 94
lactoferrin: in breast milk, 48, 65
lactose
in breast milk, 48
in formula, 63, 69
intolerance to, 68, 76, 98
latching on, 46, 53
lead toxicity, 162
leaky gut, 92–93, 99
legumes
affecting breast milk, 52
cooking, 10–11
as finger food, 159
as protein source, 237
lentils
cooking, 11*t*
as iron source, 33–34*t*
leukocytes, 86–87
lima beans: cooking, 11*t*
lipase, 48
lunches
health guidelines, 244–45
for immune boosting, 240–41
for mothers, 28–29
planning, 242–43
suggestions, 245–47
lymphocytes, 86

magnesium
for babies, 43*t*
for mothers, 21, 43*t*
maltodextrin: in formula, 63
manganese, 22
mast cells, 86–87
mastitis, 52
meals, for baby: hybrid feeding
method, 116
meals, for family
for emotional/physical
connection, 235
fermented foods, 237–39
hydration, 239
immune boosting, 240–42
and mental focus, 239–40
planning, 247–49, 248–49*t*
plant-based eating, 236
school lunches, 242–47
supplements, 250–51
with toddler in mind, 201*t*
vegetarian/vegan, 236–37
meals, for mother, 26–29
meals, for toddler, 195–96, 197, 201*t*
meat broth, 104–5, 106, 120–21
meats
about, 11–12
introducing, 123
as iron source, 33–34*t*
meconium (baby poo at birth), 46,
74, 91

RECIPE INDEX